Geriatric Medicine

Guest Editor

JOHN E. MORLEY, MB, BCh

MEDICAL CLINICS OF NORTH AMERICA

www.medical.theclinics.com

May 2011 • Volume 95 • Number 3

SAUNDERS an imprint of ELSEVIER, Inc.

W.B. SAUNDERS COMPANY
A Division of Elsevier Inc.

1600 John F. Kennedy Boulevard • Suite 1800 • Philadelphia, Pennsylvania 19103-2899

http://www.theclinics.com

MEDICAL CLINICS OF NORTH AMERICA Volume 95, Number 3
May 2011 ISSN 0025-7125, ISBN-13: 978-1-4557-0621-1

Editor: Rachel Glover
Developmental Editor: Donald Mumford

Medical Clinics of North America (ISSN 0025-7125) is published bimonthly by Elsevier Inc., 360 Park Avenue South, New York, NY 10010-1710. Months of issue are January, March, May, July, September, and November. Periodicals postage paid at New York, NY, and additional mailing offices. Subscription prices are USD 218 per year for US individuals, USD 404 per year for US institutions, USD 110 per year for US students, USD 277 per year for Canadian individuals, USD 525 per year for Canadian institutions, USD 173 per year for Canadian students, USD 336 per year for international individuals, USD 525 per year for international institutions and USD 173 per year for international students. To receive student/resident rate, orders must be accompanied by name of affiliated institution, date of term, and the *signature* of program/residency coordinator on institution letterhead. Orders will be billed at individual rate until proof of status is received. Foreign air speed delivery is included in all *Clinics* subscription prices. All prices are subject to change without notice. **POSTMASTER:** Send address changes to *Medical Clinics of North America*, Elsevier Health Sciences Division, Subscription Customer Service, 3251 Riverport Lane, Maryland Heights, MO 63043. **Customer Service: Telephone: 1-800-654-2452** (U.S. and Canada); **1-314-447-8871** (outside U.S. and Canada). **Fax: 1-314-447-8029. E-mail: journalscustomerservice-usa@elsevier.com** (for print support); **journalsonlinesupport-usa@ elsevier.com** (for online support).

Reprints. For copies of 100 or more of articles in this publication, please contact the Commercial Reprints Department, Elsevier Inc., 360 Park Avenue South, New York, NY 10010-1710. Tel.: 212-633-3812; Fax: 212-462-1935; E-mail: reprints@elsevier.com.

Medical Clinics of North America is also published in Spanish by McGraw-Hill Interamericana Editores S. A., P.O. Box 5-237, 06500 Mexico, D.F., Mexico.

Medical Clinics of North America is covered in *MEDLINE/PubMed (Index Medicus), Current Contents, ASCA, Excerpta Medica, Science Citation Index,* and *ISI/BIOMED.*

Printed and bound by CPI Group (UK) Ltd, Croydon, CR0 4YY

Transferred to Digital Print 2011

GOAL STATEMENT

The goal of *Medical Clinics of North America* is to keep practicing physicians up to date with current clinical practice by providing timely articles reviewing the state of the art in patient care.

ACCREDITATION

The *Medical Clinics of North America* is planned and implemented in accordance with the Essential Areas and Policies of the Accreditation Council for Continuing Medical Education (ACCME) through the joint sponsorship of the University of Virginia School of Medicine and Elsevier. The University of Virginia School of Medicine is accredited by the ACCME to provide continuing medical education for physicians.

The University of Virginia School of Medicine designates this educational activity for a maximum of 15 *AMA PRA Category 1 Credits*™ for each issue, 90 credits per year. Physicians should only claim credit commensurate with the extent of their participation in the activity.

The American Medical Association has determined that physicians not licensed in the US who participate in this CME activity are eligible for a maximum of 15 *AMA PRA Category 1 Credits*™ for each issue, 90 credits per year.

Credit can be earned by reading the text material, taking the CME examination online at http://www.theclinics.com/home/cme, and completing the evaluation. After taking the test, you will be required to review any and all incorrect answers. Following completion of the test and evaluation, your credit will be awarded and you may print your certificate.

FACULTY DISCLOSURE/CONFLICT OF INTEREST

The University of Virginia School of Medicine, as an ACCME accredited provider, endorses and strives to comply with the Accreditation Council for Continuing Medical Education (ACCME) Standards of Commercial Support, Commonwealth of Virginia statutes, University of Virginia policies and procedures, and associated federal and private regulations and guidelines on the need for disclosure and monitoring of proprietary and financial interests that may affect the scientific integrity and balance of content delivered in continuing medical education activities under our auspices.

The University of Virginia School of Medicine requires that all CME activities accredited through this institution be developed independently and be scientifically rigorous, balanced and objective in the presentation/discussion of its content, theories and practices.

All authors/editors participating in an accredited CME activity are expected to disclose to the readers relevant financial relationships with commercial entities occurring within the past 12 months (such as grants or research support, employee, consultant, stock holder, member of speakers bureau, etc.). The University of Virginia School of Medicine will employ appropriate mechanisms to resolve potential conflicts of interest to maintain the standards of fair and balanced education to the reader. Questions about specific strategies can be directed to the Office of Continuing Medical Education, University of Virginia School of Medicine, Charlottesville, Virginia.

The faculty and staff of the University of Virginia Office of Continuing Medical Education have no financial affiliations to disclose.

The authors/editors listed below have identified no professional or financial affiliations for themselves or their spouse/partner:

Gabor Abellan van Kan, MD; Ali Ahmed, MD, MPH; Nazwem Bassil, MD; Lenise A. Cummings-Vaughn, MD; Abhilash K. Desai, MD; Joseph H. Flaherty, MD; Julie K. Gammack, MD; Sophie Gillette, PhD; Rachel Glover, (Acquisitions Editor); Milta O. Little, DO; Alayne D. Markland, DO, MSc; Debbie Tolson, MSc, PhD, RGN; Andrew Wolf, MD (Test Author); and Jean Woo, MD, FRCP.

The authors/editors listed below identified the following professional or financial affiliations for themselves or their spouse/ partner:

Kathryn L. Burgio, PhD is an industry funded research/investigator and consultant for Pfizer, is a consultant and is on the Advisory Board for Astellas, and is a consultant for Johnson & Johnson.

Ian M. Chapman, MBBS, PhD, FRACP is on the Advisory Committee/Board for Pfizer (Australia), and is on the Speakers' Bureau for Merck (Australia) and Lilly (Australia).

Charlotte Dupuy, MS is employed by Nutricia.

Patricia S. Goode, MSN, MD is an industry funded research/investigator for Pfizer.

Theodore M. Johnson II, MD, MPH is an industry funded research/investigator and consultant for Pfizer and Vantia.

John E. Morley, MB, BCh (Guest Editor) is an industry funded research/investigator for Cardiokine, Danone, Nestle, and Numico; is a consultant for Amgen, Cytokinetics, Edunn Biotec, GSK, Healthspan, Incyte, Lilly LCC, Matteren Pharmaceuticals, and Sanofi-Aventis; owns stock in Mattern Pharmaceuticals and Edunn Biotec; and is on the Speakers' Bureau for Amgen, Mattern, and Healthspan.

Yves Rolland, MD, PhD is on the Speakers' Bureau for Lundbeck, MSD, Danone, Lilly, and Nutricia; is an industry funded research/investigator for Lactalis; and is on the Advisory Committee/Board for Cheisi and Lilly.

Alan J. Sinclair, MSc, MD, FRCP is a consultant, and is on the Speakers' Bureau and Advisory Board for Takeda, Novartis, MSD; and is on the Speakers' Bureau for Pfizer.

Camille P. Vaughan, MD, MS's spouse is employed by Kimberly-Clark Corp; is an industry funded research/investigator for Astellas Pharma, Inc.

Bruno Vellas, MD, PhD is on the Advisory Committee/Board for Astra-Zeneca, Danone/Nutricia, Eisai, Eli Lilly and Company, Exhonit, GSK, Ipsen, Nestle, and Pfizer, Inc., and is a consultant for Avid Radiopharmaceuticals, BMS, Danone, Eisai Inc, Elan Pharma, Eli Lilly and Company, Exhonit, G.S.K, Ipsen, Lundbeck, Médivation, Merck, Nestle, Pfizer, Pierre Fabre Laboratories, Roche, Sanofi-Aventis, and Servier.

Adie Viljoen, MBChB, MMed, FCPath(SA), FRCPath, MBA is an industry funded research/investigator, and is on the Speakers' Bureau and Advisory Board for Merck, Sharpe, Dohme, Takeda, Novo Nordisk, Lilly, Astra Zeneca, Pfizer, and Novartis.

Disclosure of Discussion of Non-FDA Approved Uses for Pharmaceutical Products and/or Medical Devices.

The University of Virginia School of Medicine, as an ACCME provider, requires that all faculty presenters identify and disclose any off-label uses for pharmaceutical and medical device products. The University of Virginia School of Medicine recommends that each physician fully review all the available data on new products or procedures prior to clinical use.

TO ENROLL

To enroll in the Medical Clinics of North America Continuing Medical Education program, call customer service at 1-800-654-2452 or visit us online at http://www.theclinics.com/home/cme. The CME program is available to subscribers for an additional fee of USD 228.

RELATED INTEREST

Clinics in Geriatric Medicine, February 2011 (Volume 27, Issue 1)
Frailty
Jeremy D. Walston, MD, *Guest Editor*

VISIT US ONLINE!
Access your subscription at:
www.theclinics.com

Contributors

GUEST EDITOR

JOHN E. MORLEY, MB, BCh
Dammert Professor of Gerontology, Director, Division of Geriatric Medicine, Saint Louis University Medical Center; Director, Geriatric Research, Education and Clinical Center, St Louis Veterans Affairs Medical Center, St Louis, Missouri

AUTHORS

ALI AHMED, MD, MPH
Professor of Medicine and Epidemiology, Division of Gerontology, Geriatrics and Palliative Care, and Division of Cardiovascular Disease, Department of Medicine, School of Medicine, and Department of Epidemiology, School of Public Health; Senior Scientist, Center for Aging; Scientist, Center for Heart Failure Research; Scientist, Center for Cardiovascular Biology; Director, Geriatric Heart Failure Clinic, University of Alabama at Birmingham; Staff Geriatrician, Section of Geriatrics; Director, Geriatric Heart Failure Clinic, Veterans Affairs Medical Center, Birmingham, Alabama

NAZEM BASSIL, MD
Assistant Professor of Medicine, Department of Medicine, Saint George Hospital Medical Center, Balamand University, Beirut, Lebanon

KATHRYN L. BURGIO, PhD
Professor, Division of Gerontology, Geriatrics, and Palliative Care, Department of Medicine, University of Alabama at Birmingham and Veterans Affairs Birmingham/Atlanta Geriatric Research, Education, and Clinical Center, Birmingham, Alabama

IAN M. CHAPMAN, MBBS, PhD, FRACP
Division of Medicine, Royal Adelaide Hospital, University of Adelaide, North Terrace, Adelaide, Australia

LENISE A. CUMMINGS-VAUGHN, MD
Clinical Instructor, Jefferson Barracks Division, Geriatric Research, Education, and Clinical Center, Saint Louis Veterans Affairs Medical Center; Division of Geriatric Medicine, Department of Internal Medicine, Saint Louis University School of Medicine, St Louis, Missouri

ABHILASH K. DESAI, MD
Chief, Geriatric Psychiatry; Director, Memory Clinic, Sheppard Pratt Health Systems, Baltimore, Maryland

CHARLOTTE DUPUY, MS
Inserm U1027, University of Toulouse III; PhD Student, Gérontopôle of Toulouse, CHU Purpan, Toulouse, France

JOSEPH H. FLAHERTY, MD
Geriatric Research, Education and Clinical Center, St Louis Veterans Affairs Medical Center; Division of Geriatrics, Department of Internal Medicine, Saint Louis University School of Medicine, St Louis, Missouri

JULIE K. GAMMACK, MD
Associate Professor of Medicine, Division of Geriatric Medicine, Department of Internal Medicine, Saint Louis University School of Medicine, St Louis, Missouri

SOPHIE GILLETTE, PhD
Inserm U1027, University of Toulouse III; Researcher, Gérontopôle of Toulouse, CHU Purpan, Toulouse, France

PATRICIA S. GOODE, MSN, MD
Professor, Division of Gerontology, Geriatrics, and Palliative Care, Department of Medicine, University of Alabama at Birmingham and Veterans Affairs Birmingham/Atlanta Geriatric Research, Education, and Clinical Center, Birmingham, Alabama

THEODORE M. JOHNSON II, MD, MPH
Professor, Division of Geriatric Medicine and Gerontology, Emory University and Veterans Affairs Birmingham/Atlanta Geriatric Research, Education, and Clinical Center, Atlanta, Georgia

MILTA O. LITTLE, DO
Assistant Professor of Medicine, Division of Gerontology and Geriatric Medicine, Department of Internal Medicine, Saint Louis University School of Medicine, St Louis, Missouri

ALAYNE D. MARKLAND, DO, MSc
Associate Professor, Division of Gerontology, Geriatrics, and Palliative Care, Department of Medicine, University of Alabama at Birmingham and Veterans Affairs Birmingham/Atlanta Geriatric Research, Education, and Clinical Center, Birmingham, Alabama

JOHN E. MORLEY, MB, BCh
Dammert Professor of Gerontology, Director, Division of Geriatric Medicine, Saint Louis University Medical Center; Director, Geriatric Research, Education and Clinical Center, St Louis Veterans Affairs Medical Center, St Louis, Missouri

YVES ROLLAND, MD, PhD
Inserm U1027, University of Toulouse III; Professor, Gérontopôle of Toulouse, CHU Purpan, Toulouse, France

ALAN J. SINCLAIR, MSc, MD, FRCP
Dean, Bedfordshire and Hertfordshire Postgraduate Medical School, University of Bedfordshire, Bedfordshire, United Kingdom

DEBBIE TOLSON, MSc, PhD, RGN
Scottish Centre for Evidence Based Care of Older People: A Collaborating Centre for the Joanna Briggs Institute, Glasgow Caledonian University, Glasgow, United Kingdom

GABOR ABELLAN VAN KAN, MD
Inserm U1027, University of Toulouse III; Gérontopôle of Toulouse, CHU Purpan, Toulouse, France

CAMILLE P. VAUGHAN, MD, MS
Assistant Professor, Division of Geriatric Medicine and Gerontology, Emory University and Veterans Affairs Birmingham/Atlanta Geriatric Research, Education, and Clinical Center, Atlanta, Georgia

BRUNO VELLAS, MD, PhD
Inserm U1027, University of Toulouse III; Professor, Gérontopôle of Toulouse, CHU Purpan, Toulouse, France

ADIE VILJOEN, MBChB, MMed, FCPath(SA), FRCPath, MBA
Senior Lecturer in Medicine and Consultant Chemical Pathologist, University of Bedfordshire, Bedfordshire; Department of Chemical Pathology, Lister Hospital, Stevenage, United Kingdom

JEAN WOO, MD, FRCP
Professor of Medicine, Department of Medicine and Therapeutics, The Chinese University of Hong Kong, Hong Kong, China

Contents

Treatment Strategies for Sarcopenia and Frailty   **427**

Yves Rolland, Charlotte Dupuy, Gabor Abellan van Kan, Sophie Gillette, and Bruno Vellas

> Sarcopenia is the key feature of frailty in older people and a major determinant of adverse health outcomes such as functional limitations and disability. Resistance training and adequate protein and energy intake are the key strategies for the management of sarcopenia. Management of weight loss and resistance training are the most relevant protective countermeasures to slow down the decline of muscle mass and muscle strength. The quality of amino acids in the diet is an important factor for stimulating protein synthesis. Vitamin D deficiency should be treated, and new pharmacologic approaches for sarcopenia are currently assessed.

Chronic Heart Failure in Older Adults   **439**

Ali Ahmed

> Assessment and management of heart failure (HF) in older adults may be simplified and structured by the mnemonic DEFEAT-HF: Diagnosis, Etiology, Fluid volume, Ejection fraction, And Treatment of Heart Failure. A clinical diagnosis and etiology of HF can often be established during history and physical examination. Fluid volume status must be assessed by estimating jugular venous pressure in centimeters of water by identifying the top of the jugular venous pulsation in the neck and estimating its vertical height from the right atrium. Left ventricular ejection fraction must be obtained to classify patients into systolic and diastolic HF and to guide evidence-based therapy.

Revitalizing the Aged Brain   **463**

Abhilash K. Desai

> Optimal cognitive and emotional function is vital to independence, productivity, and quality of life. Cognitive impairment without dementia may be seen in 16% to 33% of adults older than 65 years, and is associated with significant emotional distress. Cognitive and emotional well-being are inextricably linked. This article qualifies revitalizing the aged brain, discusses neuroplasticity, and suggests practical neuroplasticity-based strategies to improve the cognitive and emotional well-being of older adults.

Nutritional Strategies for Successful Aging   **477**

Jean Woo

> With increasing life expectancy in developed and developing countries, maintaining health and function in old age has become an important

goal, including avoidance or optimal control of chronic diseases; maintenance or retarding the decline of physical and cognitive function; optimizing psychological health; and maintaining independent functioning in tasks related to self-care and societal interaction. This article discusses all of those, as well as other components of successful aging such as social network and socioeconomic status.

Osteoporosis and falls are distinct conditions that share the potential clinical endpoint of fracture. This article explores the associations between osteoporosis and falls by examining the epidemiology, risk factors, risk prevention, and treatments. It outlines the evidence on falls prevention, osteoporosis diagnosis, and fracture risk assessment. It includes several studies that challenge the common view on the use of fall prevention tools, dual energy X-ray absorptiometry testing, and postfracture bisphosphonate treatment. By understanding the evidence, it becomes clearer how to target populations at risk, interpret screening methods, and promote disease prevention and treatment.

Late-onset hypogonadism is a clinical and biological syndrome associated with advancing age and characterized by typical symptoms and a deficiency in serum testosterone levels. It is a common condition but often underdiagnosed and undertreated. The main symptoms of hypogonadism are reduced libido/erectile dysfunction, reduced muscle mass and strength, increased adiposity, osteoporosis/low bone mass, depressed mood, and fatigue. Testosterone replacement therapy is only warranted in the presence of both clinical symptoms suggesting hormone deficiency and decreased hormone levels. It improves libido and sexual function, bone density, muscle mass, body composition, mood, erythropoiesis, cognition, quality of life, and cardiovascular disease.

Hypertension is a significant risk factor for cardiovascular morbidity and mortality in people older than 60 years. Isolated systolic hypertension and widened pulse pressure appear to be more important than diastolic hypertension. Very low blood pressure and orthostatic hypotension are associated with increased mortality, and should be checked for at every visit. Best evidence suggests that adjusting hypertension goals with age, and starting therapy when blood pressure is greater than 160/90 leads to improved outcomes. Therapy should start with a thiazide diuretic (best evidence) or an angiotensin-converting enzyme inhibitor.

> Urinary incontinence is a common problem among older women and men. Older adults are reluctant to seek treatment, and health care providers should inquire about symptoms. Treatment of urinary incontinence includes multiple, office-based modalities, such as behavioral approaches, medications, and devices. Older adults may also consider surgical options to improve urinary incontinence. Special consideration should be given to older adults with cognitive impairment and incontinence.

> This article reviews the pathophysiology, prevalence, incidence, and consequences of delirium, focusing on the evaluation of delirium, the published models of care for prevention in patients at risk of delirium, and management of patients for whom delirium is not preventable. Evidence on why physical restraints should not be used for patients with delirium is reviewed. Current available evidence on antipyschotics does not support the role for the general use in the treatment of delirium. An example of a restraint-free, nonpharmacologic management approach [called the TADA approach (tolerate, anticipate, and don't agitate)] is presented.

> Weight loss is common in older people. It is associated with increased morbidity and mortality, particularly when unintentional, excessive (>5% body weight), or associated with low body weight (body mass index <22 kg/m^2). It is often unrecognized, the associated adverse effects not appreciated, and underlying causes not addressed. Intentional weight loss by overweight older people is probably appropriate only when functional problems have resulted from the excess weight. It is important to include, wherever possible, exercise in weight-loss measures to preserve skeletal muscle mass.

> With the advent of the graying of the baby boomers, there is an urgent need to enhance care in the nursing home. This article focuses on the areas where high-quality care can improve outcomes.

> Diabetes is a common condition in older people. Diabetes significantly lowers the chances of successful aging, and notably increases functional limitations and impairs quality of life. Diabetes in older persons represents significant medical, human, and socioeconomic burden. Multiple

interventions are now available to treat patients with diabetes. Clinicians have to weigh the risks and benefits of the treatments available to prevent these complications. This article discusses the pathophysiology, diagnosis, and vascular complications of diabetes and summarizes the various risk factors that are the focus of clinical care.

Preface

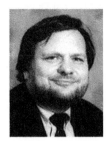

John E. Morley, MB, BCh
Guest Editor

"I offer no apology for the publication of this volume.
The subject is one of the highest importance, and yet it has been strangely
overlooked during the last half-century by the physicians of all countries."

George Edward Day
(1815–1872)

Unfortunately little has changed since George Day wrote his introduction to "Disease of Advanced Life" in 1848. My colleagues in internal medicine and family practice are continually telling me that they see so many older persons, that they really are geriatricians. Despite their belief, a large number of children bring their parents to me because they are frustrated with the inability of their physicians to solve the problem they perceive. Geriatricians differ from generalist physicians in that they focus on improving function as opposed to focusing on treating specific diseases. The tools of the geriatrician are to assess function, from basic activities of daily living to walking speed, and identify those who are frail so they can prevent them from developing disability.[1] Their treatment armamentarium consists of reducing polypharmacy; enhancing nutrition, including preventing weight loss; treating delirium, dementia, and depression; increasing exercise capacity with a focus on aerobic, resistance, and balance exercises; and providing social support for the older adult.

At present in the United States there are just over 7,000 geriatricians with an added certification of specialization. This means that there are approximately 3.8 geriatricians for 10,000 of the population 75 years and older. Clearly these numbers suggest that geriatricians should perform as subspecialists, focusing on the care of the most complex older persons. To allow this to happen, there is an urgent need to increase the basic geriatric knowledge among generalists. This issue of *Medical Clinics* is focused on increasing the basic knowledge of geriatrics.

This issue focuses on geriatric syndromes and diseases where the treatment of frail elderly with this condition often differs from that of younger persons. In addition, we review the growing need for high-quality nursing home care. The International Association of Gerontology and Geriatrics together with the World Health Organization have produced a white paper calling for increased prestige for all who work in nursing homes, and an increase in research to improve quality of life in nursing homes.[2] The

Med Clin N Am 95 (2011) xiii–xiv
doi:10.1016/j.mcna.2011.03.004
0025-7125/11/$ – see front matter
medical.theclinics.com

task force also stressed the need for increased physician presence in nursing homes. This has been justified by the finding that nursing homes with a medical director who has been trained as a Certified Medical Director by the American Medical Directors Association have better outcomes than those nursing homes with untrained physicians.[3,4]

It is hoped that as the "baby boomers" age, articles such as the ones in this issue of the *Medical Clinics* will increase the physician's awareness of the nuances of geriatric medicine, and enhance the quality of care of our aging population.

John E. Morley, MB, BCh
Division of Geriatric Medicine
Saint Louis University & GRECC VA Medical Center
1402 South Grand Boulevard, M238
St Louis, MO 63104, USA

E-mail address:
morley@slu.edu

REFERENCES

1. Abellan van Kan G, Rolland YM, Morley JE, et al. Frailty: Toward a clinical definition. J Am Med Directors Assoc 2008;9:71–2.
2. Tolson D, Rolland Y, Andrieu S, et al. The International Association of Gerontiology and Geriatrics/World Health Organization/Society Française de Gérontologie et de Gériatrie Task Force. J Am Med Directors Assoc 2011;12:184–9.
3. Morley JE. Having a CMD is associated with improved nursing home quality of care. J Am Med Directors Assoc 2008;10:515.
4. Rowland FN, Cowles M, Dickstein C, et al. Impact of medical director certification on nursing home quality of care. J Am Med Directors Assoc 2009;10:431–5.

Treatment Strategies for Sarcopenia and Frailty

Yves Rolland, MD, PhD[a,b,]*, Charlotte Dupuy, MS[a,b],
Gabor Abellan van Kan, MD[a,b], Sophie Gillette, PhD[a,b],
Bruno Vellas, MD, PhD[a,b]

KEYWORDS

- Sarcopenia • Frailty • Physical activity • Weight loss
- Testosterone • Creatine • Vitamin D

The syndrome of frailty describes older people at a higher risk for adverse health outcomes. Compared with the robust older people frail older people are characterized by a higher risk of disability, illnesses, admission to nursing home, and mortality when confronted by a stressor.[1] Frailty is usually described as a complex condition that occurs during the aging process and results from an imbalance and dysregulation of interrelated physiologic systems, such as the immune system (with cytokine over-expression) or the neuroendocrine system (with hormonal decline) and body compositional changes (with the loss of muscle mass and muscle strength or sarcopenia). Frailty often occurs in combination with chronic and acute diseases. For the clinician, frail elderly patients can be recognized by a combination of specific symptoms such as weight loss, weakness, fatigue, slow walking speed, and low physical activity. These 5 symptoms are used in research to characterize the frail elderly population.[2] These symptoms interact with each other and lead to a decrease in physiologic reserves in older adults.[2–4]

The concept of frailty is relevant, as it can provide an explanation for the considerable differences in tolerance of stress among older subjects. The recognition of frailty may be a determinant in the decision making for care in the presence of various other conditions, such as cancer. Benefit of chemotherapy or other therapeutic options may be lower in the frail than in the robust older patients with cancer. The main interest in the concept of frailty is also related to its reversible nature.[5] Frailty is a dynamic condition and can predict adverse health events. Interventions focused on the determinant factors of frailty can prevent the transition of frailty into disability.[5]

---

[a] Inserm U1027; F-31073, Avenue Jules Guesdes, University of Toulouse III, F-31073, France
[b] Gérontopôle of Toulouse, 170 avenue de Casselardit, CHU Purpan, 31300 Toulouse, France
* Corresponding author. Gérontopôle de Toulouse, Pavillon Junod, 170 avenue de Casselardit, Toulouse University Hospital, 31300 Toulouse, France.
E-mail address: rolland.y@chu-toulouse.fr

Med Clin N Am 95 (2011) 427–438
doi:10.1016/j.mcna.2011.02.008
0025-7125/11/$ – see front matter © 2011 Elsevier Inc. All rights reserved.

Sarcopenia is recognized as the key feature of frailty.[6] The feeling of tiredness, decreased strength, involuntary weight loss, slowness, and inactivity characterize frailty and can be, at least in part, related to the loss of muscle mass and muscle strength. About 20% of men aged 70 to 75 years and about 50% of the elderly men 80 years and older have sarcopenia, whereas 25% to 40% of women in the same age ranges are sarcopenic. Janssen and colleagues[7] reported that 35% and 10% of the elderly participants in the National Health and Nutrition Examination Survey were moderately and severely sarcopenic, respectively.

Sarcopenia is an important field of research in geriatrics, as it is responsible for functional limitations and disability. Lack of strength or functional limitations, such as slow walking speed, is a strong predictor of adverse health outcomes[8,9] and death.[10,11] Poor physical performances and poor strength are relevant markers of frailty. The management of sarcopenia would certainly have a major effect on limiting the frailty adverse events, so that even a modest reduction in sarcopenia would have a significant economic impact.[12]

Various conditions can result in sarcopenia and frailty. Epidemiologic and interventional studies suggest that most etiologic factors for frailty and sarcopenia are preventable or manageable. Among these factors, inactivity and poor nutritional intake and their underlying causes are the main treatable domains. Resistance training in combination with adequate protein and energy intake is currently the key strategy proposed for the management of sarcopenia.[13] However, the treatment of sarcopenia may also rely on new pharmacologic approaches.

NUTRITION

Reduced food intake, in particular of protein, results in weight loss and reduced muscle mass synthesis and hastens transition to frailty.[14] Weight loss is a frequent condition and always a serious event in older people whether the person is overweight or underweight.[15] Anorexia precedes weight loss and predicts death and institutionalization.[16–19] A high investment from the practitioner is needed to assess and treat its various causes. The Mini Nutritional Assessment is a 30-item validated scale to assess the nutritional risk.[20] The Simplified Nutrition Assessment Questionnaire is also a simple 4-question scale, validated both in the community and institutions for documenting anorexia.[21] The management of weight loss relies first on identifying its main causes in older people. The various treatable causes of weight loss in older people can easily be remembered by the mnemonic, "MEALS-ON-WHEELS," proposed by John Morley (**Box 1**).[15,22]

Caloric supplements produce a small weight gain and may reduce mortality in undernourished older people. However, a recent Cochrane collaboration reported no evidence of improvement in functional parameters with supplements.[23] There exist only weak evidences of the benefit of supplements on muscle mass and muscle strength, which may be increased by recent new approaches.

The loss of muscle mass results from an imbalance between protein degradation and synthesis rates. Recommendations for protein intake in the older population are still debated. Changes in protein metabolism observed in the muscle of older people suggest that the dietary requirement of proteins and amino acids may be higher in older people than in young adults.[24] In healthy adults, 0.83 g protein/kg/d is required and safe,[25] whereas the mean protein requirement is estimated at 0.89 g protein/kg/d for older people[26] and might be much higher (at least 1.3 g protein/kg/d) in acute conditions such as during hospitalization.[27] The need for adequate protein intake to maintain muscle mass is also supported by the

---

Box 1
MEALS-ON-WHEELS mnemonic as an easy method to screen for causes of weight loss in older persons

Medications (eg, digoxin, theophylline, cimetidine)

Emotional problems (eg, depression)

Alcoholism, elder abuse, anorexia tardive

Late life paranoia

Swallowing problems

Oral factors

Nosocomial infections (eg, tuberculosis)

Wandering and other dementia-related factors

Hyperthyroidism, hypercalcemia, hypoadrenalism

Enteral problems (eg, gluten enteropathy)

Eating problems

Low-salt, low-cholesterol, and other therapeutic diets

Stones (cholecystitis)

---

results from the Health, Aging and Body Composition study. The lesser reduction in appendicular lean body mass of older people at 3 years was found in subjects who consumed a higher amount of proteins.[28]

Current evidences show that the negative net balance of amino acids across the muscle tissue is not related only to inadequate nutritional intakes.[29] In older people, the first-pass splanchnic extraction of amino acids is increased. This harnessing of the amino acids decreases delivery to the skeletal muscle tissue and availability for muscle tissue anabolism. However, in both young and older subjects, an increased intake of a mixture of amino acids or essential amino acids can increase amino acid availability and result in the stimulation of muscle protein anabolism.[30,31] Muscle response to intake of oral essential amino acids is preserved in older people in comparison with younger people. However, other factors such as the sensitivity of muscles to hormones contribute to the imbalance in muscle tissue metabolism in the elderly. The sensitivity of the aged skeletal muscle to amino acids and insulin is also reduced. Glucose in addition to amino acids reduced muscle breakdown and stimulated muscle synthesis in the young, but the same intake resulted in a lower anabolic response in older people.[32] These results suggest that the anabolic response of muscle protein metabolism to the increased blood levels of insulin and amino acids is impaired in older adults.

Several other determinants of muscle metabolism that may influence dietary recommendation have been highlighted by recent surveys. Diets based on proteins from vegetables result in a lower inhibition of muscle protein breakdown than proteins from meat.[33] These results support the fact that proteins from different sources have different effects on muscle metabolism. The notion of fast and slow proteins refers to the speed of intestinal protein absorption.[34] In the older population, faster kinetics of the amino acids (faster appearance of the amino acids in the plasma and higher magnitude of plasma amino acids level) may contribute to counteract the decrease in muscle sensitivity to amino acids. Fast proteins, such as whey proteins are able to enhance the rate of muscle protein synthesis in healthy elderly individuals.[35]

The quality of dietary amino acids is an important factor for stimulating protein synthesis. New approaches, based on essential amino acids (such as leucine), have been recently reported to stimulate protein anabolism in the elderly, whereas nonessential amino acids (given in association to essential amino acids) added no supplementary effect.[36] Nutritional supplementation with proteins rich in leucine is proposed as a simple and safe strategy to prevent sarcopenia.[37] Muscle protein synthesis also depends on the protein supplementation schedule. A large amount of amino acid in 1 meal per day has been reported to be more efficient in increasing the anabolic effect than the same amount of amino acid spread in different meals during daytime.[38] All these results suggest that the anabolic effect of protein supplementation may be maximized with a large amount of a highly efficient nutritional supplement (such as essential amino acids, especially leucine) once a day. The beneficial effects of these approaches based on the effect of essential amino acids such as leucine on muscle protein synthesis are currently under study in older people.

The additional benefit of combining resistance training and nutritional supplementations is controversial. For this strategy, timing of the supplementation seems an important issue. Recent findings support that the response to amino acid intake depends on the timing of the supplementation after the resistance training.[39] In adults, the ingestion of essential amino acid supplements immediately before the resistance training session results in a greater muscle protein synthesis than when consumed at a distance from the exercise.[40] This strategy may be relevant to enhance the anabolic effect of resistance training programs in older people.

Vitamin D supplementation is a simple, safe, and relevant treatment of sarcopenia. The current recommendation for the management of sarcopenia is that all sarcopenic patients with a 25-hydroxyvitamin D level lower than 100 nmol/L should be given supplementation.[13] Vitamin D deficiency is a frequent condition in older people, which results in proximal muscle weakness.[41,42]

Randomized controlled trials have reported that administration of 2 to 12 months of 800 IU of vitamin D_3 significantly improves lower extremity strength or function.[43–45] This direct effect of vitamin D on muscle tissue reduces the risk of falling by 19% in older people.[46]

PHYSICAL ACTIVITY

Inactivity is an important contributor to the loss of muscle mass and strength.[47] In community-dwelling elderly subjects, the mean loss of muscle mass in a decade is estimated at 2 kg in men and 1 kg in women older than 60 years,[48] but only 10 days of bed rest results in no less than 1.5 kg of lean mass loss (mainly in the lower extremities) and 15% decline of knee extensor muscle strength in healthy elders.[49] Immobilization induces anabolic resistance,[50] mitochondrial dysfunction, and apoptosis.[51]

Resistance training is currently the most relevant protective countermeasure to slow down the decline of muscle mass and muscle strength. Strong evidences support that, even in the frail elderly, resistance training increases muscle mass and strength.[52–56] The improvement of muscle strength is related to an increase in muscle mass through myofibrillar muscle protein synthesis and an improvement of neuronal adaptation (innervations, activation pattern).[57,58] Muscle strength increases after a few days of training, whereas muscle mass increases after 6 to 8 weeks of resistance training. This difference between strength and mass gain is poorly understood.[59] Resistance training is believed to improve the underlying mechanisms that contribute to generate strength from the brain to the muscle fibers. It probably improves the excitatory drive from the cortex, excitability of the alfa-motoneuron, motor unit recruitment and neuromuscular transmission, excitation-contraction coupling processes, and muscle morphology and architecture.[60]

The current recommendations for resistance training from the American Heart Association Council For Older People is to perform 1 set of 8 to 12 repetitions and 10 to 15 repetitions at reduced levels of resistance.[61] The resistance training should be performed 2 to 3 times a week with 8 to 10 different exercises each time. These recommendations from the American Heart Association Council are similar to the guidelines proposed by the American College of Sport and Medicine[62] or the American Geriatrics Society for older adults with osteoarthritis pain.[63] These recommendations are not specific for sarcopenia. Endurance training can also stimulate muscle protein synthesis[64] and satellite cell activation and increase muscle fiber area[65] but does not contribute as much to muscle hypertrophy and improve muscle strength as resistive training. It is, therefore, not the proprietary advice to treat or prevent sarcopenia. However, in sarcopenic obese older people, endurance training may result in weight control and improve physical performances. Moreover, in older people, compliance to aerobic activities such as walking, running, cycling, or swimming may be higher than in resistance training. Then, both resistance and endurance training for the maintenance of muscle mass and strength in the elderly seem relevant. Finally, endurance training increases maximum oxygen consumption and reduces fatigue, a relevant factor of frailty. The synergic effect of physical activity and hormones has been studied in several clinical studies in older people. However, the effects of testosterone[66] or estrogens[67,68] on muscle strength and function are controversial even when combined with physical training.[66] In a study with a small sample size, the administration of testosterone in addition to resistance training produced greater muscle size and a trend toward greater muscle strength than resistance training alone. Estrogen in association with strength training does not seem to produce any additional anabolic effect on muscle mass or muscle strength.[69] However, exercise in rats may reverse the resistance of aging muscle to insulinlike growth factor 1,[70] a potential contributor to sarcopenia. Endurance and resistance training reduce insulin resistance and stimulate its anabolic effect in the presence of amino acids.[71]

PHARMACOLOGIC AGENTS

Several new pharmacologic approaches are currently assessed in sarcopenia.

Epidemiologic studies support a relationship between the decline of testosterone level with aging and the loss of muscle mass, strength, and the functional decline. The effect of testosterone administration on muscle mass, muscle strength, and decreased fat mass has been repeatedly assessed in hypogonadal elderly subjects.[72–77] Although testosterone administration in hypogonadal subjects improves body composition and muscle strength and rehabilitation outcomes, inconclusive results are reported from studies evaluating the effectiveness of testosterone in community-dwelling population. A meta-analysis performed in 2006 by Ottenbacher and colleagues[66] concluded that testosterone administration results in a moderate increase in muscle strength among men. They also noticed that among the 11 randomized studies included, 1 study influenced the mean effect size. The conflicting results on muscle mass and muscle strength may be explained by the heterogeneous characteristics of the recruited population. Testosterone administration seems all the more relevant in frail elderly subjects[78] than in healthy subjects[72] and when combined with nutritional supplement in undernourished older people.[79] Large clinical trials on testosterone supplementation in the frail elderly people are required to validate this approach.[80] Moreover, testosterone safety is an important concern. A recent survey reports that testosterone is associated with an increased risk of cardiovascular adverse events in frail older people.[81] The synthetic androgen modulators such as the selective androgen receptor modulators (SARMs) may be potential alternatives to testosterone. The SARMs have the same anabolic effect on muscle tissue as testosterone but without the undesirable sideeffects.[82]

Conflicting results have been reported during growth hormone (GH) supplementation. Most studies have failed to demonstrate that GH supplementation increases muscle mass or muscle strength even in association with resistance training.[83–86] The high prevalence of side effects such as arthralgias, gynecomastia, edema, and diabetes is a serious concern. Recent findings show that combined supplementation of GH with testosterone significantly increases lean mass by up to 7.5 kg (mean, 3 kg) and muscle strength by 30% at mean while reducing the fat mass by up to 7 kg (mean, 2.3 kg).[87] Previous studies combining GH and testosterone supplementation did not demonstrate an improvement in muscle performance.[88,89]

Other hormones such as ghrelin, a peptide hormone produced by the stomach in response to fasting, are currently assessed with promising effects to reduce wasting.[90,91] Very few clinical trials on estrogens and tibolone, a steroid with estrogenic, progestogenic, and androgenic activity, included older women.[92] The roles of these compounds on skeletal muscle in postmenopausal women are still controversial. The positive effect of tibolone on the functional performance may be related to its beneficial effect on fat mass.[93,94]

Myostatin is a recently discovered member of the transforming growth factor β family. It is expressed in skeletal muscle and inhibits its growth.[95] Several drugs that inhibit the effect of myostatin are under development.[96] Antagonizing myostatin represents an important promising therapeutic approach for sarcopenia. Recent findings report that recombinant human antibodies to myostatin tested in healthy postmenopausal women increased in lean body mass by about 2.5% after only 15 days of treatment.[97]

The beneficial effect of angiotensin II converting enzyme (ACE) inhibitors on the prognosis may be, at least in part, related to the direct effect of the ACE inhibitor on the skeletal muscle tissue.[92,98,99] People using ACE inhibitors usually have a higher lower extremity lean body mass than older people using other hypertensive drugs, even after adjustment for potential confounders.[100] Sumukadas and colleagues[101] reported in 130 elderly participants that the ACE inhibitor group performed a better 6-minute walking test relative to the placebo group.

Creatine has been recently proposed by a panel of experts as a potential medication for the prevention and management of sarcopenia.[13] Some recent clinical trials have reported that creatine increases lean mass (by 1.7 kg[102] to 3.3 kg)[103] after about 3 months of resistance training. On the other hand, other trials have failed to demonstrate any increase in lean mass.[104,105]

SUMMARY

Frailty can be attributed to multiple risk factors in older people and during the whole lifespan. These factors have been extended beyond the genetic predispositions and comorbidities and included both risk and protective factors. Most epidemiologic studies underlined the importance of nutrition and several other potential modifiable lifestyle factors such as physical exercise. At present, there is no specific recommendation to treat or avoid frailty and its distal health outcomes such as mobility disability. However, sarcopenia has a key role in the development of frailty, and recent randomized controlled trials showed promising results for mobility disability prevention in frail older adults.[106] Because of the multifactorial nature of frailty, it seems logical to propose multidomain interventions with potential synergistic effects.[107]

Even if intervention studies have shown their effectiveness in old age in several specific areas, we still observe inequalities to access to innovation for older adults. Specific studies of older adults that include only frail elderly subjects remained rare. Therefore, the prevention of functional decline in older adults has to be a priority, representing a major goal for today's research, medical practice, and public health. It is now time to develop large health care interventions and pharmacologic trials in frail older people.

REFERENCES

1. Rockwood K, Stadnyk K, MacKnight C, et al. A brief clinical instrument to classify frailty in elderly people. Lancet 1999;353:205.
2. Fried LP, Tangen CM, Walston J, et al. Frailty in older adults: evidence for a phenotype. J Gerontol A Biol Sci Med Sci 2001;56:M146.
3. Bortz WM 2nd. The physics of frailty. J Am Geriatr Soc 1993;41:1004.
4. Lipsitz LA, Goldberger AL. Loss of 'complexity' and aging. Potential applications of fractals and chaos theory to senescence. JAMA 1992;267:1806.
5. Gill TM, Gahbauer EA, Allore HG, et al. Transitions between frailty states among community-living older persons. Arch Intern Med 2006;166:418.
6. Walston J, Fried LP. Frailty and the older man. Med Clin North Am 1999;83:1173.
7. Janssen I, Baumgartner RN, Ross R, et al. Skeletal muscle cutpoints associated with elevated physical disability risk in older men and women. Am J Epidemiol 2004;159:413.
8. Abellan van Kan G, Rolland Y, Andrieu S, et al. Gait speed at usual pace as a predictor of adverse outcomes in community-dwelling older people an International Academy on Nutrition and Aging (IANA) Task Force. J Nutr Health Aging 2009;13:881.
9. Nguyen T, Sambrook P, Kelly P, et al. Prediction of osteoporotic fractures by postural instability and bone density. BMJ 1993;307:1111.
10. Cooper R, Kuh D, Hardy R. Objectively measured physical capability levels and mortality: systematic review and meta-analysis. BMJ 2010;341:c4467.
11. Studenski S, Perera S, Patel K, et al. Gait speed and survival in older adults. JAMA 2011;305:50.
12. Janssen I, Shepard DS, Katzmarzyk PT, et al. The healthcare costs of sarcopenia in the United States. J Am Geriatr Soc 2004;52:80.
13. Morley JE, Argiles JM, Evans WJ, et al. Nutritional recommendations for the management of sarcopenia. J Am Med Dir Assoc 2010;11:391.
14. Vanitallie TB. Frailty in the elderly: contributions of sarcopenia and visceral protein depletion. Metabolism 2003;52:22.
15. Rolland Y, Kim MJ, Gammack JK, et al. Office management of weight loss in older persons. Am J Med 2006;119:1019.
16. Cornali C, Franzoni S, Frisoni GB, et al. Anorexia as an independent predictor of mortality. J Am Geriatr Soc 2005;53:354.
17. Cornoni-Huntley JC, Harris TB, Everett DF, et al. An overview of body weight of older persons, including the impact on mortality. The National Health and Nutrition Examination Survey I–Epidemiologic Follow-up Study. J Clin Epidemiol 1991;44:743.
18. Ensrud KE, Ewing SK, Stone KL, et al. Intentional and unintentional weight loss increase bone loss and hip fracture risk in older women. J Am Geriatr Soc 2003; 51:1740.

19. Payette H, Coulombe C, Boutier V, et al. Nutrition risk factors for institutionalization in a free-living functionally dependent elderly population. J Clin Epidemiol 2000;53:579.

20. Rubenstein LZ, Harker JO, Salva A, et al. Screening for undernutrition in geriatric practice: developing the short-form mini-nutritional assessment (MNA-SF). J Gerontol A Biol Sci Med Sci 2001;56:M366.

21. Wilson MM, Thomas DR, Rubenstein LZ, et al. Appetite assessment: simple appetite questionnaire predicts weight loss in community-dwelling adults and nursing home residents. Am J Clin Nutr 2005;82:1074.

22. Morley JE. Anorexia, body composition, and ageing. Curr Opin Clin Nutr Metab Care 2001;4:9.

23. Milne AC, Potter J, Vivanti A, et al. Protein and energy supplementation in elderly people at risk from malnutrition. Cochrane Database Syst Rev 2009;2:CD003288.

24. Walrand S, Boirie Y. Optimizing protein intake in aging. Curr Opin Clin Nutr Metab Care 2005;8:89.

25. Rand WM, Pellett PL, Young VR. Meta-analysis of nitrogen balance studies for estimating protein requirements in healthy adults. Am J Clin Nutr 2003;77:109.

26. Campbell WW, Evans WJ. Protein requirements of elderly people. Eur J Clin Nutr 1996;50(Suppl 1):S180.

27. Gaillard C, Alix E, Boirie Y, et al. Are elderly hospitalized patients getting enough protein? J Am Geriatr Soc 2008;56:1045.

28. Houston DK, Nicklas BJ, Ding J, et al. Dietary protein intake is associated with lean mass change in older, community-dwelling adults: the Health, Aging, and Body Composition (Health ABC) Study. Am J Clin Nutr 2008;87:150.

29. Short KR, Nair KS. The effect of age on protein metabolism. Curr Opin Clin Nutr Metab Care 2000;3:39.

30. Boirie Y, Gachon P, Beaufrere B. Splanchnic and whole-body leucine kinetics in young and elderly men. Am J Clin Nutr 1997;65:489.

31. Volpi E, Mittendorfer B, Wolf SE, et al. Oral amino acids stimulate muscle protein anabolism in the elderly despite higher first-pass splanchnic extraction. Am J Physiol 1999;277:E513.

32. Volpi E, Mittendorfer B, Rasmussen BB, et al. The response of muscle protein anabolism to combined hyperaminoacidemia and glucose-induced hyperinsulinemia is impaired in the elderly. J Clin Endocrinol Metab 2000;85:4481.

33. Pannemans DL, Wagenmakers AJ, Westerterp KR, et al. Effect of protein source and quantity on protein metabolism in elderly women. Am J Clin Nutr 1998;68:1228.

34. Boirie Y, Dangin M, Gachon P, et al. Slow and fast dietary proteins differently modulate postprandial protein accretion. Proc Natl Acad Sci U S A 1997;94:14930.

35. Paddon-Jones D, Sheffield-Moore M, Katsanos CS, et al. Differential stimulation of muscle protein synthesis in elderly humans following isocaloric ingestion of amino acids or whey protein. Exp Gerontol 2006;41:215.

36. Volpi E, Kobayashi H, Sheffield-Moore M, et al. Essential amino acids are primarily responsible for the amino acid stimulation of muscle protein anabolism in healthy elderly adults. Am J Clin Nutr 2003;78:250.

37. Hayes A, Cribb PJ. Effect of whey protein isolate on strength, body composition and muscle hypertrophy during resistance training. Curr Opin Clin Nutr Metab Care 2008;11:40.

38. Arnal MA, Mosoni L, Boirie Y, et al. Protein pulse feeding improves protein retention in elderly women. Am J Clin Nutr 1999;69:1202.

39. Wolfe RR. Regulation of muscle protein by amino acids. J Nutr 2002;132:3219S.
40. Tipton KD, Rasmussen BB, Miller SL, et al. Timing of amino acid-carbohydrate ingestion alters anabolic response of muscle to resistance exercise. Am J Physiol Endocrinol Metab 2001;281:E197.
41. Braddy KK, Imam SN, Palla KR, et al. Vitamin D deficiency/insufficiency practice patterns in a veterans health administration long-term care population: a retrospective analysis. J Am Med Dir Assoc 2009;10:653.
42. Holick MF. The vitamin D deficiency pandemic and consequences for nonskeletal health: mechanisms of action. Mol Aspects Med 2008;29:361.
43. Bischoff HA, Stahelin HB, Dick W, et al. Effects of vitamin D and calcium supplementation on falls: a randomized controlled trial. J Bone Miner Res 2003;18:343.
44. Moreira-Pfrimer LD, Pedrosa MA, Teixeira L, et al. Treatment of vitamin D deficiency increases lower limb muscle strength in institutionalized older people independently of regular physical activity: a randomized double-blind controlled trial. Ann Nutr Metab 2009;54:291.
45. Pfeifer M, Begerow B, Minne HW, et al. Effects of a long-term vitamin D and calcium supplementation on falls and parameters of muscle function in community-dwelling older individuals. Osteoporos Int 2009;20:315.
46. Bischoff-Ferrari HA, Dawson-Hughes B, Staehelin HB, et al. Fall prevention with supplemental and active forms of vitamin D: a meta-analysis of randomised controlled trials. BMJ 2009;339:b3692.
47. Rolland Y, Czerwinski S, Abellan Van Kan G, et al. Sarcopenia: its assessment, etiology, pathogenesis, consequences and future perspectives. J Nutr Health Aging 2008;12:433.
48. Janssen I, Heymsfield SB, Wang ZM, et al. Skeletal muscle mass and distribution in 468 men and women aged 18–88 yr. J Appl Physiol 2000;89:81.
49. Kortebein P, Ferrando A, Lombeida J, et al. Effect of 10 days of bed rest on skeletal muscle in healthy older adults. JAMA 2007;297:1772.
50. Glover EI, Phillips SM, Oates BR, et al. Immobilization induces anabolic resistance in human myofibrillar protein synthesis with low and high dose amino acid infusion. J Physiol 2008;586:6049.
51. Marzetti E, Leeuwenburgh C. Skeletal muscle apoptosis, sarcopenia and frailty at old age. Exp Gerontol 2006;41:1234.
52. Fiatarone MA, O'Neill EF, Ryan ND, et al. Exercise training and nutritional supplementation for physical frailty in very elderly people. N Engl J Med 1994;330:1769.
53. Hagerman FC, Walsh SJ, Staron RS, et al. Effects of high-intensity resistance training on untrained older men. I. Strength, cardiovascular, and metabolic responses. J Gerontol A Biol Sci Med Sci 2000;55:B336.
54. Ivey FM, Roth SM, Ferrell RE, et al. Effects of age, gender, and myostatin genotype on the hypertrophic response to heavy resistance strength training. J Gerontol A Biol Sci Med Sci 2000;55:M641.
55. Jozsi AC, Campbell WW, Joseph L, et al. Changes in power with resistance training in older and younger men and women. J Gerontol A Biol Sci Med Sci 1999;54:M591.
56. Yarasheski KE, Pak-Loduca J, Hasten DL, et al. Resistance exercise training increases mixed muscle protein synthesis rate in frail women and men >/=76 yr old. Am J Physiol 1999;277:E118.
57. Hasten DL, Pak-Loduca J, Obert KA, et al. Resistance exercise acutely increases MHC and mixed muscle protein synthesis rates in 78–84 and 23–32 yr olds. Am J Physiol Endocrinol Metab 2000;278:E620.

58. Yarasheski KE, Zachwieja JJ, Bier DM. Acute effects of resistance exercise on muscle protein synthesis rate in young and elderly men and women. Am J Physiol 1993;265:E210.

59. Edstrom E, Altun M, Bergman E, et al. Factors contributing to neuromuscular impairment and sarcopenia during aging. Physiol Behav 2007;92:129.

60. Clark BC, Manini TM. Sarcopenia =/= dynapenia. J Gerontol A Biol Sci Med Sci 2008;63:829.

61. Williams MA, Haskell WL, Ades PA, et al. Resistance exercise in individuals with and without cardiovascular disease: 2007 update: a scientific statement from the American Heart Association Council on Clinical Cardiology and Council on Nutrition, Physical Activity, and Metabolism. Circulation 2007;116:572.

62. Medicine ACoS. ACSM's guidelines for exercise testing and prescription. Philadelphia: Medicine ACoS; 2006.

63. American Geriatrics Society Panel on Exercise and Osteoarthritis. Exercise prescription for older adults with osteoarthritis pain: consensus practice recommendations. A supplement to the AGS Clinical Practice Guidelines on the management of chronic pain in older adults. J Am Geriatr Soc 2001;49:808.

64. Sheffield-Moore M, Yeckel CW, Volpi E, et al. Postexercise protein metabolism in older and younger men following moderate-intensity aerobic exercise. Am J Physiol Endocrinol Metab 2004;287:E513.

65. Coggan AR, Spina RJ, King DS, et al. Skeletal muscle adaptations to endurance training in 60- to 70-yr-old men and women. J Appl Physiol 1992;72:1780.

66. Ottenbacher KJ, Ottenbacher ME, Ottenbacher AJ, et al. Androgen treatment and muscle strength in elderly men: a meta-analysis. J Am Geriatr Soc 2006;54:1666.

67. Rolland YM, Perry HM 3rd, Patrick P, et al. Loss of appendicular muscle mass and loss of muscle strength in young postmenopausal women. J Gerontol A Biol Sci Med Sci 2007;62:330.

68. Taaffe DR, Newman AB, Haggerty CL, et al. Estrogen replacement, muscle composition, and physical function: the Health ABC Study. Med Sci Sports Exerc 2005;37:1741.

69. Brown M, Birge SJ, Kohrt WM. Hormone replacement therapy does not augment gains in muscle strength or fat-free mass in response to weight-bearing exercise. J Gerontol A Biol Sci Med Sci 1997;52:B166.

70. Clavel S, Coldefy AS, Kurkdjian E, et al. Atrophy-related ubiquitin ligases, atrogin-1 and MuRF1 are up-regulated in aged rat tibialis anterior muscle. Mech Ageing Dev 2006;127:794.

71. Rasmussen BB, Phillips SM. Contractile and nutritional regulation of human muscle growth. Exerc Sport Sci Rev 2003;31:127.

72. Emmelot-Vonk MH, Verhaar HJ, Nakhai Pour HR, et al. Effect of testosterone supplementation on functional mobility, cognition, and other parameters in older men: a randomized controlled trial. JAMA 2008;299:39.

73. Katznelson L, Finkelstein JS, Schoenfeld DA, et al. Increase in bone density and lean body mass during testosterone administration in men with acquired hypogonadism. J Clin Endocrinol Metab 1996;81:4358.

74. Ly LP, Jimenez M, Zhuang TN, et al. A double-blind, placebo-controlled, randomized clinical trial of transdermal dihydrotestosterone gel on muscular strength, mobility, and quality of life in older men with partial androgen deficiency. J Clin Endocrinol Metab 2001;86:4078.

75. Morley JE, Perry HM 3rd, Kaiser FE, et al. Effects of testosterone replacement therapy in old hypogonadal males: a preliminary study. J Am Geriatr Soc 1993;41:149.

76. Sih R, Morley JE, Kaiser FE, et al. Testosterone replacement in older hypogonadal men: a 12-month randomized controlled trial. J Clin Endocrinol Metab 1997; 82:1661.
77. Tenover JS. Effects of testosterone supplementation in the aging male. J Clin Endocrinol Metab 1992;75:1092.
78. Srinivas-Shankar U, Roberts SA, Connolly MJ, et al. Effects of testosterone on muscle strength, physical function, body composition, and quality of life in intermediate-frail and frail elderly men: a randomized, double-blind, placebo-controlled study. J Clin Endocrinol Metab 2010;95:639.
79. Chapman IM, Visvanathan R, Hammond AJ, et al. Effect of testosterone and a nutritional supplement, alone and in combination, on hospital admissions in undernourished older men and women. Am J Clin Nutr 2009;89:880.
80. LeBrasseur NK, Lajevardi N, Miciek R, et al. Effects of testosterone therapy on muscle performance and physical function in older men with mobility limitations (The TOM Trial): design and methods. Contemp Clin Trials 2009;30:133.
81. Basaria S, Coviello AD, Travison TG, et al. Adverse events associated with testosterone administration. N Engl J Med 2010;363:109.
82. Li JJ, Sutton JC, Nirschl A, et al. Discovery of potent and muscle selective androgen receptor modulators through scaffold modifications. J Med Chem 2007;50:3015.
83. Hennessey JV, Chromiak JA, DellaVentura S, et al. Growth hormone administration and exercise effects on muscle fiber type and diameter in moderately frail older people. J Am Geriatr Soc 2001;49:852.
84. Lange KH, Andersen JL, Beyer N, et al. GH administration changes myosin heavy chain isoforms in skeletal muscle but does not augment muscle strength or hypertrophy, either alone or combined with resistance exercise training in healthy elderly men. J Clin Endocrinol Metab 2002;87:513.
85. Taaffe DR, Pruitt L, Reim J, et al. Effect of recombinant human growth hormone on the muscle strength response to resistance exercise in elderly men. J Clin Endocrinol Metab 1994;79:1361.
86. Yarasheski KE, Zachwieja JJ, Campbell JA, et al. Effect of growth hormone and resistance exercise on muscle growth and strength in older men. Am J Physiol 1995;268:E268.
87. Sattler FR, Castaneda-Sceppa C, Binder EF, et al. Testosterone and growth hormone improve body composition and muscle performance in older men. J Clin Endocrinol Metab 1991;94:2009.
88. Blackman MR, Sorkin JD, Munzer T, et al. Growth hormone and sex steroid administration in healthy aged women and men: a randomized controlled trial. JAMA 2002;288:2282.
89. Brill KT, Weltman AL, Gentili A, et al. Single and combined effects of growth hormone and testosterone administration on measures of body composition, physical performance, mood, sexual function, bone turnover, and muscle gene expression in healthy older men. J Clin Endocrinol Metab 2002;87:5649.
90. Molfino A, Laviano A, Rossi Fanelli F. Contribution of anorexia to tissue wasting in cachexia. Curr Opin Support Palliat Care 2010;4:249.
91. Nass R, Pezzoli SS, Oliveri MC, et al. Effects of an oral ghrelin mimetic on body composition and clinical outcomes in healthy older adults: a randomized trial. Ann Intern Med 2008;149:601.
92. Onder G, Della Vedova C, Landi F. Validated treatments and therapeutics prospectives regarding pharmacological products for sarcopenia. J Nutr Health Aging 2009;13:746.

93. Hanggi W, Lippuner K, Jaeger P, et al. Differential impact of conventional oral or transdermal hormone replacement therapy or tibolone on body composition in postmenopausal women. Clin Endocrinol (Oxf) 1998;48:691.

94. Jacobsen DE, Samson MM, Kezic S, et al. Postmenopausal HRT and tibolone in relation to muscle strength and body composition. Maturitas 2007;58:7.

95. Artaza JN, Bhasin S, Magee TR, et al. Myostatin inhibits myogenesis and promotes adipogenesis in C3H 10T(1/2) mesenchymal multipotent cells. Endocrinology 2005;146:3547.

96. Tsuchida K. Targeting myostatin for therapies against muscle-wasting disorders. Curr Opin Drug Discov Devel 2008;11:487.

97. Kung T, Springer J, Doehner W, et al. Novel treatment approaches to cachexia and sarcopenia: highlights from the 5th Cachexia Conference. Expert Opin Investig Drugs 2010;19:579.

98. Savo A, Maiorano PM, Onder G, et al. Pharmacoepidemiology and disability in older adults: can medications slow the age-related decline in physical function? Expert Opin Pharmacother 2004;5:407.

99. Sumukadas D, Witham MD, Struthers AD, et al. Ace inhibitors as a therapy for sarcopenia—evidence and possible mechanisms. J Nutr Health Aging 2008; 12:480.

100. Di Bari M, van de Poll-Franse LV, Onder G, et al. Antihypertensive medications and differences in muscle mass in older persons: the Health, Aging and Body Composition Study. J Am Geriatr Soc 2004;52:961.

101. Sumukadas D, Witham MD, Struthers AD, et al. Effect of perindopril on physical function in elderly people with functional impairment: a randomized controlled trial. CMAJ 2007;177:867.

102. Brose A, Parise G, Tarnopolsky MA. Creatine supplementation enhances isometric strength and body composition improvements following strength exercise training in older adults. J Gerontol A Biol Sci Med Sci 2003;58:11.

103. Chrusch MJ, Chilibeck PD, Chad KE, et al. Creatine supplementation combined with resistance training in older men. Med Sci Sports Exerc 2001;33:2111.

104. Jakobi JM, Rice CL, Curtin SV, et al. Neuromuscular properties and fatigue in older men following acute creatine supplementation. Eur J Appl Physiol 2001; 84:321.

105. Rawson ES, Wehnert ML, Clarkson PM. Effects of 30 days of creatine ingestion in older men. Eur J Appl Physiol Occup Physiol 1999;80:139.

106. Pahor M, Blair SN, Espeland M, et al. Effects of a physical activity intervention on measures of physical performance: Results of the lifestyle interventions and independence for Elders Pilot (LIFE-P) study. J Gerontol A Biol Sci Med Sci 2006;61:1157.

107. Gillette-Guyonnet S, Andrieu S, Dantoine T, et al. Commentary on "A roadmap for the prevention of dementia II. Leon Thal Symposium 2008." The Multidomain Alzheimer Preventive Trial (MAPT): a new approach to the prevention of Alzheimer's disease. Alzheimers Dement 2009;5:114.

Chronic Heart Failure in Older Adults

Ali Ahmed, MD, MPH[a,b,*]

KEYWORDS

- Geriatric heart failure • Diagnosis • Etiology
- Fluid volume assessment • Ejection fraction • Treatment

Most of the estimated 6 million heart failure (HF) patients in the United States are 65 years and older. The vast majority of the nearly 700,000 patients who are newly diagnosed with HF every year are also older adults, and the incidence of HF increases with aging, approaching 10 per 1000 persons for those 65 years and older.[1] The annual cost of HF was estimated to be $40 billion in 2010, nearly half of which was spent for inpatient care.[2] HF is the leading cause of hospitalization among Medicare beneficiaries and it is listed as the primary discharge diagnosis for an estimated 1 million hospitalizations in the United States. HF is responsible for about 60,000 deaths annually in the United States, and those 65 years and older carry most of the brunt of this mortality. HF is listed as a secondary diagnosis in more than 200,000 other deaths annually.[1]

HF is a clinical syndrome and is often difficult to diagnose, because unlike acute myocardial infarction (AMI) or stroke, there is no single test or procedure that can definitively confirm or rule out HF. The diagnosis and management of HF in older adults, who suffer from multiple morbidities and polypharmacy, are particularly difficult.[3] A typical geriatric HF patient is an older woman with diastolic HF or clinical HF with normal or near-normal left ventricular ejection fraction (LVEF), often with a history of hypertension. Often these patients have other morbidities such as coronary artery disease (CAD), atrial fibrillation, diabetes mellitus, arthritis, chronic kidney

---

Grant support: Dr Ahmed is supported by the National Institutes of Health through grants (R01-HL085561 and R01-HL097047) from the National Heart, Lung, and Blood Institute and a generous gift from Ms Jean B. Morris of Birmingham, Alabama.
The author has nothing to disclose.

[a] Divisions of Gerontology, Geriatrics and Palliative Care, and Cardiovascular Disease, Department of Medicine, School of Medicine; Department of Epidemiology, School of Public Health; Center for Aging; Center for Heart Failure Research; Center for Cardiovascular Biology; and Geriatric Heart Failure Clinic; University of Alabama at Birmingham, 1530 3rd Avenue South, CH19-219, Birmingham, AL 35294-2041, USA
[b] Section of Geriatrics and Geriatric Heart Failure Clinic, Veterans Affairs Medical Center, 700 19th Street South, Birmingham, AL 35233, USA
* UAB Center for Aging, 1530 3rd Avenue South, CH19-219, Birmingham, AL 35294-2041.
E-mail address: aahmed@uab.edu

Med Clin N Am 95 (2011) 439–461
doi:10.1016/j.mcna.2011.02.001
0025-7125/11/$ – see front matter. Published by Elsevier Inc.

medical.theclinics.com

disease (CKD), and depression, and take multiple medications. Yet, the clinical presentation of HF is similar, regardless of the LVEF.[4] The diagnosis and management of HF in an older adult is clearly more complex and challenging than in a younger HF patient, who is likely to be a man with impaired LVEF, often with a history of CAD and/or AMI. The diagnosis and management of HF in older adults is made more difficult by the fact that major randomized clinical trials (RCT) of HF have often excluded older adults and those with diastolic HF.[5,6]

However, the diagnosis and management of HF in older adults can be simplified by a clear understanding of the key facts, and following a structured protocol that covers all the key areas of the process. In this article, the author presents several cases of geriatric HF to illustrate the heterogeneity and complexity of HF in older adults, and demonstrate how the process of diagnosis and management can be simplified by the use of the mnemonic DEFEAT-HF: Diagnosis, Etiology, Fluid volume, Ejection fraction, And Treatment of Heart Failure (**Table 1**).[3,7,8]

CASE PRESENTATIONS
Case 1

A 79-year-old man without a history of HF presented with progressive dyspnea on exertion (DOE) and leg swelling for 6 months (**Table 2**). He had no history of dyspnea at rest, orthopnea, paroxysmal nocturnal dyspnea (PND), cough, wheezing, or chest pain. He was receiving lisinopril and propranolol. There was no history of emergency department (ED) visits or hospitalizations due to HF or dyspnea. His vital signs were within normal limits.

His physical examination was remarkable for mild pitting edema around his ankles and lower leg areas. He had normal jugular venous pressure (JVP), no hepatojugular reflux (HJR), no third heart sound (S3), and no pulmonary râles. His electrocardiogram and chest radiograph findings were within normal limits. His medical history revealed 2 etiologic risk factors for HF: a history of generally well-controlled hypertension and CAD with a known old AMI (**Table 3**).

At a 45° incline, no jugular pulsation could be observed in his neck. Further, when the head of his bed was lowered to at about 35°, there was no visible pulsation of his internal jugular veins (IJV). However, at this position the top of the pulsations of his external jugular veins (EJV) was visible in the lower neck area. When the head of the bed was lowered to about 30°, the pulsation of his EJV was now visible in the middle of his neck. The top of his EJV pulsation was about 2 cm vertically below his sternal angle (**Table 4**). In this near-supine position, a firm pressure on his abdomen slightly raised the top of his EJV pulsation by about 1 cm that lasted a few seconds while the abdominal pressure was maintained. An echocardiogram showed an LVEF of 35%.

Case 2

An 86-year-old woman with a history of HF (LVEF unknown) presented with a history of fatigue and DOE on minimal exertion of 1 month's duration (see **Table 2**). Her DOE was so extreme that she reported dyspnea on turning sides in bed. She was sleeping in a recliner to avoid orthopnea, and her occasional PND had ceased since she started sleeping on the recliner. She reported no chest pain. She also complained of fatigue on minimal exertion, right upper quadrant pain, nausea but no vomiting, loss of appetite, and severe leg swelling. Her clothes were wet from the oozing of clear liquid from her swollen legs, and she had multiple blisters on both legs. She was receiving digoxin, atenolol, and spironolactone. Despite her symptoms, she had not visited the ED. She also had no history of hospitalization for HF.

Table 1		
DEFEAT-HF: a simple 5-step protocol for the assessment and management of chronic HF in older adults		
D	Diagnosis	HF is a clinical diagnosis, and cannot be confirmed or ruled out by any single test or procedure. Therefore, a clinical diagnosis of HF must be made. LVEF should not be used to diagnose HF, as over half of all older adults with HF have diastolic HF or HF with normal or near-normal LVEF
E	Etiology	HF is a clinical syndrome, and not a disease, thus an underlying cause must be sought and identified. If no underlying cause can be identified, patients should be referred to a cardiologist or HF expert for further evaluation. HF patients with ongoing etiologic insults such as myocardial ischemia should also be referred for appropriate management, it may adversely affect disease progression and prognosis
F	Fluid volume	Nearly all newly diagnosed HF patients present with fluid retention, which is also a recurring problem for those with chronic HF, at times despite proper management. Careful estimation of JVP using IJV and EJV is the most reliable means to assess fluid volume status. A determination of "no fluid retention" is not enough, as many HF patients may suffer from hypovolemia, often due to overdiuresis. Therefore, JVP should be estimated in centimeters of water
E	Ejection fraction	LVEF, estimated preferably by an echocardiogram, is the single most important test after a clinical diagnosis of HF has been made. It has both prognostic and therapeutic implications. Patients with systolic HF or clinical HF with low LVEF often have poorer prognosis than those with diastolic HF, who in turn have poorer prognosis than those without HF. Although therapy with neurohormonal blockade has been shown to improve the poor outcomes in systolic HF, their effectiveness in diastolic HF has not been well established
A	And	
T	Therapy	HF therapy can be broadly divided into those directed at relieving symptoms and those directed at improving outcomes. Because HF symptoms are indistinguishable between systolic and diastolic HF, symptom-relieving therapy is also similar for all HF patients. However, life-prolonging therapy is often restricted to those with systolic HF. Although most guideline recommendations for the management of systolic HF are based on evidence from younger systolic HF patients, they can be reasonably individualized and applied to the care of older systolic HF patients

Adapted from Ahmed A. DEFEAT heart failure: clinical manifestations, diagnostic assessment, and etiology of geriatric heart failure. Heart Failure Clin 2007;4:389–402; with permission.

On physical examination she had elevated JVP, positive HJR, a right-sided S3, no pulmonary râles or wheezing, an enlarged soft tender liver, and severe bilateral lower extremity edema up to mid-thigh with brown pigmentation and induration of skin, and multiple blisters over the lower legs. An accentuated second heart sound at the left fifth intercostal space suggested pulmonary hypertension, with an estimated pulmonary artery systolic pressure of 50 to 55 mm Hg. She had a normal electrocardiogram. A chest radiograph revealed marked cardiomegaly, pulmonary venous congestion, and mild pulmonary edema. Except for a history of hypertension and atrial fibrillation, she had no other known etiologic risk factors for HF; the control status of her hypertension was not well known (see **Table 3**).

At a 45° incline, her EJV could be seen distended, but there was no visible pulsation. However, when the head of her bed was raised to about 60° incline, the top of her EJV

Table 2
Diagnosis of HF in older adults

	Cases					Comments
	1	2	3	4	5	
Dyspnea on exertion	Yes	Yes	Yes	Yes	No	DOE, although nearly always present, is a very nonspecific symptom, and by itself, without other associated symptoms and signs, is not often very helpful in making a diagnosis of HF
Orthopnea	No	Yes	Yes	Yes	No	HF patients often sleep on multiple pillows or in a recliner, or use blocks to raise the head of their bed to avoid orthopnea, and may report negatively when asked
Paroxysmal nocturnal dyspnea	No	Yes	No	No	No	PND is uncommon, as chronic HF patients often sleep with their head elevated to avoid orthopnea, which also reduces the occurrence of PND
Dyspnea at rest	No	No	No	No	No	Constitutes NYHA Class IV or most severe symptom. Rare
Fatigue on exertion	Yes	Yes	Yes	Yes	No	Exertional fatigue often is more common in older adults with HF than exertional dyspnea. As opposed to exertional dyspnea, which tends to occur when things are done in a hurry, like rushing to pick up the ringing phone at the end of the room, exertional fatigue often occurs when a patient does things, like walking two city blocks, at his/her own pace
Chest pain	No	No	No	No	No	Not a common presenting or associated symptom in geriatric HF patients
Cough	No	No	No	Yes	No	Rare. In some older adults with HF cough may precede dyspnea, while in others it may accompany or follow dyspnea
Swelling of foot/leg	Yes	Yes	Yes	Yes	No	Extremely common. It is more useful in the diagnosis process if the leg swelling in bilateral and the onset of leg swelling and dyspnea on exertion are contemporary. However, leg swelling often may not correlate with dyspnea, as venous insufficiency is common in older adults, which may be unilateral
Gastrointestinal symptoms	No	Yes	No	No	No	Usually uncommon, except in those with prolonged fluid retention leading to congestive hepatopathy. A more prolonged and severe fluid retention may also result in congestive gastropathy, which may cause nausea, vomiting, anorexia, and poor absorption and response to drugs, such as diuretics

Finding					Comments
Chronic obstructive pulmonary disease (COPD)	No	No	No	No	The diagnosis of HF may be difficult in the presence of COPD as dyspnea is rather similar in both HF and COPD. Patients with COPD may also report PND, in which cough may precede dyspnea. Often HF and COPD may coexist, which may further complicate the diagnosis process. An elevated JVP is probably the most important physical finding in establishing a diagnosis of HF in this context. A normal BNP, especially in the presence of a normal JVP or when JVP cannot be estimated, would likely rule out HF
Deconditioning	No	Yes	No	No	Exertional dyspnea and fatigue associated with deconditioning may be distinguished by the lack of associated orthopnea, PND, leg edema, or other evidence of fluid retention
Depression	No	Yes	No	Yes	Somatization is common in older adults with depression and symptoms are often not physiologically plausible; for example, dyspnea or chest pain at rest that is not worsened by physical activities. Also, lack of associated symptoms and signs of fluid retention may help distinguish somatization from HF
HF risk factors present	Yes	Yes	Yes	Yes	When traditional risk factors such as hypertension and coronary artery disease are absent, referral to cardiologists should be considered for confirmation of diagnosis and identification of an underlying etiologic risk factor
Jugular venous pressure elevated	No	Yes	Yes	No	Almost always present during initial presentation and acute exacerbation of HF, but chronic stable patients may have normal JVP, and may even be low in overdiuresed patients
Jugular venous waveforms	?	?	?	?	Not needed to estimate JVP or make a diagnosis of HF. However, familiarity with the double undulation of the IJV pulsation may help distinguish it from carotid pulsation
Third heart sound	No	Yes	Yes	No	Often present in acute HF but its presence is not necessary to establish a diagnosis of HF. An S3 can also be present in a chronic HF patient who is euvolemic
Pulmonary crackles and wheezing	No	No	Yes	No	Rare in chronic HF because of the hyperefficient pulmonary lymphatic drainage system. However, a more rapid fluid build up may overwhelm the system and result in pulmonary edema
Abdominal tenderness	No	Yes	No	No	Right upper quadrant tenderness may results from congestive hepatopathy secondary to prolonged fluid retention
Hepatojugular reflux	No	Yes	No	No	It also helps in identifying the position and patency of external jugular veins in neck When present in those with normal JVP, it may indicate early fluid retention

(continued on next page)

Table 2
(continued)

	Cases					Comments
	1	2	3	4	5	
Lower extremity edema	Yes	Yes	No	Yes	No	Pitting edema in those with normal JVP may indicate chronic venous insufficiency, often unilateral and may be accompanied by skin discoloration and stasis dermatitis. Prolonged venous insufficiency may lead to secondary lymphedema and nonpitting edema
Cardiomegaly	No	Yes	Yes	Yes	No	Cardiomegaly by chest radiograph may help support a clinical diagnosis of HF
Pulmonary venous congestion	No	Yes	No	Yes	No	Uncommon in chronic HF, but when present on radiograph may support diagnosis
Pulmonary edema	No	Yes	No	No	No	Rare in chronic HF. Radiographic evidence of pulmonary edema suggests acute fluid buildup or severe HF
Pleural effusion	No	No	No	No	No	Not uncommon, usually bilateral, often more severe on right side, rarely massive
B-type natriuretic peptides (BNP)	Not done	Not done	400	<50	No	Elevated BNP and the N-terminal portion of BNP (NT-pro-BNP) levels may support the diagnosis of HF. HF is unlikely if BNP <100 pg/mL and NT pro-BNP <300 pg/mL. However, their role in older adults with HF has not been well studied
Left ventricular ejection fraction	35%	55%	25%	55%	55%	A low LVEF *may* support a diagnosis of HF when clinical presentation is atypical or insufficient. However, a normal LVEF *should not* be used to rule out a diagnosis of HF
Response to diuretics	N/A	Yes	Yes	Yes	N/A	A therapeutic response to diuretic may help confirm the diagnosis of HF when clinical presentation is atypical or insufficient

Case 1: Had no clinical evidence of HF, and the diagnosis was facilitated by his low LVEF.
Case 2: Had a classic text book presentation of HF, and the diagnosis could not be confounded by her normal LVEF.
Case 3: Although he was overdiuresed and hypovolemic in his initial presentation, he had historical evidence of clinical HF and a low LVEF.
Case 4: Despite clear evidence to clinical HF, a diagnosis of HF may have been previously confounded by his normal LVEF and BNP.
Case 5: Dyspnea at rest but not during exertion suggested somatization. Therapy with antidepressant completely resolved her symptoms.

Table 3
Etiology of HF in older adults

	Cases 1	2	3	4	5	Comments
Coronary artery disease	Yes	No	No	Yes	No	CAD is a rather strong risk factor for HF, and the risk is further increased for those with a prior AMI. The presence or absence of CAD can often be established during history and physical examination
Hypertension	Yes	Yes	Yes	Yes	Yes	Hypertension is probably the most common risk factor for HF among older adults, especially for diastolic HF. The presence or absence can be established during history and physical examination. Persons with hypertension have a lower relative risk for HF than those with CAD, but hypertension contributes to more cases of new HF, as hypertension is more common in older adults
Diabetes mellitus	No	No	Yes	No	No	The risk of HF among those with diabetes is nearly similar to that among those with CAD
Valvular heart disease	No	No	No	No	No	May coexist with other risk factors. Diagnosed by echocardiography
Cardiomyopathy	No	No	No	No	No	While dilated and hypertrophic cardiomyopathies are less common in older adults, restrictive cardiomyopathies may be more common in older adults
Chronic kidney disease	No	Yes	No	Yes	No	Has long been known as a risk factor; the independent risk may not increase until the chronic kidney disease is advanced
Smoking	No	No	Yes	No	No	Heavy smokers may have increased risk despite many years of cessation
Atrial fibrillation	No	Yes	No	Yes	No	Uncontrolled ventricular rate is probably more important than the presence atrial fibrillation itself
Hyperthyroidism	No	No	No	No	No	Rare
Peripheral arterial disease	No	No	No	No	No	Probably as a marker of overall atherosclerosis
Anemia	No	No	No	No	No	Rarely a risk factor, and often not until anemia is very severe
Left ventricular hypertrophy	No	Yes	No	No	No	A very strong risk factor
Asymptomatic left ventricular systolic dysfunction	No	No	No	No	No	A very strong risk factor. The low LVEF and slowly progressive symptoms of Case 1 suggest that he may have had asymptomatic left ventricular systolic dysfunction

Table 4
Fluid volume status evaluation in older adults with HF

	Cases					Comments
	1	2	3	4	5	
Internal jugular vein	No	No	No	Yes	No	IJV lies behind the sternocleidomastoid muscle for most of its course in the neck and thus not visible. The IJV pulsation is also often not seen over this area. However, the pulsation can be seen in the triangular area at the base of the neck in between the 2 heads of the muscle where the IJV is subcutaneous, and in the upper part of the neck where the IJV emerges from under the sternocleidomastoid muscles (as the muscle ascends laterally to its insertion on the mastoid). In some chronic HF patients, the IJV pulsation may not be seen
External jugular vein	Yes	Yes	Yes	Yes	Yes	The contour of the EJV can be seen in the neck like the veins on the dorsum of the hand. If the vein is patent, the pulsation is also clearly visible. When EJV is visible on either side of the neck and have different heights, the one with the higher height should be used. When both IJV and EJV pulsations are visible, the JVP based on the IJV should be used. At times, the top of EJV pulsation may be lower than the top of the IJV pulsation, likely due to narrow lumen of the former
Hepatojugular reflux	No	Yes	No	Yes	No	Often present in patients with elevated JVP, but not necessary for diagnosis
Degrees of incline of the head of the bed at which top of the jugular pulsation visible in neck	30	80	10	45	30	The incline of the head of the bed or examination table is irrelevant as the goal is to make the top of the jugular venous pulsation visible in the middle of the neck. The top of jugular pulsation for a patient with low JVP may only be visible in a supine position and that for a patient with high JVP in a sitting position. However, it is important to make a note of the degree of the head elevation so that the appropriate "right atrium to the sternal angle" distance can be added to the "sternal angle-to-top of the jugular pulsation" distance

Estimated distance in centimeters from sternal angle to top of jugular pulsation	-2	8	-2	6	-2	When the top of the jugular pulsation is below the sternal angle, then one needs to *subtract* the "sternal angle-to-top of the jugular pulsation" (a negative value) from the "right atrium to sternal angle" distance to obtain the JVP. Of note, the "sternal angle-to-top of the jugular pulsation" distance is the vertical distance, not horizontal. This is especially important to remember in patients with low JVP who often would need to be in a supine or near-supine position
Estimated distance in centimeters from right atrium to sternal angle	8	10	5	10	8	Unlike what is taught in many old text books, the distance is not 5 cm regardless of body position. Findings based on CT scan images of chest suggest that it varies by body position (head elevation). Remember 3 numbers: 5, 8 and 10 cm at 0, 30 and $\geq$45 degrees of inclines, respectively. The distance may be higher for individuals with large chest. For example, at a 45 degree incline, it would be 10 cm for a male patient with an average anteroposterior chest diameter of 25 cm (~10 inches). However, it would be 12 cm for a patient with a 35 cm chest diameter (rule of thumb: add ~1 cm for every 5 cm increase in anteroposterior chest diameter)
Estimated JVP	6	18	3	16	6	A JVP of 6–8 cm of water may be considered normal in HF. Some HF patients may tolerate a JVP of 8–10 cm of water. Most HF patients with JVP greater than 10 cm of water would be symptomatic, and achieving euvolemia in these patients may improve breathing. However, a JVP of 4–5 cm of water in a symptomatic patient may indicate overdiuresis and hypovolemia, and should be avoided
How JVP was estimated	8 – 2 = 6	10 + 8 = 18	5 – 2 = 3	10 + 6 = 16	8 – 2 = 6	Two key points to remember: (1) the "sternal angle-to-top of the jugular pulsation" distance is *vertical* and varies with the position of the patient, (2) the "sternal angle-to-top of the jugular pulsation" distance must be *subtracted* from the "right atrium to the sternal angle" distance, when the JVP is low and the top of jugular pulsation is below the sternal angle

pulsations was visible in her upper neck area. When the head of her bed was further raised to a near-sitting position, the top of her EJV was visible in the middle of her neck (see **Table 4**). At this position, the top of her EJV pulsation was vertically nearly 8 cm above her sternal angle. A firm pressure on her abdomen made her EJV be more distended and the top of her EJV pulsation to rise by about 3 cm and be invisible behind the angle of her jaws, and remained so for about 10 seconds as the abdominal pressure was maintained. She had no visible pulsation of her IJV on either side of her neck. An echocardiogram later showed an LVEF of greater than 55%.

Case 3

An 84-year-old man presented with worsening DOE and fatigue of 2 months' duration (see **Table 2**). He had occasional orthopnea but no PND. He had no chest pain but reported dizziness. He was recently hospitalized with a syncopal episode. Before that hospitalization, he was physically active. On further questioning, he admitted some mild DOE prior to hospitalization, but denied any dyspnea at rest, orthopnea, PND, or chest pain. A workup during hospitalization demonstrated an enlarged heart by chest radiograph, an LVEF of 25% by echocardiogram, but a normal coronary angiogram. He was discharged on furosemide, 80 mg daily. His DOE subsequently worsened, and his furosemide was increased to 160 mg daily. Over the next 2 weeks he lost more than 20 lbs (9 kg) and his symptoms improved. His serum B-type natriuretic peptide (BNP) level was about 400 (normal <100) pg/mL. He continued on a diuretic regimen of furosemide, 160 mg a day. Four weeks later he presented with worsening fatigue and DOE. His physical examination was remarkable for a systolic blood pressure of 95 mm Hg and a low JVP. His medical history revealed hypertension and diabetes, but he had no other known etiologic risk factors for HF, including CAD (see **Table 3**). He said his hypertension had generally been well controlled. He quit smoking about 15 years ago after about 35 pack-years of smoking.

At a 45° incline, he had no visible IJV or EJV pulsation in his neck. However, when the head of the examination table was lowered to a supine position, the top of his EJV pulsations was visible in his mid-neck, which was vertically nearly 2 cm below his sternal angle (see **Table 4**). A firm pressure on his abdomen raised the top of his EJV by about 1 cm for about 2 second. He had no visible IJV pulsation. As already mentioned, an echocardiogram a few months earlier had shown an LVEF of 25%.

Case 4

A 76-year-old man presented with history of persistent chronic DOE and cough of more than 5 years' duration that had become worse in recent months (see **Table 2**). He slept on a couch to avoid orthopnea, but denied dyspnea at rest or PND. The swelling of his feet, ankles, and lower leg had also worsened in recent months. He stated that he had to cut a split in the top of his socks so that he could wear them. He was not aware of a history of HF and denied any HF-related hospitalization. He was receiving furosemide 80 mg every morning. He also received bronchodilator inhalation for suspected emphysema. However, his pulmonary function test showed no obstructive lung disease and was remarkable for only mild restrictive lung disease. A review of his medical record revealed 3 values of BNP levels over the past 12 months, all of which were less than 50 (normal <100) pg/mL.

His physical examination was remarkable for elevated JVP, positive HJR, rare pulmonary râles, and severe bilateral lower extremity edema, surrounded by socks with cut edges. His electrocardiogram showed atrial fibrillation with controlled ventricular rate. His chest radiograph revealed mild cardiomegaly and pulmonary congestion but no pulmonary edema. In addition to atrial fibrillation, he also had hypertension and CAD, 2 key etiologic risk factors for HF (see **Table 3**).

At a 45° incline, he had both his IJV and EJV visible in upper neck area. The top of his EJV pulsation was vertically 4 cm above his sternal angle and the top of his IJV was vertically 6 cm above his sternal angle. A firm pressure on his abdomen raised both IJV and EJV pulsation by 3 cm, which remained elevated for about 12 seconds as the abdominal pressure was sustained. According to a recent echocardiogram, his LVEF was greater than 55%.

Case 5

An 82-year-old woman presented with a 1-year history of dyspnea, chest tightness, and dizziness, all of which occurred at rest (see **Table 2**). She denies orthopnea, PND, or leg swelling, and more importantly she reported no DOE. She visited the ED 3 times during the previous 12 months, and was hospitalized each time. Extensive tests and procedures during these hospitalizations included echocardiogram, cardiac catheterization, and magnetic resonance imaging of brain, none of which revealed any pathology. A review of her medical record revealed a history of hypertension (see **Table 3**). Her physical examination was unremarkable. She had no evidence of clinical HF, and specifically, she had no JVP elevation or HJR.

At a 45° incline, neither her IJV nor her EJV was visible in the neck. When her head was lowered to about 30°, the top of her EJV pulsation could be seen at the base of her neck, which was 2 cm below her sternal angle (see **Table 4**). The top of her EJV pulsation briskly moved up for a second when a firm pressure was applied on her abdomen. A repeat echocardiogram revealed normal LVEF.

DIAGNOSIS OF HEART FAILURE

HF is a clinical syndrome that is characterized by dyspnea, fatigue, and swelling, most of which are manifestations of a reduced cardiac output, the hallmark pathology of HF (**Table 5**). Because there is no single test or procedure that can definitively diagnose or rule out HF, it is imperative that clinicians become familiar with the symptoms and signs of HF. It is also important to remember that the diagnosis of chronic HF may be a process that can span over days to months. A clinical diagnosis of HF should ideally be made before ordering an echocardiogram, as nearly half of all geriatric HF

Table 5
A simplified illustration demonstrating how patients with diastolic HF may have similar symptoms as those with systolic HF, despite normal LVEF

	End-Diastolic Volume (mL)	Left Ventricular Ejection Fraction (%)	Left Ventricular Stroke Volume (mL)	Heart Rate (beats/min)	Cardiac Output (L/min)	Symptoms
Normal	150	55%	75	72	5.4	None
Systolic heart failure	200	25%	50	72	3.6	Dyspnea, fatigue, edema
Diastolic heart failure	100	55%	50	72	3.6	Dyspnea, fatigue, edema

Adapted from Ahmed A. DEFEAT heart failure: clinical manifestations, diagnostic assessment, and etiology of geriatric heart failure. Heart Failure Clin 2007;4:389–402; with permission.

patients have normal LVEF.[9–11] However, not infrequently, a patient may present with mild DOE and a normal LVEF from a recent echocardiogram performed in another hospital or clinic. In those circumstances, the key is to not rule out HF because the LVEF is normal. With that understanding in mind, it may be appropriate to order an echocardiogram so that LVEF data can be incorporated into the diagnostic process.

For example, Case 1 had insufficient symptoms and signs of HF to make a clinical diagnosis of HF (see **Table 3**). However, in the context of a low LVEF, his presentation was sufficient to establish the clinical diagnosis of HF. An advantage of this approach was that it allowed early initiation of therapy with life-saving drugs such as an angiotensin-converting enzyme (ACE) inhibitor and a β-blocker. A clinical diagnosis of HF probably could not be made until months later, by which time his HF would have further progressed and he would have developed more classic symptoms and signs of HF. Because HF is a clinical syndrome, it is almost inevitable that all HF patients will at some point in time develop overt HF. However, the nature and duration of this process is often difficult to predict. Case 2 had nearly all textbook symptoms and signs of HF. However, most HF patients fall somewhere between these two cases in their clinical presentations. Because diagnosis of HF may be difficult, it is possible that HF may have been misdiagnosed in the past. Therefore, it is important to confirm the diagnosis of HF during initial evaluation of a patient with known chronic HF. For patients who are currently euvolemic and have no clinical HF, this can often be done by reviewing symptoms and signs of HF in the past, response to diuretics, hospitalization due to HF, and the use of current HF medications.

Dyspnea or fatigue on exertion is the most common early symptoms of HF, often accompanied by some degree of lower extremity edema (Case 1). However, both are rather nonspecific symptoms, even when jointly present, and are often not sufficient to make a clinical diagnosis of HF. Case 1 was a very active person before his dyspnea began, and as such he was bothered by his dyspnea. However, many older adults attribute their early mild symptoms of dyspnea or fatigue to older age, and respond by restricting their physical activities, which may result in delayed diagnosis, or delayed care, as in Case 2.

Orthopnea and PND are more specific HF symptoms. However, patients often sleep with their head raised to avoid orthopnea, which may also reduce the occurrence of PND. Therefore, asking about the number of pillows currently used, whether currently sleeping on a couch or in a recliner, and past episodes of orthopnea may help elicit otherwise underreported orthopnea. Orthopnea and PND are 2 major Framingham criteria for the diagnosis of HF, and their presence suggests a diagnosis of HF. However, an analysis of the Cardiovascular Health Study (CHS) suggested that many older adults with both these symptoms may not have HF.[12] In that study, 7% (388/5771) of the community-dwelling adults 65 years or older had both orthopnea and PND, yet only 20% (76/388) of those with both orthopnea and PND had centrally adjudicated HF.

Lower extremity edema is often present in HF but needs to be distinguished from pitting edema due to venous insufficiency, which may be unilateral and may predate the onset of dyspnea. Unpublished data based on the analysis by this author of the public-use copy of the CHS data obtained from the National Heart, Lung, and Blood Institute suggest that only about one-third of community-dwelling older adults with orthopnea, PND, and lower extremity edema had centrally adjudicated HF. These findings suggest that the diagnosis of HF may not be made merely on the basis of a few symptoms or signs, even if they appear rather specific or suggestive of HF, and that a clinical diagnosis of HF at times may be an ongoing process whereby an initial diagnosis may need to be reevaluated based on other accumulating evidence of HF.

An evidence of fluid volume retention in the context of classic symptoms of HF such as dyspnea and fatigue on exertion, orthopnea, PND, and lower extremity edema is most helpful in making an early clinical diagnosis of HF. An elevated JVP is the most specific sign of fluid retention in HF and is likely the most important physical examination in the process of diagnosis of HF in older adults.[13] While most textbooks of physical examination suggest that IJV should be used for JVP estimation, many clinicians find this difficult to appreciate. In part this is because for the most part of its course in the neck, the IJV lies behind the large sternocleidomastoid muscles. Because unlike the carotid pulsation, the jugular pulsation is relatively much weaker (10 cm of water = 7.4 mm Hg), IJV pulsations often are not transmitted well for JVP estimation. This finding is confirmed by the results from several studies that suggest underestimation of the prevalence of JVP elevation in HF.

Findings from nearly 10,000 chronic systolic HF patients enrolled in 2 major RCTs and examined by cardiologists demonstrated that slightly more than 10% had elevated JVP.[14,15] One might argue that the low prevalence of JVP in those patients is likely attributable to the fact that most of those patients with chronic HF were euvolemic. However, the prevalence of JVP elevation was similar in a group of older adults with dyspnea who presented at the ED.[16] The prevalence of JVP elevation would be expected to be higher in those patients. One would expect that nearly all hospitalized acute HF patients would have elevated JVP. However, findings from the OPTIMIZE-HF registry demonstrated that only about one-third of more than 40,000 hospitalized older adults with acute decompensated HF had JVP elevation.[4] This systematic underestimation of the prevalence of JVP elevation in chronic HF may in part be attributed to reliance on IJV for JVP estimation.

Therefore, when a clear IJV pulsation cannot be seen, EJV pulsation should be used to estimate JVP.[17] The key limitation of the EJV in estimating JVP is that it is a superficial vein, and as such it is vulnerable to external pressure (eg, contraction of the overlying platysma muscle) or internal obstruction (thrombosis or sclerosis of valves). Therefore, a distended EJV should never be used as a marker of JVP elevation or to estimate JVP. However, at times a patent EJV may also look distended, which can happen if the JVP is very high and the patient is at a 45° incline. The top of the EJV pulsation may be behind the angle of mandible. In that case, raising the head of the bed or sitting the patient make the EJV pulsation visible in the middle of the neck. Using both IJV and EJV and proper techniques, JVP can be estimated in 90% to 95% of all HF patients.

Although popularized in the medical literature and promoted by the industry, serum BNP and N-terminal pro-BNP (NT-proBNP) are rarely needed by skilled clinicians to establish a clinical diagnosis of chronic HF in older adults. These neurohormones are secreted by the failing ventricle in HF in response to myocardial wall stress. However, they may also be elevated in many conditions other than HF including aging, infection, and renal insufficiency.[18] In one prospective study of 1586 patients (mean age, 64 years) with acute dyspnea, clinical diagnosis of HF was adjudicated in 744 (47%) patients by 2 independent cardiologists.[19] In that study, bedside BNP data were collected on all participants in the ED, and values of less than 100 and less than 50 pg/mL were shown to have negative predictive values of 89% and 96%, respectively.[19] However, currently there are no standard cutoffs for these neurohormones to confirm or rule out HF in general, and even less is known about their usefulness in older adults.[18,20] In the aforementioned study, BNP was observed to be more accurate than physical signs in identifying HF in patients presenting with acute dyspnea. However, only 22% of patients in that study had JVP elevation, whereas 47% of the patients had adjudicated HF.[19] This finding underscores the importance of proper estimation of JVP in older adults with HF. The limitations of the use of BNP are also illustrated in Cases 3 and 4. Therefore, a careful and proper clinical estimation of JVP is indispensible for a clinical diagnosis of HF.

ETIOLOGY OF HEART FAILURE

Because HF is a syndrome, an underlying etiology for HF must be established for all HF patients. In older adults, more than one etiologic factor may be involved. CAD and hypertension are the 2 most common risk factors (see **Table 4**), and can often be identified during history and physical examination, sometimes with the help of a few additional tests. This identification has important secondary prevention values, as the ongoing presence of an underlying cause, such as myocardial ischemia or uncontrolled hypertension, may lead to continuing myocardial damage, thus adversely affecting disease progression and prognosis. The presence of one or more risk factors does not necessarily mean that they have caused HF or that other factors did not play any etiologic role. However, the absence of any known risk factors mandates that HF patients be referred to a cardiologist for additional investigations. As a diagnosis of fever is not sufficient for the proper management of fever, a diagnosis of HF must be accompanied by the identification and management of potential etiologic risk factors.

FLUID VOLUME ASSESSMENT IN HEART FAILURE

As already mentioned, the documentation of an elevated JVP is essential in making a clinical diagnosis of HF. An elevated JVP is also the most specific sign of fluid overload in patients with established HF. The estimation of JVP is probably the most important physical examination in HF, during both initial and subsequent visits. Yet physicians often find it challenging, and traditional textbook and bedside teaching have not been helpful. To understand the problem of underestimation of the prevalence of JVP elevation in HF,[4,14–16] one needs to recognize the 3 myths associated with the traditional approach to JVP estimation: (1) the IJV myth, (2) the 45° myth, and (3) the 5 cm myth. As mentioned earlier, the singular use of IJV to determine JVP is likely to substantially underestimate the prevalence of JVP elevation in HF.[4,14–16] Therefore, both IJV and EJV should be used to estimate JVP in HF, and JVP should be estimated even when it seems normal. For example, Case 3 had a JVP of 3 cm of water. At a 45° incline, there would be no IJV or EJV pulsation in his neck, and it would be correct to state that he had no JVP elevation. While that may be enough in most healthy individuals and even in those presenting with new-onset HF, it is not sufficient for patients with established HF. Therefore, EJV or IJV pulsation should be looked for at lower inclines (including the supine position if necessary) to identify low JVP. Clinicians need to remember one key point when estimating low JVP in HF. The top of the jugular venous pulsation visible in the middle of the neck in a near-supine position would likely be below the level of the sternal angle. Therefore, the "sternal angle to top of the jugular pulsation" distance would be negative, and as such, when estimating JVP, the "sternal angle to top of the jugular pulsation" distance should be subtracted from the "right atrium to sternal angle" distance.

Proper estimation of JVP requires identification of the jugular venous pulsation in the middle of the neck (**Fig. 1**). The examination can begin in any position, but the neck should be examined for venous pulsation in all possible positions between supine and sitting until the jugular pulsation is visualized. EJV's, like the veins on the dorsum of one's hands, are superficial and subcutaneous, and thus clearly visible without any tangential light. The position of the EJV's in the neck may be identified by lowering the

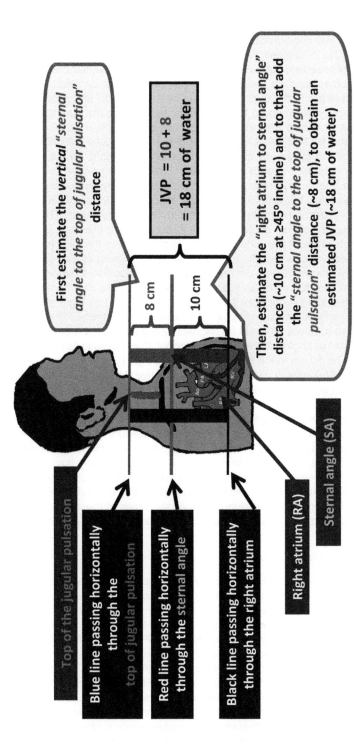

Fig. 1. The jugular venous pressure (JVP, *marked by the black bar*) is the vertical height of the top of the jugular venous pulsation from the right atrium (RA), expressed in centimeters of water. To estimate JVP, one needs to use the sternal angle (SA) as a landmark. After first estimating the "SA to the top of the jugular venous pulsation" distance (8 cm in this case, *marked by the blue bar*), one needs to add this number to the "RA to SA" distance (10 cm in this case, *marked by the brown bar*). Of note, the top of the jugular venous pulsation would be vertically lower than the SA when the JVP is low, in which case the "SA to the top of the jugular pulsation" distance needs to be subtracted from the "RA to SA" distances (**Fig. 2**), which would vary depending on the body position. It is helpful to remember 3 "RA to SA" distances: about 5 cm in supine position, about 8 cm at a 30 degree incline, and about 10 cm at ≥45 degree inclines.

head of the bed, eliciting the HJR, or exerting a gentle pressure at the root of the neck with a finger. In some older adults, EJV's may be stiff and their contours are visible without those maneuvers. For optimal visualization of EJV pulsation, the head needs to be turned slightly (10 to 20 degrees) to the opposite direction. This allows the skin folds in the neck to be straightened enough for visualization but not tight enough to obliterate it.

The IJV's, on the other hand, lie deep and their contours cannot be seen. The IJV pulsation is best visualized in the upper neck area, when the head of the patient is turned laterally (optimally between 50 to 80 degrees) to the opposite direction. The IJV pulsation can be confused with that of the carotid artery, which can be easily distinguished from the latter by several observations: (1) the jugular pulsation has double undulation (vs the single upward stroke of carotid pulsation), (2) the jugular pulsation cannot be palpated, and (3) the jugular pulsation is responsive to gravity (body positions) and abdominal pressure. Once the top of the jugular pulsation has been identified in the middle of the neck, the vertical "sternal angle to top of the jugular pulsation" distance should be estimated in centimeters (see **Fig. 1; Fig. 2**). Then, the estimated "right atrium to sternal angle" distance appropriate for the body position should be added (subtracted if the vertical "sternal angle to top of the jugular pulsation" distance is negative; see **Fig. 2**). The "right atrium to sternal angle" distance has been traditionally thought to be 5 cm regardless of body position. However, estimates based on computer tomographic scans of chest suggest that the "right atrium to sternal angle" varies with the position of the body (see **Fig. 2**).[21] The "right atrium to sternal angle" is 5 cm only during supine position. It increases to 8 at about 30 degrees of head elevation, and to about 10 cm at 45 degrees of head elevation (see **Fig. 2**).[21] The "right atrium to sternal angle" distance remains about 10 cm despite further elevation, so that it would be 10 cm in the sitting position (see **Fig. 1**).

HJR is often positive in patients with clinical HF. A positive HJR is one in which the JVP rises by 2 to 3 cm and remains elevated for about 10 seconds when a firm sustained pressure is applied to the upper to middle abdomen area. The cause of the positive HJR is poorly understood, and is believed to reflect right ventricular noncompliance. In one study, a positive HJR predicted right atrial pressure greater than 9 mm Hg, with high sensitivity (100%) and specificity (85%).[22] A positive HJR is often more helpful in identifying EJV and determining its patency than establishing fluid volume retention, as those with positive HJR usually will also have an elevated JVP. Not infrequently, HJR may be positive in HF patients who have normal or low JVP, which may indicate early fluid retention or mild residual fluid overload. Many of these patients are stable and have no bothersome dyspnea, and thus maybe be clinically insignificant.

EJECTION FRACTION IN HEART FAILURE

Estimation of LVEF by an echocardiogram is the most important test after a clinical diagnosis of HF has been made, as it has both prognostic and therapeutic implications. Patients with clinical HF have diastolic HF if they a normal or near-normal LVEF and systolic HF if they have reduced HF (see **Table 5**). Although various LVEF cutoffs have been used to define systolic and diastolic HF, an LVEF of greater than 55% is often considered normal and an LVEF of less than 45% is often considered reduced. Baseline characteristics and prognosis of HF patients with LVEF between 45% and 55% are more similar to those with normal LVEF than reduced LVEF.[4] In general, older adults with systolic HF are at higher risk of mortality and hospitalization than those with diastolic HF.[23] Despite poor outcomes, systolic HF patients are more likely to benefit from life-prolonging therapy using neurohormonal blockade. On the other hand, the benefit of these drugs in diastolic HF has not been well established.

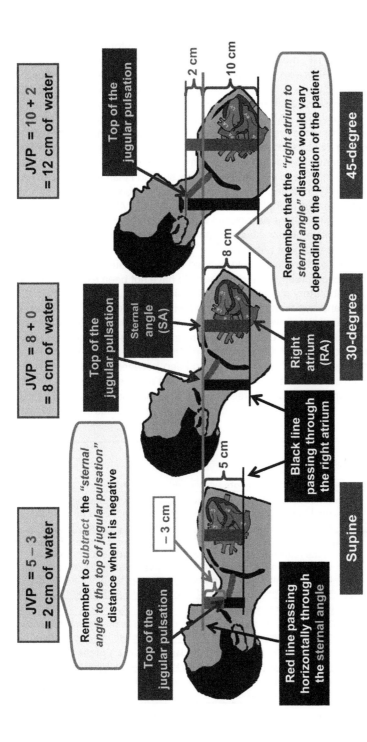

Fig. 2. To estimate the jugular venous pressure (JVP, *marked by the black bar*), the jugular venous pulsation must be visualized in the middle of the neck. This requires positioning patients at various inclines, depending on the JVP level. Note that the "RA to SA" distance (*marked by the brown bar*) varies with the body position and when the JVP is low (*left panel*), the "SA to the top of jugular pulsation" distance (*marked by the blue bar*) is negative and must be *subtracted* from the "RA to SA" distance to obtain the estimated JVP in cm of water. (*Adapted from Ahmed A, Jones L, Hays CI. DEFEAT heart failure: assessment and management of heart failure in nursing homes made easy. J Am Med Dir Assoc 2008;9:386.*)

TREATMENT OF HEART FAILURE

Treatment of HF can be summarized into two broader groups: symptom-relieving therapy and life-prolonging therapy (**Table 6**). Because symptoms of HF are similar in systolic and diastolic HF, therapy to relieve symptoms and prevent hospitalization because of worsening HF is also rather similar. This therapy is primarily based on judicial use of diuretics and digoxin. Most HF patients with symptoms need loop diuretics to stay euvolemic. Furosemide is the most popular loop diuretic, followed by torsemide and bumetenide. Furosemide 40 mg is equivalent to torsemide 20 mg and bumetenide 1 mg. It is preferable to use diuretics as a single morning dose to avoid sleep disturbances. Large doses of diuretics (eg, furosemide 480 mg daily) may be given twice a day: morning and early afternoon. The long-term effects of prolonged loop diuretic therapy on outcomes in HF patients have not been studied in large RCTs. However, findings from propensity-matched studies suggest that prolonged diuretic use may be associated with increased mortality and hospitalization.[24,25] Although these findings may represent bias by indications associated with the use of diuretics, they have also been attributed to hypokalemia and neurohormonal activation, both of which are associated with diuretic use and poor outcomes.[26–29] Therefore, after euvolemia has been achieved, lower doses of diuretics should be tried to maintain euvolemia.

Although the effects of torsemide and furosemide have not been examined in large RCT, findings from laboratory studies and small clinical trials suggest that the neurohormonal activation and hypokalemia associated with torsemide may be milder and that its use may be associated with better outcomes.[30–32] Therefore, torsemide may be preferred over furosemide, especially when large doses are used. However, despite being generic for many decades, torsemide is more expensive than furosemide. Serum potassium should be monitored to keep between 4 and 5 mEq/L.[26,33] Whereas potassium supplement may be used to correct hypokalemia, spironolactone may be preferable for patients with persistent hypokalemia who need chronic potassium supplement to remain normokalemic.[34,35] Because judicious use of diuretics

Table 6
Pharmacotherapy in older adults with HF

Symptom-relieving therapy (applicable to both systolic and diastolic HF)	
Diuretics	After euvolemia has been achieved, lower doses of diuretics should be tried to maintain euvolemia. Serum potassium should be periodically monitored to keep between 4 and 5 mEq/L
Digoxin	Applicable to both systolic and diastolic HF. The main benefit of digoxin is in the reduction of hospitalization due to worsening HF. However, when used in low doses (0.125 mg or less per day), digoxin may also lower mortality, which is especially important for older adults with systolic HF who cannot afford or tolerate ACE inhibitors or β-blockers
Life-prolonging therapy (applicable to systolic HF only)*	
ACE inhibitors or ARBs	ACE inhibitors are the drugs of first choice. ARBs should only be used in those who cannot tolerate ACE inhibitors (often because of cough)
β-Blockers	Unlike ACE inhibitors, there is no class effect, and 1 of the 3 approved β-blockers (carvedilol, metoprolol succinate, bisoprolol) should be used
Aldosterone antagonist	Limited indication. Avoid use in patients with renal insufficiency and monitor serum potassium to avoid hyperkalemia

Abbreviations: ACE, angiotensin-converting enzyme; ARB, angiotensin receptor blocker.
 * Although many life-prolonging drugs also reduce the risk of hospitalization, most HF patients require diuretics to remain euvolemic.

plays an important role in achieving euvolemia, clinicians should be familiar with the use of all 3 loop diuretics. Although not clearly understood why, when response to a particular diuretic is poor, a better response may be observed with another diuretic. Finally, there is no evidence suggesting that a large dose of a loop diuretic (eg, furosemide 320 mg daily) is superior to a combination of a lower dose of diuretic (eg, furosemide 160 mg) and a thiazide-like diuretic (eg, metolazone 2.5 mg daily). However, the combination regimen has been suggested to cause more electrolyte imbalance, requiring a closer monitoring of serum electrolytes, and may also be more inconvenient for older adults.

Digoxin has been shown to reduce HF hospitalization in both systolic and diastolic HF.[36–40] However, in diastolic HF, the use of digoxin was also associated with a significant increase in hospitalization due to unstable angina.[38] Because these patients were not receiving beta-blockers, it is not unknown if hospitalization due to unstable angina would be lower in contemporary HF patients, many of whom receive beta-blockers. In systolic HF, when used in low doses (0.125 mg or less per day), leading to low serum digoxin concentrations (0.5–0.9 ng/ml), digoxin has also been associated with reduction in mortality.[37,39,40] When used in low doses, there is no need to routinely check serum digoxin concentration, though it may be checked if there is clinical evidence of digoxin toxicity and if an increase in the dose of digoxin is being considered in a symptomatic patient unresponsive to lower doses. Digoxin should be prescribed to systolic HF patients with or without atrial fibrillation who continue to remain symptomatic despite therapy with ACE inhibitors or angiotensin receptor blockers (ARBs), and β-blockers, or for those who cannot afford or tolerate these drugs.[37] Digoxin should also be tried before considering cardiac resynchronization therapy (CRT), which is invasive, costly, and indicated for systolic HF patients a wide QRS complex, but the response is often unpredictable.[37]

Life-prolonging therapy for HF is limited to the use of an ACE inhibitor or an ARB for patients who cannot tolerate an ACE inhibitor (mostly due to cough, but allergic reactions are not uncommon), and any of the 3 β-blockers approved for use in HF (carvedilol, metoprolol succinate long-acting, and bisoprolol) in patients with systolic HF (see **Table 6**). There is no evidence of additional mortality reduction from the addition of an ARB to systolic HF patients receiving ACE inhibitors. In addition, patients receiving both an ACE inhibitor and an ARB are more likely to experience adverse side effects such as worsening kidney function and hyperkalemia.[41] There is no need to maximize the dose of ACE inhibitors before β-blocker therapy is initiated.[42] Because metoprolol succinate is a β-1 selective blocker and has little effect on blood pressure, it may be preferred as the β-blocker of initial choice over carvedilol, a nonselective β-blocker with a potential antihypertensive effect.[43] However, in older adults with systolic HF and uncontrolled hypertension, switching metoprolol succinate to carvedilol should be considered before adding another antihypertensive agent. The indication of aldosterone antagonists such as spironolactone is limited to symptomatic patients with advanced systolic HF without renal insufficiency or hyperkalemia.[35] Eplerenone may be prescribed to HF patients who cannot tolerate spironolactone (mostly because of painful gynecomastia).[44,45]

There is little evidence from RCT's that therapy with ACE inhibitors or ARBs or β-blockers reduces all-cause mortality in diastolic HF.[46–51] However, candesartan and digoxin have been shown to reduce HF hospitalization, and may be considered in symptomatic diastolic HF patients with frequent hospitalizations as a result of worsening HF.[38,50,52]

Device-based and surgical therapy for older adults with HF needs to be individualized based on comorbidities and functional status. CRT has been shown to reduce mortality and hospitalization in symptomatic systolic (LVEF <30%) HF patients with a wide QRS complex (>120 ms).[53] The advantage of CRT devices in combination with defibrillator function versus pacemaker function in older adults with HF remains unclear. Considering the risk of sudden cardiac death in HF, many prefer an implantable cardioverter with defibrillator (ICD) function over one with pacemaker function. However, the effectiveness of ICD's in older adults with multiple morbidities has not been well established.[54–56]

Finally, older adults with end-stage HF should be considered for hospice and palliative care referral. Because most acutely decompensated HF patients become asymptomatic when euvolemic and many apparently stable HF patients may die of sudden cardiac death, predicting 6-month life expectancy may be difficult in older adults with end-stage HF. However, clinicians familiar with HF patients may use a subjective criterion of asking themselves if they would be surprised if their HF patients died within the next 6 months. If the answer is no, such patients could be considered for possible hospice and palliative care referrals. The issue of deactivation of ICD and other cardiac devices should be discussed with patients and family members of older adults with HF being considered for hospice and end-of-life care.[57]

SUMMARY

Most of the HF patients are older adults, and HF is the leading cause of hospitalization among older adults. The assessment and management of HF in older adults can be challenging. However, it can be structured and simplified by using the mnemonic DEFEAT-HF: Diagnosis (clinical, and must not be ruled out based on normal LVEF), Etiology (CAD and hypertension being the most common), Fluid volume (must be assessed by estimating JVP using IJV or EJV), Ejection fraction (LVEF has both prognostic and therapeutic implications), And Treatment of Heart Failure (symptom-relieving therapy using diuretic and digoxin for systolic and diastolic HF, and life-prolonging therapy using neurohormonal blockade in systolic HF). Device and surgical therapy must be individualized, and hospice and palliative care should be considered for those with terminal HF.

REFERENCES

1. Roger VL, Go AS, Lloyd-Jones DM, et al. Heart disease and stroke statistics—2011 update: a report from the American Heart Association. Circulation 2010;123(4):e18–209.
2. Lloyd-Jones D, Adams RJ, Brown TM, et al. Executive summary: heart disease and stroke statistics—2010 update: a report from the American Heart Association. Circulation 2010;121:948–54.
3. Ahmed A. Clinical manifestations, diagnostic assessment, and etiology of heart failure in older adults. Clin Geriatr Med 2007;23:11–30.
4. Fonarow GC, Stough WG, Abraham WT, et al. Characteristics, treatments, and outcomes of patients with preserved systolic function hospitalized for heart failure: a report from the OPTIMIZE-HF Registry. J Am Coll Cardiol 2007;50:768–77.
5. Aronow WS. Drug treatment of systolic and of diastolic heart failure in elderly persons. J Gerontol A Biol Sci Med Sci 2005;60:1597–605.
6. Ahmed A. American College of Cardiology/American Heart Association chronic heart failure evaluation and management guidelines: relevance to the geriatric practice. J Am Geriatr Soc 2003;51:123–6.

7. Ahmed A. DEFEAT heart failure: clinical manifestations, diagnostic assessment, and etiology of geriatric heart failure. Heart Fail Clin 2007;3:389–402.
8. Ahmed A, Jones L, Hays CI. DEFEAT heart failure: assessment and management of heart failure in nursing homes made easy. J Am Med Dir Assoc 2008;9:383–9.
9. Gottdiener JS, McClelland RL, Marshall R, et al. Outcome of congestive heart failure in elderly persons: influence of left ventricular systolic function. The cardiovascular health study. Ann Intern Med 2002;137:631–9.
10. Kitzman DW, Gardin JM, Gottdiener JS, et al. Importance of heart failure with preserved systolic function in patients > or = 65 years of age. CHS research group. Cardiovascular health study. Am J Cardiol 2001;87:413–9.
11. Kitzman DW, Little WC, Brubaker PH, et al. Pathophysiological characterization of isolated diastolic heart failure in comparison to systolic heart failure. JAMA 2002; 288:2144–50.
12. Ekundayo OJ, Howard VJ, Safford MM, et al. Value of orthopnea, paroxysmal nocturnal dyspnea, and medications in prospective population studies of incident heart failure. Am J Cardiol 2009;104:259–64.
13. Butman SM, Ewy GA, Standen JR, et al. Bedside cardiovascular examination in patients with severe chronic heart failure: importance of rest or inducible jugular venous distension. J Am Coll Cardiol 1993;22:968–74.
14. Drazner MH, Rame JE, Stevenson LW, et al. Prognostic importance of elevated jugular venous pressure and a third heart sound in patients with heart failure. N Engl J Med 2001;345:574–81.
15. Curtis JP, Selter JG, Wang Y, et al. The obesity paradox: body mass index and outcomes in patients with heart failure. Arch Intern Med 2005;165:55–61.
16. Mueller C, Scholer A, Laule-Kilian K, et al. Use of B-type natriuretic peptide in the evaluation and management of acute dyspnea. N Engl J Med 2004;350: 647–54.
17. Vinayak AG, Levitt J, Gehlbach B, et al. Usefulness of the external jugular vein examination in detecting abnormal central venous pressure in critically ill patients. Arch Intern Med 2006;166:2132–7.
18. Dickstein K, Cohen-Solal A, Filippatos G, et al. ESC Guidelines for the diagnosis and treatment of acute and chronic heart failure 2008: the task force for the diagnosis and treatment of acute and chronic heart failure 2008 of the European Society of Cardiology. Developed in collaboration with the Heart Failure Association of the ESC (HFA) and endorsed by the European Society of Intensive Care Medicine (ESICM). Eur Heart J 2008;29:2388–442.
19. Maisel AS, Krishnaswamy P, Nowak RM, et al. Rapid measurement of B-type natriuretic peptide in the emergency diagnosis of heart failure. N Engl J Med 2002;347:161–7.
20. Nieminen MS, Bohm M, Cowie MR, et al. Executive summary of the guidelines on the diagnosis and treatment of acute heart failure: the task force on acute heart failure of the European Society of Cardiology. Eur Heart J 2005;26:384–416.
21. Seth R, Magner P, Matzinger F, et al. How far is the sternal angle from the mid-right atrium? J Gen Intern Med 2002;17:852–6.
22. Sochowski RA, Dubbin JD, Naqvi SZ. Clinical and hemodynamic assessment of the hepatojugular reflux. Am J Cardiol 1990;66:1002–6.
23. Ahmed A. Association of diastolic dysfunction and outcomes in ambulatory older adults with chronic heart failure. J Gerontol A Biol Sci Med Sci 2005;60:1339–44.
24. Ahmed A, Husain A, Love TE, et al. Heart failure, chronic diuretic use, and increase in mortality and hospitalization: an observational study using propensity score methods. Eur Heart J 2006;27:1431–9.

25. Ahmed A, Young JB, Love TE, et al. A propensity-matched study of the effects of chronic diuretic therapy on mortality and hospitalization in older adults with heart failure. Int J Cardiol 2008;125:246–53.
26. Alper AB, Campbell RC, Anker SD, et al. A propensity-matched study of low serum potassium and mortality in older adults with chronic heart failure. Int J Cardiol 2009;137:1–8.
27. Ahmed A, Zannad F, Love TE, et al. A propensity-matched study of the association of low serum potassium levels and mortality in chronic heart failure. Eur Heart J 2007;28:1334–43.
28. Bowling CB, Pitt B, Ahmed MI, et al. Hypokalemia and outcomes in patients with chronic heart failure and chronic kidney disease: findings from propensity-matched studies. Circ Heart Fail 2010;3:253–60.
29. Francis GS, Benedict C, Johnstone DE, et al. Comparison of neuroendocrine activation in patients with left ventricular dysfunction with and without congestive heart failure. A substudy of the Studies of Left Ventricular Dysfunction (SOLVD). Circulation 1990;82:1724–9.
30. Lopez B, Querejeta R, Gonzalez A, et al. Effects of loop diuretics on myocardial fibrosis and collagen type I turnover in chronic heart failure. J Am Coll Cardiol 2004;43:2028–35.
31. Cosin J, Diez J, TORIC investigators. Torasemide in chronic heart failure: results of the TORIC study. Eur J Heart Fail 2002;4:507–13.
32. Murray MD, Deer MM, Ferguson JA, et al. Open-label randomized trial of torsemide compared with furosemide therapy for patients with heart failure. Am J Med 2001;111:513–20.
33. Ahmed MI, Ekundayo OJ, Mujib M, et al. Mild hyperkalemia and outcomes in chronic heart failure: a propensity matched study. Int J Cardiol 2010;144:383–8.
34. Ekundayo OJ, Adamopoulos C, Ahmed MI, et al. Oral potassium supplement use and outcomes in chronic heart failure: a propensity-matched study. Int J Cardiol 2010;141:167–74.
35. Pitt B, Zannad F, Remme WJ, et al. The effect of spironolactone on morbidity and mortality in patients with severe heart failure. Randomized aldactone evaluation study investigators. N Engl J Med 1999;341:709–17.
36. The Digitalis Investigation Group. The effect of digoxin on mortality and morbidity in patients with heart failure. N Engl J Med 1997;336:525–33.
37. Ahmed A, Rich MW, Love TE, et al. Digoxin and reduction in mortality and hospitalization in heart failure: a comprehensive post hoc analysis of the DIG trial. Eur Heart J 2006;27:178–86.
38. Ahmed A, Rich MW, Fleg JL, et al. Effects of digoxin on morbidity and mortality in diastolic heart failure: the ancillary digitalis investigation group trial. Circulation 2006;114:397–403.
39. Ahmed A, Pitt B, Rahimtoola SH, et al. Effects of digoxin at low serum concentrations on mortality and hospitalization in heart failure: a propensity-matched study of the DIG trial. Int J Cardiol 2008;123:138–46.
40. Ahmed A. Digoxin and reduction in mortality and hospitalization in geriatric heart failure: importance of low doses and low serum concentrations. J Gerontol A Biol Sci Med Sci 2007;62:323–9.
41. McMurray JJ, Ostergren J, Swedberg K, et al. Effects of candesartan in patients with chronic heart failure and reduced left-ventricular systolic function taking angiotensin-converting-enzyme inhibitors: the CHARM-Added trial. Lancet 2003;362:767–71.

42. Hunt SA, Abraham WT, Chin MH, et al. ACC/AHA 2005 guideline update for the diagnosis and management of chronic heart failure in the adult: a report of the American College of Cardiology/American Heart Association Task force on practice guidelines (Writing Committee to Update the 2001 Guidelines for the Evaluation and Management of Heart Failure): developed in collaboration with the American College of Chest Physicians and the International Society for Heart and Lung Transplantation: endorsed by the Heart Rhythm Society. Circulation 2005;112:e154–235.
43. Ahmed A, Dell'Italia LJ. Use of beta-blockers in older adults with chronic heart failure. Am J Med Sci 2004;328:100–11.
44. Pitt B, Remme W, Zannad F, et al. Eplerenone, a selective aldosterone blocker, in patients with left ventricular dysfunction after myocardial infarction. N Engl J Med 2003;348:1309–21.
45. Zannad F, McMurray JJ, Krum H, et al. Eplerenone in patients with systolic heart failure and mild symptoms. N Engl J Med 2011;364:11–21.
46. Massie BM, Carson PE, McMurray JJ, et al. Irbesartan in patients with heart failure and preserved ejection fraction. N Engl J Med 2008;359:2456–67.
47. Zile MR, Gaasch WH, Anand IS, et al. Mode of death in patients with heart failure and a preserved ejection fraction: results from the Irbesartan in heart failure with preserved ejection fraction study (I-Preserve) trial. Circulation 2010;121:1393–405.
48. Cleland JG, Tendera M, Adamus J, et al. Perindopril for elderly people with chronic heart failure: the PEP-CHF study. The PEP investigators. Eur J Heart Fail 1999;1:211–7.
49. Cleland JG, Tendera M, Adamus J, et al. The perindopril in elderly people with chronic heart failure (PEP-CHF) study. Eur Heart J 2006;27:2338–45.
50. Yusuf S, Pfeffer MA, Swedberg K, et al. Effects of candesartan in patients with chronic heart failure and preserved left-ventricular ejection fraction: the CHARM-Preserved trial. Lancet 2003;362:777–81.
51. Flather MD, Shibata MC, Coats AJ, et al. Randomized trial to determine the effect of nebivolol on mortality and cardiovascular hospital admission in elderly patients with heart failure (SENIORS). Eur Heart J 2005;26:215–25.
52. Ahmed A, Young JB, Gheorghiade M. The underuse of digoxin in heart failure, and approaches to appropriate use. CMAJ 2007;176:641–3.
53. Tang AS, Wells GA, Talajic M, et al. Cardiac-resynchronization therapy for mild-to-moderate heart failure. N Engl J Med 2010;363:2385–95.
54. Swindle JP, Rich MW, McCann P, et al. Implantable cardiac device procedures in older patients: use and in-hospital outcomes. Arch Intern Med 2010;170:631–7.
55. Kusumoto F. Best clinical practice: art, science, or both?: comment on "implantable cardiac device procedures in older patients". Arch Intern Med 2010;170: 638–9.
56. Nichol G, Kaul P, Huszti E, et al. Cost-effectiveness of cardiac resynchronization therapy in patients with symptomatic heart failure. Ann Intern Med 2004;141: 343–51.
57. Zellner RA, Aulisio MP, Lewis WR. Should implantable cardioverter-defibrillators and permanent pacemakers in patients with terminal illness be deactivated? Deactivating permanent pacemaker in patients with terminal illness. Patient autonomy is paramount. Circ Arrhythm Electrophysiol 2009;2:340–4.

Revitalizing the Aged Brain

Abhilash K. Desai, MD

KEYWORDS

• Cognition • Fitness • Memory • Brain • Health • Older

In the last decade, interest in staying sharp has taken central stage in the minds of older adults.[1] More and more older adults are asking primary care providers (PCPs) to give them advice regarding how to prevent Alzheimer disease (AD) and ways to fix the day-to-day forgetfulness they are experiencing. Optimal cognitive and emotional function is vital to independence, productivity, and quality of life.[2] New research has shown that age-related decline in memory and thinking abilities is smaller than previously believed and is reversible with lifestyle modification.[3] At the same time, new research has also found that even senior moments may be the earliest signs of neurodegenerative disorders.[4] Also, cognitive impairment without dementia may be seen in 16% to 33% of adults older than 65 years and is associated with significant emotional distress.[5,6] PCPs need to be able to give their patients practical guidance in ways to revitalize their aging brain.

The Cognitive and Emotional Health Project commissioned by the National Institutes of Health defined successful cognitive and emotional aging as "the development and preservation of the multidimensional cognitive structures that allows the older adult to maintain social connectedness, an ongoing sense of purpose, and the abilities to function independently, to permit functional recover from illness or injury, and to cope with residual functional deficits."[7] Thus, cognitive and emotional well-being are inextricably linked. This article uses this definition to qualify revitalizing the aged brain, discuss neuroplasticity, and suggest practical neuroplasticity-based strategies to improve cognitive and emotional well-being of older adults.

NEUROPLASTICITY

Neuroplasticity is the capacity of the brain to change with experience. The brain has a remarkable capacity to change with experience at all ages, and neuroplasticity is dynamic and flexible.[8] Because experiences can be positive (health promoting) or negative (harming our health), in tandem, neuroplastic changes in the brain can be positive (eg, increased dendritic arborization, synaptogenesis, neurogenesis, stronger

Financial disclosure: Nothing to disclose.
Memory Clinic, Department of Geriatric Psychiatry, Sheppard Pratt Health Systems, 6501 North Charles Street, Baltimore, MD 21204-6815, USA
E-mail address: adesai@sheppardpratt.org

Med Clin N Am 95 (2011) 463–475
doi:10.1016/j.mcna.2011.03.002

signals during neurotransmission) or negative (eg, suppression of neurogenesis, debranching of dendrites, decreased dendritic connections between neurons, weaker signals during neurotransmission).[3,9] Various factors that promote positive and negative neuroplasticity are listed in **Box 1**.[3,10–19]

Cognitive reserve (ability of an adult brain to sustain normal function despite disease or injury to the brain) is probably set early in life (in the first or second decade) and reflects positive neuroplastic changes in the brain caused by an enriched environment during the early years.[20] Older persons who are highly educated have higher cognitive reserve (both functional and structural). Older adults with high cognitive reserve are at an advantage in terms of having bigger and more efficient neural networks and thus may have more efficient neuroplasticity late into their lives. Compensation is another aspect of neuroplasticity and typically involves undamaged neural networks compensating for damaged neural areas involved not only in language and movement but also cognitive functions of attention and memory.

Many cognitive scientists believe that our neglect of intensive learning as we age causes decline in efficiency of various neuronal networks involved in attention and memory function as well as other cognitive functions.[21] Many older adults, after having completed school, rarely engaged in tasks for prolonged periods (months to years) that required focused attention to learn new vocabulary or master a new skill. This situation may have resulted in loss of efficiency of neural networks required for attention. Attention networks are crucial for all forms of learning at all ages. Thus, normal cognitive aging (NCA) may be influenced not only by our genes but also our lifestyle.

Neuroplasticity informs us about the importance of practice (repetitive engagement in activities that enhance brain health) if one wants to improve brain function

---

Box 1
Common factors that influence neuroplasticity

Positive Neuroplasticity	Comments
Physical activity	Even light exercise (eg, walking) promotes cognitive function
Challenging cognitive activities	Learning something new that is interesting and requires intense focus for prolonged periods has the most dramatic effects
Socially active lifestyle	Intergenerational activities may be particularly beneficial
Healthy nutrition	Diet rich in fruits, vegetables, whole grains, and fatty fish along with adequate amount of water is recommended
Nutritional supplements	Omega 3 supplements (for older adults who do not eat fish) and vitamin B_{12} and vitamin D (for older adults who are deficient in these vitamins) may promote positive neuroplasticity
Negative Neuroplasticity	Comments
Chronic psychosocial stress	Meditation and psychotherapy may mitigate effects of stress
Chronic insomnia	Adequate sleep (in quantity and quality) is important for synaptic neuroplasticity and thus, learning and memory
Cardiovascular risk factors (CRFs)	CRFs (eg, hypertension, obesity, smoking, diabetes, dyslipidemia) in middle age have been associated with increased risk of AD in later years
Air pollution	Besides accelerating atherosclerosis, air pollution may have a direct toxic effect on brain function

noticeably. As the brain networks and neurons get activated repetitively, they become more efficient and can process faster. They also require less initial stimulus to fire up the action potential (the initial neuronal activity that starts communication between different cells and eventually between different networks). Revitalizing the brain involves replacing unhealthy habits with healthy habits. Each time we engage in unhealthy habits, it activates certain brain networks. As we engage in these habits, the networks strengthen and require less and less stimulation from the environment to get activated. When we try to engage in healthy habits to replace unhealthy habits, more energy is required because these new networks have not yet become as strong and efficient as networks of unhealthy habits. For this reason unhealthy habits are difficult to break or unlearn. Thus, persistence is key in an effort to replace neural networks that support unhealthy habits with neural networks that support healthy habits.

Although chronic severe psychosocial stress is neurotoxic (hampers neuroplasticity), animal studies have found that a little daily stress may enhance neuronal and synaptic function, promote neurogenesis in the hippocampus, and improve cognitive performance in certain tasks.[22] This finding is not surprising because emotional arousal (associated with stress) can enhance learning and memory via synaptic plasticity of limbic pathways. Stress hormones (eg, glucocorticoids) have an inverted U-shaped dose-response curve in which low to moderate levels of adrenal steroids enhance acquisition of tasks that involve the hippocampus, whereas high levels of glucocorticoids disrupt task acquisition.[23] This finding may explain why many older adults experience a decline in cognitive functioning after they retire from work: work was providing these older adults with an optimum amount of stress and this in turn helped the brain function better.

A PRACTICAL APPROACH TO REVITALIZING THE AGED BRAIN

Three key steps are recommended to PCPs in helping older adults achieve and maintain cognitive and emotional vitality.

Step 1: Comprehensive Physical and Mental Health Assessment

A comprehensive assessment of health to identify and treat medical and psychiatric conditions that are prevalent in older adults and can cause current or future cognitive impairment is recommended.[2–4,11–13,24,25] Please refer to **Box 2**. If these conditions are recognized and treated early, much of the negative effect of these conditions on cognitive and emotional well-being can be prevented or reversed. Observational studies strongly support a link between CRFs (especially hypertension, diabetes, smoking, obesity) and future cognitive impairment and depression.[10] Thus, optimal control of CRFs and secondary prevention of stroke are also recommended to promote brain health. Many older adults (especially if they have subjective cognitive complains and some functional decline) may need neuropsychological testing to clarify severity of cognitive impairment (whether it is subjective cognitive impairment, mild cognitive impairment [MCI] or mild dementia [AD and related disorders]).[4] Neuropsychological testing also provides assessment of preserved cognitive abilities, and this information may help guide appropriate cognitive strategies.

During such a comprehensive assessment, patients can also be counseled regarding the risk and potential benefits of over-the-counter (OTC) brain enhancers. In general, the risks are not insignificant (eg, drug-supplement interaction) and benefits are not proved for any of the currently available OTC supplements and herbal remedies. Drugs approved by the US Food and Drug Administration for treatment of AD and Parkinson disease (eg, cholinesterase inhibitors, memantine) are not

---

Box 2
Common reversible causes of cognitive impairment in older adults

Causes	Comments
Medications	Benzodiazepines and drugs with anticholinergic activity are common culprits. Cognitive impairment is not the hallmark of all anticholinergic drugs. For example, darifenacin, solifenacin, and tolterodine may not have a significant effect on cognition in cognitively intact healthy older adults
Harmful alcohol use	Excessive alcohol not only causes direct neurotoxicity but also interacts with many commonly prescribed medications
Sleep disorders	Chronic primary insomnia, obstructive sleep apnea, and restless leg syndrome are common culprits
Malnutrition	Dehydration, protein energy malnutrition, vitamin deficiencies (eg, vitamin B12, D) and celiac disease are prevalent in older adults, especially frail older adults (eg, nursing home population)
Electrolyte imbalance	Hypernatremia or hyponatremia can cause cognitive impairment and are often associated with malnutrition, diuretic use, and being secondary to some medications
Depression and anxiety	May directly cause cognitive impairment through increase in stress hormones and indirectly by impairing nutrition and engagement in physical and social activity. Severe depression may be misdiagnosed as dementia
Hearing and vision deficits	Optimizing hearing and vision (eg, with aids and environmental changes [eg, increased lighting]) is recommended before any cognitive testing
Hormonal deficiency	Hyperthyroidism, hypothyroidism, and testosterone deficiency are the most common endocrine disorders associated with cognitive impairment
Diabetes	Hypoglycemic episodes and sever hyperglycemia are commonly associated with cognitive impairment
Hypertriglyceridemia	High levels of triglycerides are associated with cognitive impairment
Chronic severe pain	Chronic pain is associated with cognitive impairment, and this association may be mediated through negative neuroplasticity caused by severe and chronic emotional stress as well as cognitive adverse effects of medications given to treat pain (eg, opiates)
Congestive heart failure (CHF)	Association of CHF with cognitive impairment may be related to decreased ejection fraction, resulting in decreased cerebral blood flow
Blood pressure dyscontrol	Excessively high or low blood pressure may impair cognition by reducing cerebral blood flow

---

recommended for treatment of NCA or to improve cognition in patients who do not have these conditions. Vitamins are also not recommended if the primary goal is to improve cognition unless there is documented vitamin deficiency. In addition, vitamin supplements in some individuals may prevent health-promoting effects of physical exercise.[26]

During initial assessment, evaluation for substance abuse (prescription and illicit street drugs and alcohol) and smoking is also recommended. All drugs with potential for abuse have negative effects on the brain and these effects can be permanent depending on severity and duration of abuse. The need for substance abuse treatment among Americans older than 50 years is projected to double by 2020, according to a report by the Substance Abuse and Mental Health Services Administration (SAMHSA). As baby boomers age, illicit drug use among the population older than 50 years also is rising. Illicit drugs include marijuana and the nonmedical use of prescription drugs. An estimated 4.3 million adults aged 50 years or older used an illicit drug in the past year, according to SAMHSA. Age-related physiologic and social changes make older adults more vulnerable to the harmful effect of illicit drug use. Counseling regarding harmful effects of illicit drug use, prescription drug abuse, excessive alcohol intake (more than 1–2 drinks per day) and smoking can be initiated by the PCP and followed up by the nurse.

Step 2: Counseling Patients About Practical, Individually Tailored Lifestyle Modification Strategies to Promote Cognitive and Emotional Health

In general, what is good for the heart is good for the brain. Thus, lifestyle modification strategies involve stress reduction strategies, physical activity and exercise, nutritional strategies, and a socially active lifestyle. Stressing the benefits of a brain-healthy lifestyle may work better than emphasizing the negative effects of an unhealthy lifestyle (eg, sedentary lifestyle, regular intake of fast foods). This information can be provided by a nurse, and a patient handout (refer to **Box 3**) may facilitate patient participation.

Stress reduction strategies

Psychosocial stress suppresses neurogenesis, causes dendritic shrinkage, and may accelerate the cognitive decline and synaptic loss in individuals at risk for AD.[27] Routine engagement in strategies to reduce stress and promote emotional

---

Box 3
Patient handout: to improve brain health, all you need is "SLEEP N Pills"

S: Adequate daily sleep is essential to recharge the brain and maintain good thinking skills and memory. New information gets processed and new memories get consolidated during different phases of sleep.

L: Lose it or use it. Brain is a plastic organ, meaning that it constantly changes with experience and activity. Brain functions and skills not used are lost rapidly. Age-related decline in brain function may be more related to decline in our time spent learning new skills and activities after age 30 years rather than decline because of aging.

E: Excess disability such as memory problems caused by nutritional deficiencies, sleep disorders, medication adverse effects, depression, anxiety disorder, chronic pain, chronic stress, attention-deficit/hyperactivity disorder (ADHD) and other conditions should be identified and treated for other strategies to have their beneficial effect.

E: Exercising regularly and leading a physically active lifestyle are also crucial to preserving brain function. Exercise not only boosts blood supply to the brain but also helps create new brain cells, even late in life.

P: Positive emotions (eg, relaxation, joy, serenity, happiness, laughter, optimism, feeling connected to others) not only prevent negative effects of stress on the brain but may directly improve the capacity of the brain to learn new things and remember day-to-day events.

N: Nutrition that is brain healthy (eg, a Mediterranean diet) is crucial to preserve brain function.

Pills: Nutritional supplements (eg, omega 3, vitamins [only if there is vitamin deficiency]) and medications for cardiovascular (eg, hypertension, diabetes) and neuropsychiatric disorders (eg, ADHD medications, antidepressants) may be necessary for some people to maximize the effects of other strategies mentioned earlier.

well-being promotes positive neuroplasticity in a variety of ways. For example, meditation and other mindfulness-based strategies (eg, yoga) have been found to increase white-matter connectivity and gray-matter volumes (especially in hippocampal and frontal lobes).[28,29] One of the simple stress reduction strategies is daily practice of relaxation exercises (eg, breath-awareness exercises, progressive muscle relaxation, relaxation using biofeedback and neurofeedback). Please refer to **Box 4** for a patient handout for breath-awareness exercises. During relaxation exercises, the brain rearranges itself so that the 2 cerebral hemispheres communicate better. This characteristic helps the brain better able to solve day-to-day problems. Another neurophysiologic effect of relaxation exercises is quieting down of limbic networks but an increase in activity in certain networks in the frontal lobe that are involved with attention and decision making. Thus, if an individual engages in the daily practice of relaxation training, gradually the capacity to pay attention (and thus remember) and problem solve improves. The calming response induced by relaxation exercises also releases nitric oxide, which in turn enhances dopaminergic and endorphin neurotransmission. The latter has the effect of enhancing a general sense of well-being. Humor is another strategy that not only reduces stress but may also promote the health of diverse brain and body functions such as insight, the capacity to problem solve, and the immune system.

Physical activity and exercise
A large body of research has shown the beneficial effects of physical activity and exercise (especially aerobic but also strength training) on many aspects of brain function and have suggested that they may even increase brain volume in aging humans.[14,30,31] The benefits have been seen at the molecular as well as at the behavioral level in all age groups including frail elderly people. Executive function (ability to plan, organize, and learn from previous experience) and attention has been found to improve with regular

---

Box 4
Patient handout

Breath-awareness Exercises To Improve Memory and Promote Resilience

Find a quiet spot. Sit on a flat but comfortable surface. Close your eyes and begin to pay attention to your breathing. Inhale through your nose. Slow down your breathing as you feel your breath enter and leave your body. Feel your lungs expand with the inhalation, retain the breath for a few seconds, and then exhale gently. As you continue to breathe, try and keep your attention on all 3 aspects of breathing (inhalation, pause, exhalation). The slower the breathing, the greater are the benefits. Whenever possible, exhalation should be longer than inhalation. During exhalation, the heart slows down, the blood pressure drops and stress hormone levels also drop. Also, try and do abdominal breathing/diaphragmatic breathing. Thus, during inhalation, your tummy should bulge outwards and during exhalation, your tummy should go toward the spine. Count your breaths. If you notice that you have lost count of your breaths, gently bring your attention to breathing and start counting again. Continue this for at least 2 minutes. Try and increase it to 20 minutes twice a day (early morning and before sleep). Alternatively, one can engage in this for 2 minutes several times a day. Find your own rhythm, frequency and duration. This exercise is best done when you are not tired. When you are doing this for the first time, you may experience dizziness. Generally, it is mild and transient and passes quickly.

Potential benefits of breath-awareness exercises

Improved memory (through improved capacity to focus, pay attention, be aware), improved capacity to tolerate negative emotions (anxiety, anger, resentment, guilt, grief, sadness) and improved ability to manage stress and problem solve in creative and healthy ways.

moderate physical activity in middle-aged as well as older adults, even those in their 80s. Mechanisms postulated for the beneficial effects of exercise on brain function include not only direct effects (eg, increased cerebral blood flow, increased synaptogenesis and neurogenesis) but also indirect effects (eg, reversing the negative effects of high-fat diets on neurotrophic factors in the brain that are needed for neuroplasticity and learning). "Achieving a physically active lifestyle requires effective time management, with a particular focus on reducing sedentary activities such as screen time (eg, watching television, surfing the Web, playing computer games) and making daily choices to move rather than be moved (eg, taking the stairs instead of the elevator)," is recommended by the American Heart Association (AHA) guidelines as a lifestyle modification strategy to improve cardiovascular health. These recommendations may also improve cognitive and emotional well-being.[2]

Nutritional strategies
A healthy diet may reduce fatty buildup in arteries (atherosclerosis) and counteract the neurotoxicity mediated by toxic protein(s) (eg, Aβ amyloid, hyperphosphorylated τ) that is believed to be the underlying mechanism of AD.[15] The Mediterranean diet has been associated with lower risk of future AD. The Mediterranean diet is characterized by high consumption of fruits, vegetables, legumes, nuts, and fish; a low intake of meats and poultry; the use of olive oil as the main source of fat; and a low to moderate intake of wine. Lowering intake of saturated fat to less than 7% and limiting trans fats to less than 1% is recommended by the AHA to promote cardiovascular health. These dietary changes may also improve neuronal function through improved cerebrovascular function and decreased neurodegeneration and thus may promote cognitive and emotional well-being. In individuals with limited life expectancy (eg, elderly people living in nursing homes, frail elderly people living in the community), liberalization of diet may do more to promote emotional well-being and improved nutritional status and thus cognitive performance than following therapeutic diets (eg, heart-healthy diet, diabetic diet, low-sodium diets).

Socially active lifestyle
An active and socially integrated lifestyle may protect against cognitive decline caused by aging and late-life dementias.[32] A socially active lifestyle may not only benefit cognitive functioning by providing mental stimulation (through increased use of language during conversations and increased engagement in pleasurable activities) but also by providing a buffer against negative effects of day-to-day stress. In addition, enriched social environment may also promote synaptogenesis and neurogenesis.[33] Rats in an enriched environment (eg, more social contact and novel stimuli) were found to complete a maze task faster than rats assigned to the standard environmental condition.[34] Thus, social activities have the potential to also promote problem-solving abilities.

Step 3: Counseling Patients Regarding Cognitive Strategies
Nurses can also take a leadership role in providing counseling to patients regarding cognitive strategies to improve memory and other cognitive problems. Please refer to **Box 5** for a list of strategies a nurse can use to counsel older adults who reports mild memory problems. Cognitive strategies (including cognitive training, engagement in mentally stimulating and challenging activities, brain exercises, and computer games) are necessary to optimally revitalize an aged brain because neuroplasticity is totally dependent on engaging the neural networks (ie, use it or lose it).[16,35] Cognitive strategies have been found to increase gray matter in the nucleus accumbens and

---

Box 5
Counseling patients regarding practical strategies to improve memory

1. *Use of imagination*: visual memory is stored at a different place than verbal memory. Storing memory in multiple places increases the likelihood of recalling the information. Patients can be encouraged to use all of their senses to imagine a particular scene or conversation they would like to remember.

2. *Use of mnemonics* may help some patients improve their memory by associating (chunking) information with easy-to-remember alphabets or words.

3. *Importance of cross-training*: exercising brain networks not involved in memory enhances the functioning of memory pathways in the brain. For example, learning a new language improves one's ability to remember words of one's own language. Singing, reading aloud, writing an autobiography, writing a poem, doing calculation/arithmetic with a child, solving puzzles (crosswords, sudoku, jigsaw puzzles), joining a book club, or taking a dance class are other examples of exercising nonmemory networks that may improve memory.

4. *Importance of repetition and rehearsal:* repetition is a key step to consolidate memory. Thus, encouraging patients to repeat the information in their mind (one can add visualization to this) is important.

5. *Keeping the stress down:* mild stress enhances attention but excessive stress not only impairs attention but also ability to recall information. Thus, one needs to be patient with oneself during one's attempt to remember.

6. *Importance of being present and attentive:* patients can be encouraged to focus (concentrate) with all their senses on the situation (eg, a conversation with a friend), paying attention to not only what the person is saying but their emotional intensity, and paying attention to their facial expressions. Multitasking involves splitting attention and thus is not good for remembering well. It is also important to minimize distractions (such as turning off music/TV, moving out of a noisy room to a quiet room) because with aging, one is more easily distracted. Also, full attention activates a larger area of the brain than paying less attention.

7. *Using tools:* taking notes (eg, checklist of things to do today, names of new people one meets, information obtained during visit to one's health care provider) and using a personal digital assistant are useful as memory aids. Our current hypercognitive culture can quickly overwhelm the best of us with information, and hence this strategy is used by even younger adults with normal memory.

8. *Creating a context:* giving the content emotional meaning and having an internal dialog to create the context in which information needs to be remembered promotes consolidation of memory. For example, we are more likely to remember names and events that had an emotional effect.

---

hippocampus but this effect is temporary, and once engagement in cognitive activity is stopped, these benefits are lost.[36] Engagement in cognitive activities such as reading, doing puzzles (crossword puzzles, sudoku), and playing bridge or chess provide a good brain workout. Engaging in learning new skills that are interesting/fun, especially in a social setting (eg, learning line dancing) or along with another individual (eg, learning a new language) have the potential to provide an even better brain workout, because learning something new requires an intense focus for prolonged periods of time and repetition, the 3 key ingredients to revitalize the brain. Older adults are encouraged to try new technologies (eg, texting) because it may not only provide a cognitive challenge but may enhance their social life (eg, increased contact with grandchildren).

Engaging in brain exercises to improve one's capacity to focus (pay attention) is also essential to improve brain function (especially memory). To remember something we have recently heard, first we must hear it clearly (with our full attention) because the memory can be only as clear as its original signal. Reward is also crucial to learning new things. When we reward ourselves for engaging in a challenging task, our brain releases certain neurotransmitters such as dopamine and acetylcholine. These neuro-transmitters are crucial in consolidating changes at the molecular and synaptic level that occur during learning. Engagement in creative activities may improve cognitive health directly by exercising neural networks not engaged routinely and also through psychosocial benefits.[17] Every person at all ages has at least 1 unique creative skill or talent. Engaging in this skill can reignite a passion that can not only improve cognition in that older person but may also reestablish their zest for life.

Simple strategies such as doing 1 task at a time (ie, avoiding multitasking), doing things slowly, and reminding oneself that the activity is completed (eg, locking the door and reminding oneself that one has locked the door so that one does not have to return to check if the door was locked), taking in one's surrounding before proceeding (eg, when parking, making a mental note as to where the car is parked), taking notes and visualizing the information all have the potential to mitigate senior moments and prevent associated emotional distress. High-technology strategies can involve engaging in computer-based brain exercises that are designed to enhance a specific group of cognitive functions (eg, ability to detect patterns, reaction time/pro-cessing speed) as well as engagement in computer games that promote physical fitness (eg, Wii games).

There is no one cognitive activity, or combination of activities, that is uniquely beneficial.[16] Cognitive activities that use multiple sensory systems (eg, tactile and auditory during dancing; gustatory and olfactory during cooking) may magnify the cognitive benefits of a challenging task. Nurses can help the older person create a personal program of cognitive fitness that is focused on their strengths and preserved abilities.

REALISTIC EXPECTATIONS

None of the research to date is conclusive that lifestyle modification or control of CRFs prevents dementia. Nevertheless, the benefits of the strategies described here have been proved to reduce one's risk of heart attacks and strokes, improve longevity, and in general have minimal downside and considerable potential to promote healthy brain aging.[2] Our experience and research have shown that the effect of these strategies is variable, with most seeing at least modest cognitive bene-fits and a small subgroup showing dramatic benefits. The latter group typically has multiple reversible causes of cognitive impairment (eg, depression, alcoholism, nutri-tional deficiencies, chronic pain, obstructive sleep apnea, drug-induced cognitive impairment), and on correction of these problems, show a dramatic improvement in cognitive function.

The capacity for the brain to revitalize depends on cognitive reserve and physical health. Thus, starting an individualized cognitive fitness plan as early as possible is important for optimal outcomes. Also, the brain retains capacity to improve even in the ninth decade and beyond. Thus, it is never too late to start making brain health a priority. Investments by communities, businesses, and government in creating fundamental changes in the food supply (access to affordable, tasty, and healthier options), technology that is easier for older adults to use, and social infrastructure (eg, a social environment that promotes physical activity and socialization) are neces-sary if healthy cognitive aging for all older adults is to be a reality. Please refer to **Box 6**

Box 6
Suggested resources for clinicians and patients

For Clinicians

Desai AK. Guest editor. Healthy brain aging: evidence based methods to preserve brain function and prevent dementia. Clinics of Geriatric Medicine 2010;26:1–170.

Vance DE, Roberson AJ, McGuinness TM, Fazeli PL. Now neuroplasticity and cognitive reserve protect cognitive functioning. Journal of Psychosocial Nursing 2010;48(4):23–30.

For Patients

Audio CD:

1. Weil A, Small G. The Healthy Brain Kit. Audio CDs, brain-training cards, and workbook. Boulder, CO: Sound True.

Books

2. Norman Doidge. *The Brain That Changes Itself.* New York: Penguin Books; 2007.

3. Gary Small. *The Memory Prescription: Dr. Gary Small's 14-day plan to keep your brain and body young.* New York: Hyperion; 2004.

4. *Improving memory. Understanding age-related memory loss. A special report from Harvard Medical School.* Boston: Harvard Health Publications; 2006. http://www.health.harvard.edu/

Web sites for information on brain fitness, brain training games, and software

5. http://www.positscience.com/

6. http://www.sharpbrains.com/

---

for a list of resources for both PCPs and patients. Such resources can be made available at the local library for all older adults in the community and their family.

The strategies to revitalize the aged brain are most effective in patients with NCA. In patients with MCI, these strategies if tailored to the patients' strengths may help improve cognitive function, but in patients with mild to moderate dementia, some of the cognitive interventions (eg, cognitive training, cognitive exercises using computers) may cause considerable stress and thus may do more harm than good.

A personal cognitive fitness program should be adapted to the particular strengths and limitations of each person and also his/her preferences. Consequently, instead of implementing ready-made programs, tailoring programs to the individual and resources available is recommended. Group training programs can also be considered, although mixing patients with NCA and patients with mild dementia may need to be avoided. Strategies mentioned here may not only revitalize the aged brain but also reduce risk of future stroke and may delay onset of dementia in at-risk individuals. Many older adults who engage in optimal behaviors to enrich their brain may nevertheless experience cognitive decline at some later point in their life. Thus, as McFadden and Basting[17] have commented, "this discussion turns eventually toward enduring existential and spiritual questions about life meaning and its roots in individual lives and in community." Cognitive fitness should be part of a holistic approach that also addresses patient's physical, emotional, and spiritual well-being.

FUTURE RESEARCH

One of the promising implications of neural plasticity is that many changes that occur in response to experience and aging may be reversible, including neuronal atrophy and cell loss. Future research needs to clarify to what extent this finding can be exploited in older adults. As the fundamental mechanisms of neural plasticity are discovered and understood, new targets and paradigms for enhancing cognitive function will be revealed and will lead to more effective and faster-acting intervention strategies. Future research needs to clarify to what extent cognition can be promoted by exploiting endogenous permissive neuroplasticity factors, such as neuro-modulators.[37] Future research may identify drugs that selectively target certain receptors (eg, N-methyl-D-aspartate) and thus influence components of synaptic remodeling (eg, second-messenger signaling, neurotransmitter trafficking and function) and thereby enhance cognitive function and prevent cognitive decline.[38] Large, prospective, multicenter, randomized controlled studies regarding strategies to promote cognitive health in older adults have involved aerobic exercise and cognitive training but lacking for other interventions discussed in this article. Prospective studies evaluating interventions for CRFs for the outcomes of cognition and depression have either been negative or inconclusive (except for control of blood pressure).[10] Thus, future research needs to address these gaps in research.

Cerebrovascular disease (caused by atherosclerosis and arteriosclerosis) and neurodegeneration may cause a subtle decline in cognitive function and mood. It seems possible to improve at least some aspects of cognitive and emotional functioning in older adults through various strategies described in this article. However, the effect of these interventions on quality of life and autonomy in everyday activities needs to be studied in more detail. Future research may guide us to optimally use the knowledge of mirror neurons to gain skills by observation and indirect experience. In the future, healthy older adults at high risk for AD and or other neurodegenerative disorders (assessed through calculation of dementia risk scores) may be prescribed neuroprotective agents to prevent cognitive decline.[10,39]

SUMMARY

A high level of cognitive and emotional well-being for most older adults is possible, but to achieve this, older adults need to engage in challenging cognitive, sensory, and motor activities on an intensive basis. The brain has a remarkable capacity to improve its function at all ages. Now we have increasing (although not definitive) evidence that many older adults may be able to preserve their cognitive function into their later years by adding neuroplasticity-based simple and practical cognitive strategies to their daily routine of physical activity, good sleep habits, and healthy nutrition.

REFERENCES

1. Centers for Disease Control and Prevention, Alzheimer's Association. The healthy brain initiative: a national public health road map to maintaining cognitive health. Chicago: Alzheimer's Association; 2007.
2. Desai AK, Grossberg GT, Chibnall JT. Healthy brain aging: a road map. Clin Geriatr Med 2010;26:1–26.
3. Vance DE, Roberson AJ, McGuinness TM, et al. How neuroplasticity and cognitive reserve protect cognitive functioning. J Psychosoc Nurs Ment Health Serv 2010;48(4):23–30.
4. Desai AK, Schwarz L. Subjective cognitive impairment: when to be concerned about 'senior moments'. Current Psychiatry 2010;10(4):31–44.
5. Graham JE, Rockwood K, Beattie BL, et al. Prevalence and severity of cognitive impairment with and without dementia in an elderly population. Lancet 1997;349: 1793–6.

6. Low LF, Brodaty H, Edwards R, et al. The prevalence of "cognitive impairment no dementia" in community-dwelling elderly: a pilot study. Aust N Z J Psychiatry 2004;38:725–31.

7. Hendrie HC, Albert MS, Butters MA, et al. The NIH Cognitive and Emotional Health Project: report of the critical Evaluation Study Committee. Alzheimers Dement 2006;2:12–32.

8. Ottersen OP. How hardwired is the brain? Technological advances provide new insight into brain malleability and neurotransmission. Nutr Rev 2010; 68(Suppl 2):S60–4.

9. Vance DE, Crowe M. A proposed model of neuroplastic and cognitive reserve in older adults. Activities Adaptation Aging 2006;30(3):61–79.

10. Flicker L. Cardiovascular risk factors, cerebrovascular disease burden, and healthy brain aging. Clin Geriatr Med 2010;26:17–28.

11. Kumar V, Kinsella LJ. Healthy brain aging: effect of head injury, alcohol and environmental toxins. Clin Geriatr Med 2010;26:29–44.

12. Malhotra RK, Desai AK. Healthy brain aging: what has sleep got to do with it? Clin Geriatr Med 2010;26:45–56.

13. Bassil N, Morley JE. Endocrine aspects of healthy brain aging. Clin Geriatr Med 2010;26:57–74.

14. Rolland Y, Abellan van Kan G, Vellas B. Healthy brain aging: role of exercise and physical activity. Clin Geriatr Med 2010;26:75–88.

15. Morley J. Nutrition and the brain. Clin Geriatr Med 2010;26:89–98.

16. La Rue A. Healthy brain aging: role of cognitive reserve, cognitive stimulation, and cognitive exercises. Clin Geriatr Med 2010;26:99–112.

17. McFadden SH, Basting AD. Healthy aging persons and their brains: promoting resilience through creative engagement. Clin Geriatr Med 2010;26:149–62.

18. Bierman EJ, Comijs HC, Rijmen F, et al. Anxiety symptoms and cognitive performance in later life: results from the Longitudinal Aging Study Amsterdam. Aging Ment Health 2008;12:517–23.

19. Comijs HC, Jonker C, Beekman AT, et al. The association between depressive symptoms and cognitive decline in community-dwelling elderly persons. Int J Geriatr Psychiatry 2001;16:361–7.

20. Stern Y. Cognitive reserve. Psychologia 2009;47:2015–28.

21. Mahncke HW, Bronstone A, Merzenich MM. Brain plasticity and functional losses in the aged: scientific bases for a novel intervention. Prog Brain Res 2006;157: 81–109.

22. Lyons DM, Buckmaster PS, Lee AG, et al. Stress coping stimulates hippocampal neurogenesis in adult monkeys. Proc Natl Acad Sci U S A 2010;107:14823–7.

23. Diamond DM, Bennett MC, Fleshner M, et al. Inverted-U relationship between the level of peripheral corticosterone and the magnitude of hippocampal primed burst potentiation. Hippocampus 1992;2:421–30.

24. Kamat SM, Kamat AS, Grossberg GT. Dementia risk prediction: are we there yet? Clin Geriatr Med 2010;26:113–24.

25. Issa MM, Fenter TC, Black L, et al. An assessment of the diagnosed prevalence of diseases in men 50 years of age or older. Am J Manag Care 2006;12:S83–9.

26. Ristow M, Zarse K, Oberbach A, et al. Antioxidants prevent health-promoting effects of physical exercise in humans. Proc Natl Acad Sci U S A 2009;106: 8665–70.

27. Tran TT, Srivareerat M, Alkadhi KA. Chronic psychosocial stress triggers cognitive impairment in a novel at-risk model of Alzheimer's disease. Neurobiol Dis 2009; 37(3):756–63.

28. Tang YY, Lu Q, Geng X, et al. Short-term meditation induces white matter changes in the anterior cingulated. Proc Natl Acad Sci U S A 2010;107:15649–52.
29. Luders E, Toga AW, Lepore N, et al. The underlying anatomical correlates of long-term meditation: larger hippocampal and frontal volumes of gray matter. Neuroimage 2009;45:672–8.
30. Hillman CH, Erickson KI, Kramer AF. Be smart, exercise your heart: exercise effects on brain and cognition. Nature 2008;9:58–65.
31. Colcombe SJ, Erickson KI, Scalf PE, et al. Aerobic exercise training increases brain volume in aging humans. J Gerontol A Biol Sci Med Sci 2006;61:1166–70.
32. Fratiglioni L, Paillard-Borg S, Winblad B. An active and socially integrated lifestyle in late life might protect against dementia. Lancet Neurol 2004;3:343–53.
33. Lu L, Bao G, Chen H, et al. Modification of hippocampal neurogenesis and neuro-plasticity by social environments. Exp Neurol 2003;183(2):600–9.
34. Kobayashi S, Ohashi Y, Ando S. Effects of enriched environment with different durations and starting times on learning capacity during aging in rats assessed by a refined procedure of the Hebb-Williams maze task. J Neurosci Res 2002;70: 340–6.
35. Ball K, Berch DB, Helmers KE, et al. Effects of cognitive training interventions with older adults: a randomized controlled trial. JAMA 2002;288:2271–81.
36. Boyke J, Driemeyer J, Gaser C, et al. Training-induced brain structure changes in the elderly. J Neurosci 2008;28:7031–5.
37. Bavelier D, Levi DM, Li RW, et al. Removing brakes on adult brain plasticity: from molecular to behavioral interventions. J Neurosci 2010;30(45):14964–71.
38. Bibb JA, Mayford MR, Tsien JZ, et al. Cognition enhancement strategies. J Neurosci 2010;30(45):14987–92.
39. Tarawneh R, Galvin JE. Potential future neuroprotective therapies for neurode-generative disorders and stroke. Clin Geriatr Med 2010;26:125–48.

Nutritional Strategies for Successful Aging

Jean Woo, MD, FRCP

KEYWORDS

- Nutritional strategies • Aging
- Psychological health • Chronic disease

With increasing life expectancy in many developed and developing countries, maintaining health and function in old age has become an important goal, including avoidance or optimal control of chronic diseases common with aging, maintenance or retarding the decline of physical and cognitive function, and optimizing psychological health. Common diseases include cardiovascular diseases (hypertension, ischemic heart disease, and stroke), diabetes mellitus, osteoporosis, neurodegenerative diseases (dementia and Parkinson disease), and cancer. Maintaining independent functioning in tasks related to self-care and societal interaction and avoidance of cognitive decline are also important. Avoidance of psychological morbidity, such as depression, and poor health-related quality of life, such as the geriatric syndromes of sarcopenia and frailty, are also desirable goals in successful aging. Other components of successful aging include social network and socioeconomic status. This article discusses some nutritional strategies toward reducing the risk of common chronic diseases, retarding the decline of physical and cognitive function, and optimizing psychological health. These strategies include optimizing body weight, dietary intake of some key nutrients, role of functional foods, and dietary intake patterns. The influence of social network and socioeconomic status on these nutritional strategies is also described.

OPTIMAL BODY WEIGHT
Undernutrition

A body mass index (BMI) value of less than 18.5 kg/m^2 is generally used as an indicator for undernutrition. Even in societies where obesity exists, undernutrition has been documented in institutional settings, the prevalence ranging from 15% to 65%.[1] The consequences of undernutrition include increased susceptibility to infection, loss of muscle strength (predisposing to falls), functional decline, increased health care use, and increased mortality.[2]

Department of Medicine & Therapeutics, The Chinese University of Hong Kong, Hong Kong, China

Med Clin N Am 95 (2011) 477–493
doi:10.1016/j.mcna.2011.02.009
0025-7125/11/$ – see front matter © 2011 Elsevier Inc. All rights reserved.

Overnutrition

High BMI has been shown a risk factor for cardiovascular diseases, diabetes, cancer, and dementia.[3] Optimal values for BMI and waist circumference, an indicator of central obesity, have been derived for the general adult population and are widely used in the clinical setting as well as in health promotion (**Table 1**).[4]

There has been an assumption, however, that these values also apply to all the elderly population. In the past decade, there have been reports suggesting that the adoption of these criteria to older age groups (such as those ages 70 years and older) may not be appropriate. The relationship between BMI and mortality has been shown to be U-shaped[5–8] and better health outcomes are observed for those falling into the overweight category using existing definitions. A normal reference range for waist circumference, an indicator of central obesity, is particularly problematic, in view of the age-related neuroendocrine changes with decline in growth hormone, insulinlike growth factor (IGF) 1, and sex steroids that result in inevitable changes to body shape. Body fat increases, lean mass decreases, and waist circumference increases. It has been shown that although a BMI range of 25 to 30 kg/m^2 may correspond to waist circumference ranges of 85 to 98 cm in men and 78 to 88 cm in women, in the general adult population, for people ages 70 years and older, the values of the waist circumference corresponding to the same BMI ranges are considered in the at-risk range—90 to 102 cm for men and 88 to 98 cm for women.[9] The practical implication of this observation is that many people over age 70 are advised to adopt weight control measures. The definition of optimal anthropometric values, however, should be in relation to health outcomes. Current definitions of these values have been guided by large population studies of the general adult population rather than by studies of elderly populations (ages 70 years and above, with mean age 80 years). Even for such studies of the general adult population (ages 30–74), it has been observed that obesity as a risk factor for adverse health outcomes is attenuated by age, such that the relative risk for mortality with increasing BMI among those in the 74 and older age group was not greater than 1, even following a falling trend.[10]

When a population with a mean age of 80 years was followed prospectively to document mortality and development of hypertension and diabetes, mortality was inversely associated with increasing BMI whereas hypertension and diabetes were associated with higher BMI values. The BMI value at the intersection point between the mortality curve and the curves for development of disease falls into the overweight range for women.[9] In another longitudinal study, weight loss of greater than 2 kg over a 24-month period increased the relative risk for mortality nearly 5-fold,

Table 1
Normal anthropometric values

	Normal	At Risk
BMI (kg/m^2)	<25	25–29.9 (overweight); ≥30 (obese)
WC (cm)	—	—
Men	—	>102 cm (40″)
Women	—	>88 cm (35″)
WHR (cm/cm)	—	—
Men	≤0.9	≥1.0
Women	≤0.8	≥1.0

Abbreviations: WC, waist circumference; WHR, waist-to-hip ratio.

whereas weight gain did not confer excess risk, after adjusting for age, reported health status, number of health conditions, place of residence, income, and baseline BMI.[11] A BMI of less than 0 kg/m^2 versus BMI 20 to 24 kg/m^2 increased the risk of mobility decline nearly 2-fold[12] and the risk of falls by 30% after adjusting for age, gender, number of diseases, activities of daily living score, physical activity level, and medication use.[13] Adjusted for age and gender, per-unit increase in BMI had a weak protective effect on 18-month mortality and ischemic heart disease morbidity, although there was an increase risk for rise in systolic blood pressure.[14] A 3-year longitudinal study of 2032 subjects ages 70 years and older showed that in the absence of disease, lower anthropometric values were associated with greater mortality, dependency, and poorer physical performance measures. Waist-to-hip ratio was not associated with any health outcomes. Weight loss, rather than weight gain, seems more important in this population. Therefore, promotion of lifestyle interventions targeted at weight maintenance is an important strategy for successful aging.[15]

These observations were confirmed by a more recent population study of 4000 people in similar age groups, again demonstrating a U-shaped relationship between BMI and mortality. The lowest mortality was observed among those with BMI in the fourth quintile (24–26 kg/m^2), a value considered overweight. Similar observations apply to waist-to-hip ratio and relative truncal fat as measured using dual-energy absorptiometry (DEXA). Furthermore, survival became more favorable with increasing general adiposity, measured by DEXA.[7] With respect to physical functioning, although increasing BMI and fat mass and decreasing appendicular muscle mass were associated with functional impairments, there is a U-shaped relationship between BMI and grip strength and walking speed, after adjusting for age, physical activity, and number of chronic diseases.[16]

The role of cardiorespiratory fitness may partly account for this obesity paradox. In a US population of ages 65 to 88 years, fitness ameliorated the adverse outcomes of obesity, such that health outcomes may have been better among those who were fat but fit compared with those who were not fat and not fit. The lowest mortality occurred in the highly fit but obese group.[17]

With respect to body weight in the very old, the strategy for successful ageing is placing the emphasis on weight maintenance rather than weight reduction and to avoid applying evidence obtained from studies of adult population of all ages to the elderly population to determine desirable anthropometric values. Optimal body weight should also be considered in the context of maintaining cardiorespiratory fitness.

INTAKE OF KEY NUTRIENTS
Macronutrients

Adequate protein intake is needed for the maintenance of muscle and bone mass and is important to counter the development of sarcopenia and osteoporosis, the recommended daily intake being 12% to 14% of calories (or <0.75 g/kg/d) to maintain balance.[18] The recommended daily intake value of 0.8 g/kg may not be adequate for the maintenance of muscle mass for adults ages 55 to 77,[19] and values in excess of 1 g/kg may be needed to retard the loss of muscle mass with aging.[20,21] Preservation of muscle mass may not translate directly into improved muscle function,[21] however, suggesting that adequate protein intake is only a partial strategy for the treatment of sarcopenia. Replacement of saturated fatty acids with polyunsaturated fatty acids rather than monounsaturated fatty acids or carbohydrates has been shown to prevent coronary heart disease over a wide range of intakes.[22] The lower consumption of dietary fat in the Chinese population may be a contributory factor to the lower incidence of coronary heart disease among such populations.[23] Recent studies have suggested a link between consumption of high fat diets and brain aging.[24] High dietary fat has also been suggested as a risk factor for Alzheimer disease.[25]

Micronutrients

Cations: sodium, potassium, calcium, and magnesium

It has been documented that the age-related rise in blood pressure is seldom observed in societies where the sodium intake is less than 100 mmol per day.[26] The prevalence of hypertension is high in societies with a high salt intake,[27] and reducing salt consumption reduces blood pressure.[28] A reduction of 83 mmol of salt per day in older people, ages 6 to 78 years, was associated with a reduction of 7.2 mm Hg in systolic blood pressure and 3.2 mm Hg in diastolic blood pressure in both normotensive and hypertensive subjects.[29] Because hypertension is a major risk factor for stroke, reducing salt intake is an important goal in the prevention of stroke, and resultant physical dependency.[30] The adverse effect of sodium intake on blood pressure may be partly countered by increasing the intake of potassium and magnesium.[31–33] Apart from the adverse effect on blood pressure, a high salt intake may also increase the risk of osteoporosis, through the increased obligatory urinary excretion of calcium.[34] Adequate intake of calcium is important for reducing the risk of osteoporosis; this effect is more marked among populations, such as the Chinese, with low calcium intake as a result of low consumption of dairy products.[35] Calcium intake may need to be increased as a result of high salt intake. The recommended daily intake of calcium in the elderly is at least 800 mg per day, whereas a calcium balance study in Chinese postmenopausal women required a mean intake of 735 mg per day to achieve zero balance, with a higher value of 900 to 1000 mg for reducing the rate of bone loss.[36]

Vitamins

Vitamin C and other antioxidant vitamins have been shown to promote vascular health. A vitamin C intake achieving a blood level of greater than 60 mmol per day has been shown one of four simple health behaviors associated with a 4-fold difference in mortality in European men and women ages 40 to 79 years.[37] In a study of 4000 Chinese men and women ages 65 years and older, a vitamin C intake between 141 and190 mg per day is associated with a reduced risk of atherosclerosis using the ankle-brachial index as an indicator, after adjusting for age, gender, smoking habit, and alcohol intake.[38] Antioxidant vitamins have a possible role in the preservation of cognitive function[39] and the prevention of Alzheimer disease.[25] Vitamins B_6 and B_{12} and folate are needed for the metabolism of homocysteine, because there is an inverse relationship between blood levels of these vitamins and homocysteine. The latter has been shown an independent risk factor for coronary heart disease, stroke, and cognitive impairment, likely mediated by endothelial dysfunction. Chinese vegetarians who have low vitamin B_{12} intake and blood levels have higher serum homocysteine, higher mean carotid intimal thickness, and greater forearm flow-mediated dilatation.[40] Low vitamin B status and high homocysteine levels have been linked to key pathomechanisms of dementia and also observed in patients with Parkinson disease, especially those receiving levodopa, and depression, suggesting a possible role for supplementation in these neurodegenerative diseases.[41] There may be a role for folate supplementation in depression and dementia,[42] although evidence from randomized controlled trials is lacking.[43,44] A recent 3-year randomized controlled trial of folate treatment among healthy subjects age 60 years, however, showed improved memory, better information, and sensorimotor processing speed compared with controls.[45]

Vitamin D is involved in many physiologic processes, such as muscle function, cardiovascular and bone health, immunity, cancer prevention, and metabolic signaling. It is increasingly implicated in mental health and cognition of older adults.[46,47] Vitamin deficiency or insufficiency has an adverse impact on these processes. Vitamin D deficiency is not uncommon worldwide[48,49] and is particularly common among older people. This is a result of age-related changes giving rise to reduced dietary intake, reduced sunlight exposure accompanying reduced outdoor physical activity, less efficient cholecalciferol synthesis in the skin after sun exposure, and increase in fat mass resulting in a larger distribution volume for the fat-soluble 25-hydroxyvitamin D (25OHD), which in turn decreases the bioavailability of 25OHD. Available findings suggest that serum 25OHD levels between 70 and 80 nmol/L are regarded as sufficient for multiple health outcomes. There is consensus that serum 25OHD levels of less than 25 nmol/L are considered deficient whereas those of less than 50 nmol/L are considered insufficient based on the effects of parathyroid hormone levels and bone turnover.[50–52] When other health benefits of vitamin D are taken into account, such as lower extremity function, dental health, and risk of falls, fractures, and colorectal cancer, concentrations of serum 25OHD between 70 and 80 nmol/L are regarded as sufficient and between 90 and 150 nmol/L are considered best.[53–55] In elderly populations where vitamin D status is replete, there is little association between vitamin D levels and fracture risk, physical performance measures, or psychological health.[56,57] In view of the high prevalence of vitamin D insufficiency among community-living older people,[58,59] and even higher prevalence among those living in institutions, vitamin D supplementation seems to be the only effective strategy to achieve adequate blood levels because the concentration of vitamin D in foods is low. Oral vitamin D supplementation has been shown to reduce the risk of fractures and[60] falls, improve physical performance,[61,62] and reduce colorectal cancer risk.[63] No effect on supplementation on blood pressure, however, has been demonstrated to date.[64] Low vitamin D levels have been associated with depression and poor cognitive function.[46] Results of supplementation trials, however, have been conflicting. The dose of vitamin D used generally ranges from 800 to 1000 IU per day. In general, mobile, white, community-dwelling elderly who have a varied diet need daily vitamin D supplementation of 800 to 1000 IU reach serum vitamin D levels between 70 and 80 nmol/L, whereas frail or institutionalized elderly are suggested as needing up to 2200 IU a day.[54,65]

Long-chain ω-3 fatty acids

ω-3 Fatty acids, the common dietary source of which is oily fish, have been shown to be beneficial for cardiovascular health and reducing the risk of sudden cardiac deaths.[66] A recent study of supplementation with eicosapentaenoic acid and docosahexaenoic acid (in margarine) in patients who have had myocardial infarction, however, did not reduce the risk of major cardiovascular events.[67] ω-3 Fatty acids are also postulated as affecting brain function and hence cognition and mental health, via neurotrophic and neuroendocrine factors (brain-derived neurotrophic factor and IGF-1), which act on cell signaling and neural pathways, which in turn affect neuronal function, synaptic plasticity, and adult neurogenesis.[68] A recent review of the possible neuroprotective properties against dementia shows that although ω-3 fatty acids may have an effect in slowing cognitive decline in elderly people without dementia, there is no evidence that they have a role in the prevention or treatment of dementia. Data were only available, however, from only four small clinical trials.[69]

FOOD CATEGORIES
Low–Glycemic Index Foods

Consumption of low–glycemic index (GI) foods results in a less rapid rise in blood glucose than consumption of high-GI foods, the GI of foods being calculated by the incremental area under the blood glucose response curve after a standard amount of a control food (either white bread or glucose) is consumed.[70] High-GI diets predispose to obesity, the metabolic syndrome, diabetes, and cardiovascular diseases.[4,71–73] Replacement of saturated fat with high–GI value carbohydrates significantly increases the risk of myocardial infarction.[74]

Fruits and Vegetables

An increase in intake of 50 g per day is associated with a 20% mortality from any cause, cancer, and cardiovascular diseases,[75] whereas four simple health behaviors (one of which includes 5 servings of fruits and vegetables a day to attain a blood vitamin C level of >60 mmol/L) has been shown associated with a 4-fold difference in mortality in men and women ages 40 to 79 years.[37] Recently, there has been intense interest in the potential of phytochemical-rich foods in the prevention of age-related neurodegeneration and cognitive decline. Three specific subgroups have been shown to have the greatest potential: the flavanols, anthocyanins, and flavanones, commonly found in citrus fruits, apples, and berries.[76] The beneficial effect of these compounds on neurodegeneration seem not to be mediated via the antioxidant action but by the ability to protect vulnerable neurons, enhance neuronal function, stimulate brain blood flow, and induce neurogenesis.[77] The underlying mechanism is possibly mediated through the induction of neuronal and glial signaling pathways involved in synaptic plasticity.[78–80]

FUNCTIONAL FOODS

The term, *functional foods*, refers to foods that function as modifiers of chronic disease risk factors or as compounds that augment naturally occurring physiologic processes, with overall beneficial effects on health. Many have cultural-specific origins, and some examples of such foods traditionally consumed by Chinese communities are soy, mushrooms, green tea, and black rice.

Soy

Soy is composed of 30% to 40% protein, essential amino acids, and phytoestrogens (genistin, daidzin, and glycitein). It is low in saturated fats and contains no cholesterol. Beneficial effects have been documented in blood lipid profile, bone density, glycemic control, and reduced breast cancer risk. A meta-analysis of 23 randomized controlled trials showed that soy protein was associated with modest but significant decreases in serum total cholesterol and low-density lipoprotein (LDL) cholesterol and increases in high-density lipoprotein (HDL) cholesterol, particularly with intake of isoflavones greater than 80 mg per day.[81] Possible mechanisms of action include the action of soy isoflavones as estrogen receptor modulators, their effect on hepatic lipase activity, upregulation of LDL receptors, and induced gene expression of enzymes and proteins important in lipid metabolism. Soy isoflavones have also been shown to decrease bone turnover and reduce bone loss, when intake of isoflavones exceeds 90 mg per day.[82,83] A dose-response relationship with bone mineral density in postmenopausal women has also been shown; possible underlying mechanisms are their effect on estrogen receptors in bone, enhancement of IGF-1 synthesis, enhancement of calcium absorption, and reduction of urinary calcium excretion.[84,85]

Soy intake has been shown to increase insulin sensitivity by increasing glucose uptake preferentially in skeletal muscles.[86] An intake of soy isoflavones of 40 mg per day resulted in a significant reduction in fasting glucose concentration.[87] A meta-analysis of 18 epidemiologic studies examining soy consumption and breast cancer risk showed a small reduction in breast cancer risk in the high compared with the low soy intake group, but the association was not significant among women in Asian countries.[88] Examples of foods containing approximately 40 mg of isoflavones include 456 g of soymilk (2 cups), 120 g of uncooked tofu, 73 g of uncooked green soybeans, 20 g of soy flour (one-quarter cup), and 20 g of roasted soybeans.[81]

Mushrooms

Mushrooms are high in protein and fiber and low in fat. They also contain vitamins B_1, B_2, B_{12}, C, and D, and several minerals (calcium, potassium, magnesium, sodium, phosphorus, copper, iron, manganese, and selenium). Several common mushrooms have functional properties in modulating the immune system and blood lipid profile and in inhibition of tumor formation and inflammatory processes.[89] The active ingredients are mushroom polysaccharides, β-glucans, eritadenine and phenolic compounds.[90] Proposed mechanisms by which mushrooms exert antitumor activity include prevention of oncogenesis, enhancement of immunity against tumor cells, and direct antitumor activity by inducing apoptosis of tumout cells.[91] The phenolic compounds in mushrooms are a good source of antioxidants,[92] whereas the β-glucans also have LDL cholesterol-lowering effects, possibly mediated through the leptin pathway.[93]

Green Tea

Green tea constitutes approximately 20% of tea production and is principally consumed in China, Japan, Korea, and Morocco. The main difference in the composition between green and black tea lies in the 6-fold higher concentration in green tea of phenolic compounds.[94] Potential mechanisms for beneficial effects on cardiovascular risk factors, cancer, diabetes and glucose control, weight control, bone health, and neurodegenerative diseases are suggested from in vitro and animal studies. With respect to cardiovascular risk factors, green tea polyphenols reduce LDL oxidation[95]; catechins lower cholesterol by upregulating the LDL receptor and increasing fecal bile acid and cholesterol excretion,[96] and they also have antihypertensive properties by acting as angiotensin-converting enzyme inhibitors, increasing endothelial nitric oxide production, and inducing endothelium-dependent relaxation.[97] Reduction in cancer risk is also thought to be due to catechins acting as antioxidants, antiangiogenic agents, and stimulators stimulators of tumor cell apoptosis and to their antibacterial action—relevant for *Helicobacter pylori*–associated gastric cancer.[98] Green tea catechins decrease carbohydrate absorption and hepatic glucose production and increase insulin sensitivity.[99,100] The antiobesity effect may be mediated through several mechanisms of action of catechins: inhibition of adipocyte differentiation and proliferation, reduction of fat absorption, and inhibition of catechol *O*-methyltransferase in brown adipose tissue resulting in reduction of fat mass, triacylglycerides, free fatty acids, and total cholesterol.[99] Green tea is postulated to decrease the risk of fractures by improving bone mineral density through stimulating osteoblasts and inhibiting osteoclasts. Possible underlying mechanisms include antioxidative and anti-inflammatory properties.[101] Green tea polyphenols show neuroprotective activity in cell cultures and animal models of neurotoxin-induced cell injury.

Studies in humans show that green tea consumption may be associated with reduced cardiovascular risks,[99] atherosclerosis,[102] and stroke[103] and possibly reduced cancer risk.[98,103] There have been limited and inconclusive studies in humans with respect to glucose and weight control and bone health. Tea drinking may be protective for Parkinson disease.[94]

All Tea

There are several studies in humans where no distinctions have been made between green tea or black tea. A meta-analysis of tea consumption and stroke showed that individuals consuming greater than or equal to 3 cups per day had a 21% lower risk of stroke, stroke volume, and mortality compared with those consuming less than 1 cup per day.[104] Those who consume more than 3 cups per day also had a 20% lower risk of developing diabetes.[105] Studies of cancer and vascular function have conflicting results.[106,107] A study of 2006 Chinese men and women, ages 65 years and older, showed that in men, Chinese tea consumption was positively associated with telomere length after adjustment for multiple confounding factors. The mean difference in telomere length in those consuming more than 3 cups or 750 mL per day compared with those consuming less than or equal to 0.28 cups per day, or less than or equal to 70 mL, was 0.46 kilobases, corresponding to approximately 5 years of life.[56]

Black Rice

Black rice is rich in anthocyanins and has been regarded as a health-promoting food and widely consumed since ancient times in China and other Eastern Asian countries. It is also rich in phenolic compounds and minerals. In vitro and animal studies suggest that the health beneficial effects may be mediated through its antioxidant, anti-inflammatory, antiatherogenic and insulin-enhancing properties.[108–110] There are few studies in humans. A study comparing black rice with white rice for 6 weeks in overweight premenopausal Korean women showed reduction in weight, BMI, and body fat and increase in HDL cholesterol and glutathione peroxidase activity in the black rice group.[111] In a trial of black versus white rice in 60 patients with coronary heart disease, ages 45 to 75 years, over 6 months, a more favorable cardiovascular risk profile was observed, in that plasma levels of soluble vascular adhesion molecule-1, soluble CD40 ligand, and sensitive C-reactive protein were reduced, whereas plasma total antioxidant capacity was increased.[112] In view of the possible action of anthocyanins on memory and cognition,[76] it would be interesting to repeat these studies using memory and other psychological tests as outcome measures.

DIETARY PATTERNS

Recent studies examining the relationship between nutrition and health outcomes have used dietary patterns rather than focusing on the consumption of individual nutrients or single foods. For example, studies have examined dietary variety; dietary patterns from different regions, such as the Mediterranean diet or the Chinese diet; the vegetarian diet; and a composite measure of the health-related characteristics of diets, such as the dietary quality index (DQI). Dietary variety has been shown to be associated with obesity. This measure is derived from the percentage of different food types consumed within each food group, regardless of the frequency with which they are consumed. In a US study, controlling for age and gender, variety from sweets, snacks, and carbohydrates was positively associated with body fat percentage whereas variety from vegetables was negatively associated.[113] Such an association between dietary variety and body fat was also demonstrated in populations taking a Chinese diet. There were some differences in dietary components, however. Obesity indices were positively correlated with snack variety, as in US populations, but negatively correlated with grains and meat variety. Food variety was a stronger predictor of body fat than dietary fat.[114]

Another pattern is the Mediterranean diet, which is characterized by high intake of fruits and nuts, vegetable, legumes, cereals, fish, monounsaturated lipid to saturated lipid ratio, and low intake of meat and dairy products. Populations consuming the traditional Mediterranean diets have better survival,[115] whereas those adopting such a diet post–myocardial infarction have better outcomes.[116] The Mediterranean diet has been shown to reduce the risk of Alzheimer disease and Parkinson disease (by 13%)[117] and of conversion of mild cognitive impairment to Alzheimer disease.[118] Physical activity, however, may be a confounding factor.

The Chinese diet has many similarities to the Mediterranean diet, using the Mediterranean diet score to compare characteristics. In view of the fact that coronary heart disease mortality in Hong Kong Chinese is approximately one quarter that in the United States, the traditional Chinese diet may have similar benefits.[119] Other than the relationship between snack variety and the development of overweight in a prospective study, however, no significant association was observed with other measures of dietary pattern, after adjusting for age, gender, education, and physical activity.[120]

Surveys among vegetarians in white populations show lower mortality than omnivores from ischemic heart disease.[121] There are cultural differences in types of vegetarian diet, however. For example, the Chinese vegetarian diet is predominantly based on soy products, with low consumption of dairy products. Dietary intake among Chinese vegetarians shows that they have lower intakes of total energy, fat and protein calories, and many B vitamins, but the intake of carbohydrates, vitamin C, and calcium are higher, and they have better lipid profiles. Approximately 30% have nutritional anemias due to vitamin B_{12} deficiency.[122] Although older Chinese women on a vegetarian diet have lower serum cholesterol concentration and a lower prevalence of ischemic heart disease,[123] Chinese vegetarians have higher mean carotid intimal thickness and greater endothelial dysfunction as measured by forearm flow-mediated dilatation. They also have higher blood pressure, serum triglycerides, homocysteine, and lower vitamin B_{12}.[40]

The health properties of any diet may also be measured using the DQI. This is a composite measure developed in the United States for global monitoring and exploration of dietary quality across countries.[124,125] The major categories cover variety, adequacy, moderation, and overall balance. A recent prospective study of 4000 Chinese men and women ages 65 years and older examined the relationship between DQI and some health outcomes relevant to the older population in addition to mortality, such as health-related quality of life and frailty. Frailty was measured using an index derived from the summation of multiple deficits. Adjustment for age, gender, and socioeconomic and other lifestyle factors (smoking, alcohol intake, and physical activity) as well as geographic factors was performed. DQI was positively associated with both the physical and mental components of health-related quality-of-life measures and negatively associated with frailty and mortality.[126]

INFLUENCE OF SOCIAL FACTORS ON NUTRITIONAL STRATEGIES

Nutritional strategies are affected by socioeconomic status and social networks. Adoption of a healthy eating pattern may depend on adequate income, because in some countries, such a pattern, consisting of fish, fruits, and vegetables, may not be affordable because fruits and vegetables cost more than foods high in saturated fats, sugar, and salt.[127–136] People with lower incomes tend to adopt a diet higher in fat and lower in fruit and vegetable consumption.[137,138] Older people tend to have lower incomes and, therefore, may not be able to afford healthy foods. In other countries where such foods are plentiful and cheap, it may be easier to adopt a healthy eating pattern. Education level is also important for understanding of health promotion messages. The method of promotion should be adapted to groups with different levels of health literacy to be widely disseminated effectively. Interactive methods, such as supermarket tours, healthy eating sessions at restaurants, and cooking classes, are likely to be more effective than passive methods, such as distribution of pamphlets or talks.

Because eating is to an extent a social activity, food intake may be better in a group setting rather than when eating alone. In both nursing home and acute hospital settings, food intake is improved in a dining room setting with other people.[139] In this context, having a large social network where eating together is one of the social activities may facilitate the adoption of nutritional strategies for successful aging. The living environment may also affect the adoption of a healthy diet, through neighborhood factors, such as proximity to markets, availability of transport, and safety issues. A study has shown that DQI is positively associated with higher socioeconomic status but also independently affected by the district of residence.[126]

Nutritional strategies are an important part of a healthy lifestyle to promote successful aging. Other than diet, avoidance of smoking, alcohol consumption in moderation, and physical activity are important components and should complement nutritional strategies. For example, there are additive effects of diet and exercise on synaptic plasticity and cognition, mediated through brain-derived neurotrophic factors.[140,141] Adoption of a healthy lifestyle pattern essentially involves behavior change, and promotion should adopt techniques that are effective.[142,143] Because change in behavior may be more difficult in older people, the adoption of a healthy lifestyle is all the more important in middle age. The current recommendations promoted by the food pyramid are simple to understand; they are effective in the prevention of many chronic diseases common with aging and in weight maintenance as well as functional and cognitive decline.

REFERENCES

1. Arvantakis M, Beck A, Coppens P, et al. Nutrition in care homes and home care: how to implement adequate strategies. In (report of the Brussels Forum) 2007.
2. Elia M. The economics of malnutrition. Nestle Nutr Workshop Ser Clin Perform Programme 2009;12:29–40.
3. Brown WV, Fujioka K, Wilson PW, et al. Obesity: why be concerned? Am J Med 2009;122:S4–11.
4. Obesity: preventing and managing the global epidemic. WHO Technical report series 894. Geneva (Switzerland): World Health Organization; 2000.
5. Corrada MM, Kawas CH, Mozaffar F, et al. Association of body mass index and weight change with all-cause mortality in the elderly. Am J Epidemiol 2006;163: 938–49.
6. Kulminski AM, Arbeev KG, Kulminskaya IV, et al. Body mass index and nine-year mortality in disabled and nondisabled older U.S. individuals. J Am Geriatr Soc 2008;56:105–10.
7. Auyeung TW, Lee JS, Leung J, et al. Survival in older men may benefit from being slightly overweight and centrally obese—a 5-year follow-up study in 4,000 older adults using DXA. J Gerontol A Biol Sci Med Sci 2010;65:99–104.

8. Flicker L, McCaul KA, Hankey GJ, et al. Body mass index and survival in men and women aged 70 to 75. J Am Geriatr Soc 2010;58:234–41.
9. Woo J, Ho SC, Yu AL, et al. Is waist circumference a useful measure in predicting health outcomes in the elderly? Int J Obes Relat Metab Disord 2002;26: 1349–55.
10. Stevens J, Cai J, Pamuk ER, et al. The effect of age on the association between body-mass index and mortality. N Engl J Med 1998;338:1–7.
11. Ho SC, Woo J, Sham A. Risk factor change in older persons, a perspective from Hong Kong: weight change and mortality. J Gerontol 1994;49:M269–72.
12. Ho SC, Woo J, Yuen YK, et al. Predictors of mobility decline: the Hong Kong old-old study. J Gerontol A Biol Sci Med Sci 1997;52:M356–62.
13. Ho SC, Woo J, Chan SS, et al. Risk factors for falls in the Chinese elderly population. J Gerontol A Biol Sci Med Sci 1996;51:M195–8.
14. Woo J, Ho SC, Yuen YK, et al. Cardiovascular risk factor and 18-month mortality in an elderly Chinese population aged 70 years and over. Gerontology 1997;44:51–5.
15. Woo J, Ho SC, Sham A. Longitudinal changes in body mass index and body composition over 3 years and relationship to health outcomes in Hong Kong Chinese age 70 and older. J Am Geriatr Soc 2001;49:737–46.
16. Woo J, Leung J, Kwok T. BMI, body composition, and physical functioning in older adults. Obesity (Silver Spring) 2007;15:1886–94.
17. McAuley P, Pittsley J, Myers J, et al. Fitness and fatness as mortality predictors in healthy older men: the veterans exercise testing study. J Gerontol A Biol Sci Med Sci 2009;64:695–9.
18. Munro HN, Young VR. Protein metabolism and requirements. In: Exton-Smith AN, Caird, FI, editors. Metabolic and nutritional disorders in the elderly. Bristol (UK): John Wright & Sons Ltd; 1980. p. 13–25.
19. Campbell WW, Trappe TA, Wolfe RR, et al. The recommended dietary allowance for protein may not be adequate for older people to maintain skeletal muscle. J Gerontol A Biol Sci Med Sci 2001;56:M373–80.
20. Houston DK, Nicklas BJ, Ding J, et al. Dietary protein intake is associated with lean mass change in older, community-dwelling adults: the Health, Aging, and Body Composition (Health ABC) Study. Am J Clin Nutr 2008;87:150–5.
21. Scott D, Blizzard L, Fell J, et al. Associations between dietary nutrient intake and muscle mass and strength in community-dwelling older adults: the Tasmanian Older Adult Cohort Study. J Am Geriatr Soc 2010;58:2129–34.
22. Jakobsen MU, O'Reilly EJ, Heitmann BL, et al. Major types of dietary fat and risk of coronary heart disease: a pooled analysis of 11 cohort studies. Am J Clin Nutr 2009;89:1425–32.
23. Woo J, Leung SS, Ho SC, et al. Is there a typical Chinese diet and what are the health implications? Ecol Food Nutr 1999;38:491–503.
24. Uranga RM, Bruce-Keller AJ, Morrison CD, et al. Intersection between metabolic dysfunction, high fat diet consumption, and brain aging. J Neurochem 2010; 114:344–61.
25. Morris MC. The role of nutrition in Alzheimer's disease: epidemiological evidence. Eur J Neurol 2009;16(Suppl 1):1–7.
26. Stamler J. Dietary salt and blood pressure. Ann N Y Acad Sci 1993;676:122–56.
27. MacGregor GA, de Wardener HE. Populations, slat and blood pressure. Salt, diet, and health. Cambridge (UK): Cambridge University Press; 1998. p. 100–26.
28. Law MR, Frost CD, Wald NJ. By how much does dietary salt reduction lower blood pressure? III–Analysis of data from trials of salt reduction. BMJ 1991; 302:819–24.

29. Cappuccio FP, Markandu ND, Carney C, et al. Double-blind randomised trial of modest salt restriction in older people. Lancet 1997;350:850–4.
30. Bibbins-Domingo K, Chertow GM, Coxson PG, et al. Projected effect of dietary salt reductions on future cardiovascular disease. N Engl J Med 2010;362:590–9.
31. Appel LJ, Moore TJ, Obarzanek E, et al. A clinical trial of the effects of dietary patterns on blood pressure. DASH Collaborative Research Group. N Engl J Med 1997;336:1117–24.
32. Whelton PK, He J, Cutler JA, et al. Effects of oral potassium on blood pressure. Meta-analysis of randomized controlled clinical trials. JAMA 1997;277: 1624–32.
33. Khaw KT, Barrett-Connor E. Dietary potassium and stroke-associated mortality. A 12-year prospective population study. N Engl J Med 1987;316:235–40.
34. Woo J, Kwok T, Leung J, et al. Dietary intake, blood pressure and osteoporosis. J Hum Hypertens 2009;23:451–5.
35. Lau EM, Woo J, Lam V, et al. Milk supplementation of the diet of postmenopausal Chinese women on a low calcium intake retards bone loss. J Bone Miner Res 2001;16:1704–9.
36. Chen YM. Calcium requirement study in Chinese postmenopausal women. [PhD thesis]. Hong Kong: The Chinese University of Hong Kong; 2003.
37. Khaw KT, Wareham N, Bingham S, et al. Combined impact of health behaviours and mortality in men and women: the EPIC-Norfolk prospective population study. PLoS Med 2008;5:e12.
38. Woo J, Lynn H, Wong SY, et al. Correlates for a low ankle-brachial index in elderly Chinese. Atherosclerosis 2006;186:360–6.
39. Gomez-Pinilla F. Brain foods: the effects of nutrients on brain function. Nat Rev Neurosci 2008;9:568–78.
40. Kwok T, Chook P, Tam L, et al. Vascular dysfunction in Chinese vegetarians: an apparent paradox? J Am Coll Cardiol 2005;46:1957–8.
41. Obeid R, McCaddon A, Herrmann W. The role of hyperhomocysteinemia and B-vitamin deficiency in neurological and psychiatric diseases. Clin Chem Lab Med 2007;45:1590–606.
42. D'Anci KE, Rosenberg IH. Folate and brain function in the elderly. Curr Opin Clin Nutr Metab Care 2004;7:659–64.
43. Balk EM, Raman G, Tatsioni A, et al. Vitamin B6, B12, and folic acid supplementation and cognitive function: a systematic review of randomized trials. Arch Intern Med 2007;167:21–30.
44. Jia X, McNeill G, Avenell A. Does taking vitamin, mineral and fatty acid supplements prevent cognitive decline? a systematic review of randomized controlled trials. J Hum Nutr Diet 2008;21:317–36.
45. Durga J, van Boxtel MP, Schouten EG, et al. Effect of 3-year folic acid supplementation on cognitive function in older adults in the FACIT trial: a randomised, double blind, controlled trial. Lancet 2007;369:208–16.
46. Cherniack EP, Troen BR, Florez HJ, et al. Some new food for thought: the role of vitamin D in the mental health of older adults. Curr Psychiatry Rep 2009;11:12–9.
47. Cherniack EP, Florez H, Roos BA, et al. Hypovitaminosis D in the elderly: from bone to brain. J Nutr Health Aging 2008;12:366–73.
48. Mithal A, Wahl DA, Bonjour JP, et al, Group ObotICoSACNW. Global vitamin D status and determinants of hypovitaminosis D. Osteoporos Int 2009;20: 1807–20.
49. Harris S. Emerging roles of vitamin D: more reasons to address widespread vitamin D insufficiency. Mol Aspects Med 2008;29:359–60.

50. McKenna MJ, Freaney R. Secondary hyperparathyroidism in the elderly: means to defining hypovitaminosis D. Osteoporos Int 1998;8(Suppl 2):S3–6.

51. Holick MF. Vitamin D deficiency. N Engl J Med 2007;357:266–81.

52. Bordelon P, Ghetu MV, Langan RC. Recognition and management of vitamin D deficiency. Am Fam Physician 2009;80:841–6.

53. Dawson-Hughes B, Heaney RP, Holick MF, et al. Estimates of optimal vitamin D status. Osteoporosis Int 2005;16:713–6.

54. Bischoff-Ferrari HA, Giovannucci E, Willett WC, et al. Estimation of optimal serum concentrations of 25-hydroxyvitamin D for multiple health outcomes. Am J Clin Nutr 2006;84:18–28.

55. Garland CF, Gorham ED, Mohr SB, et al. Vitamin D for cancer prevention: global perspective. Ann Epidemiol 2009;19:468–83.

56. Chan R, Chan D, Woo J, et al. Association between serum 25-hydroxyvitamin D and psychological health in older Chinese men in a cohort study. J Affect Disord 2010. [Epub ahead of print]. DOI:10.1016/j.jad.2010.10.029.

57. Chan R, Chan D, Woo J, et al. Serum 25-hydroxyvitamin D and parathyroid hormone levels in relation to blood pressure in a cross-sectional study in older Chinese men. J Hum Hypertens 2011. [Epub ahead of print]. DOI:10.1038/jhh.2010.126.

58. Ovesen L, Andersen R, Jakobsen J. Geographical differences in vitamin D status, with particular reference to European countries. Proc Nutr Soc 2003;62:813–21.

59. Hirani V, Tull K, Ali A, et al. Urgent action needed to improve vitamin D status among older people in England! Age Ageing 2010;39:62–8.

60. Bischoff-Ferrari HA, Willett WC, Wong JB, et al. Prevention of nonvertebral fractures with oral vitamin D and dose dependency: a meta-analysis of randomized controlled trials. Arch Intern Med 2009;169:551–61.

61. Pfeifer M, Begerow B, Minne HW, et al. Effects of a long-term vitamin D and calcium supplementation on falls and parameters of muscle function in community-dwelling older individuals. Osteoporos Int 2009;20:315–22.

62. Kalyani RR, Stein B, Valiyil R, et al. Vitamin D treatment for the prevention of falls in older adults: systematic review and meta-analysis. J Am Geriatr Soc 2010;58:1299–310.

63. Zhou G, Stoitzfus J, Swan BA. Optimizing vitamin D status to reduce colorectal cancer risk: an evidentiary review. Clin J Oncol Nurs 2009;13:E3–17.

64. Margolis KL, Ray RM, Van Horn L, et al. Effect of calcium and vitamin D supplementation on blood pressure: the Women's Health Initiative Randomized Trial. Hypertension 2008;52:847–55.

65. Heaney RP. The Vitamin D requirement in health and disease. J Steroid Biochem Mol Biol 2005;97:13–9.

66. Streppel MT, Ocke MC, Boshuizen HC, et al. Long-term fish consumption and n-3 fatty acid intake in relation to (sudden) coronary heart disease death: the Zutphen study. Eur Heart J 2008;29:2024–30.

67. Kromhout D, Giltay EJ, Geleijnse JM. n-3 fatty acids and cardiovascular events after myocardial infarction. N Engl J Med 2010;363:2015–26.

68. Dauncey MJ. New insights into nutrition and cognitive neuroscience. Proc Nutr Soc 2009;68:408–15.

69. Fotuhi M, Mohassel P, Yaffe K. Fish consumption, long-chain omega-3 fatty acids and risk of cognitive decline or Alzheimer disease: a complex association. Nat Clin Pract Neurol 2009;5:140–52.

70. Jenkins DJ, Wolever TM, Taylor RH, et al. Glycemic index of foods: a physiological basis for carbohydrate exchange. Am J Clin Nutr 1981;34:362–6.

71. Krishnan S, Rosenberg L, Singer M, et al. Glycemic index, glycemic load, and cereal fiber intake and risk of type 2 diabetes in US black women. Arch Intern Med 2007;167:2304–9.
72. Villegas R, Liu S, Gao YT, et al. Prospective study of dietary carbohydrates, glycemic index, glycemic load, and incidence of type 2 diabetes mellitus in middle-aged Chinese women. Arch Intern Med 2007;167:2310–6.
73. Kong AP, Chan RS, Nelson EA, et al. Role of low-glycemic index diet in management of childhood obesity. Obes Rev 2010. [Epub ahead of print]. DOI: 10.1111/j.1467-1789X.2010.00768.x.
74. Hu FB. Are refined carbohydrates worse than saturated fat? Am J Clin Nutr 2010;91:1541–2.
75. Khaw KT, Bingham S, Welch A, et al. Relation between plasma ascorbic acid and mortality in men and women in EPIC-Norfolk prospective study: a prospective population study. European Prospective Investigation into Cancer and Nutrition. Lancet 2001;357:657–63.
76. Spencer JP. The impact of fruit flavonoids on memory and cognition. Br J Nutr 2010;104(Suppl 3):S40–7.
77. Spencer JP. Food for thought: the role of dietary flavonoids in enhancing human memory, learning and neuro-cognitive performance. Proc Nutr Soc 2008;67:238–52.
78. Williams RJ, Spencer JP, Rice-Evans C. Flavonoids: antioxidants or signalling molecules? Free Radic Biol Med 2004;36:838–49.
79. Spencer JP. The impact of flavonoids on memory: physiological and molecular considerations. Chem Soc Rev 2009;38:1152–61.
80. Vauzour D, Vafeiadou K, Rodriguez-Mateos A, et al. The neuroprotective potential of flavonoids: a multiplicity of effects. Genes Nutr 2008;3:115–26.
81. Zhan S, Ho SC. Meta-analysis of the effects of soy protein containing isoflavones on the lipid profile. Am J Clin Nutr 2005;81:397–408.
82. Ma DF, Qin LQ, Wang PY, et al. Soy isoflavone intake inhibits bone resorption and stimulates bone formation in menopausal women: meta-analysis of randomized controlled trials. Eur J Clin Nutr 2008;62:155–61.
83. Ma DF, Qin LQ, Wang PY, et al. Soy isoflavone intake increases bone mineral density in the spine of menopausal women: meta-analysis of randomized controlled trials. Clin Nutr 2008;27:57–64.
84. Ho SC, Woo J, Lam S, et al. Soy protein consumption and bone mass in early postmenopausal Chinese women. Osteoporos Int 2003;14:835–42.
85. Ho SC, Chan SG, Yip YB, et al. Change in bone mineral density and its determinants in pre- and perimenopausal Chinese women: the Hong Kong Perimenopausal Women Osteoporosis Study. Osteoporos Int 2008;19:1785–96.
86. Cederroth CR, Nef S. Soy, phytoestrogens and metabolism: a review. Mol Cell Endocrinol 2009;304:30–42.
87. Ho SC, Chen YM, Ho SS, et al. Soy isoflavone supplementation and fasting serum glucose and lipid profile among postmenopausal Chinese women: a double-blind, randomized, placebo-controlled trial. Menopause 2007;14:905–12.
88. Trock BJ, Hilakivi-Clarke L, Clarke R. Meta-analysis of soy intake and breast cancer risk. J Natl Cancer Inst 2006;98:459–71.
89. Chang R. Functional properties of edible mushrooms. Nutr Rev 1996;54:S91–3.
90. Wasser SP. Medicinal mushrooms as a source of antitumor and immunomodulating polysaccharides. Appl Microbiol Biotechnol 2002;60:258–74.

91. Zhang M, Cui SW, Cheung PC, et al. Antitumor polysaccharides from mushrooms: a reivew on isolation process, structural characteristics and antitumor activity. Trends Food Sci Tech 2007;18:4–19.

92. Cheung LM, Cheung CK, Ooi EC. Antioxidant activity and total phenolics of edible mushroom extracts. Food Chem 2003;81:249–55.

93. Rop O, Mlcek J, Jurikova T. Beta-glucans in higher fungi and their health effects. Nutr Rev 2009;67:624–31.

94. Cabrera C, Artacho R, Gimenez R. Beneficial effects of green tea—a review. J Am Coll Nutr 2006;25:79–99.

95. Basu A, Lucas EA. Mechanisms and effects of green tea on cardiovascular health. Nutr Rev 2007;65:361–75.

96. Chen ZY, Jiao R, Ma KY. Cholesterol-lowering nutraceuticals and functional foods. J Agric Food Chem 2008;56:8761–73.

97. Chen ZY, Peng C, Jiao R, et al. Anti-hypertensive nutraceuticals and functional foods. J Agric Food Chem 2009;57:4485–99.

98. Carlson JR, Bauer BA, Vincent A, et al. Reading the tea leaves: anticarcinogenic properties of (-)-epigallocatechin-3-gallate. Mayo Clin Proc 2007;82:725–32.

99. Thielecke F, Boschmann M. The potential role of green tea catechins in the prevention of the metabolic syndrome - a review. Phytochemistry 2009;70:11–24.

100. Cheng TO. All teas are not created equal: the Chinese green tea and cardiovascular health. Int J Cardiol 2006;108:301–8.

101. Shen CL, Yeh JK, Cao JJ, et al. Green tea and bone metabolism. Nutr Res 2009; 29:437–56.

102. Yung LM, Leung FP, Wong WT, et al. Tea polyphenols benefit vascular function. Inflammopharmacology 2008;16:230–4.

103. Schneider C, Segre T. Green tea: potential health benefits. Am Fam Physician 2009;79:591–4.

104. Arab L, Liu W, Elashoff D. Green and black tea consumption and risk of stroke: a meta-analysis. Stroke 2009;40:1786–92.

105. Huxley R, Lee CM, Barzi F, et al. Coffee, decaffeinated coffee, and tea consumption in relation to incident type 2 diabetes mellitus: a systematic review with meta-analysis. Arch Intern Med 2009;169:2053–63.

106. Sharma V, Rao LJ. A thought on the biological activities of black tea. Crit Rev Food Sci Nutr 2009;49:379–404.

107. Garden EJ, Ruxton CH, Leeds AR. Black tea—helpful or harmful? a review of the evidence. Eur J Clin Nutr 2007;61:3–18.

108. Chiang AN, Wu HL, Yeh HI, et al. Antioxidant effects of black rice extract through the induction of superoxide dismutase and catalase activities. Lipids 2006;41: 797–803.

109. Xia X, Ling W, Ma J, et al. An anthocyanin-rich extract from black rice enhances atherosclerotic plaque stabilization in apolipoprotein E-deficient mice. J Nutr 2006;136:2220–5.

110. Guo H, Ling W, Wang Q, et al. Cyanidin 3-glucoside protects 3T3-L1 adipocytes against H2O2- or TNF-alpha-induced insulin resistance by inhibiting c-Jun NH2-terminal kinase activation. Biochem Pharmacol 2008;75:1393–401.

111. Kim JY, Kim JH, Lee da H, et al. Meal replacement with mixed rice is more effective than white rice in weight control, while improving antioxidant enzyme activity in obese women. Nutr Res 2008;28:66–71.

112. Wang Q, Han P, Zhang M, et al. Supplementation of black rice pigment fraction improves antioxidant and anti-inflammatory status in patients with coronary heart disease. Asia Pac J Clin Nutr 2007;16(Suppl 1):295–301.

113. McCrory MA, Fuss PJ, McCallum JE, et al. Dietary variety within food groups: association with energy intake and body fatness in men and women. Am J Clin Nutr 1999;69:440–7.
114. Sea MM, Woo J, Tong PC, et al. Associations between food variety and body fatness in Hong Kong Chinese adults. J Am Coll Nutr 2004;23:404–13.
115. Trichopoulou A, Kouris-Blazos A, Wahlqvist ML, et al. Diet and overall survival in elderly people. BMJ 1995;311:1457–60.
116. de Lorgeril M, Salen P, Martin JL, et al. Mediterranean diet, traditional risk factors, and the rate of cardiovascular complications after myocardial infarction: final report of the Lyon Diet Heart Study. Circulation 1999;99:779–85.
117. Sofi F, Cesari F, Abbate R, et al. Adherence to Mediterranean diet and health status: meta-analysis. BMJ 2008;337:a1344.
118. Scarmeas N, Stern Y, Mayeux R, et al. Mediterranean diet and mild cognitive impairment. Arch Neurol 2009;66:216–25.
119. Woo J, Woo KS, Leung SS, et al. The Mediterranean score of dietary habits in Chinese populations in four different geographical areas. Eur J Clin Nutr 2001;55:215–20.
120. Woo J, Cheung B, Ho S, et al. Influence of dietary pattern on the development of overweight in a Chinese population. Eur J Clin Nutr 2008;62:480–7.
121. Key TJ, Davey GK, Appleby PN. Health benefits of a vegetarian diet. Proc Nutr Soc 1999;58:271–5.
122. Woo J, Kwok T, Ho SC, et al. Nutritional status of elderly Chinese vegetarians. Age Ageing 1998;27:455–61.
123. Kwok TK, Woo J, Ho S, et al. Vegetarianism and ischemic heart disease in older Chinese women. J Am Coll Nutr 2000;19:622–7.
124. Stookey JD, Wang Y, Ge K, et al. Measuring diet quality in china: the INFH-UNC-CH diet quality index. Eur J Clin Nutr 2000;54:811–21.
125. Kim S, Haines PS, Siega-Riz AM, et al. The Diet Quality Index-International (DQI-I) provides an effective tool for cross-national comparison of diet quality as illustrated by China and the United States. J Nutr 2003;133:3476–84.
126. Woo J, Chan R, Leung J, et al. Relative contributions of geographic, socioeconomic, and lifestyle factors to quality of life, frailty, and mortality in elderly. PLoS One 2010;5:e8775.
127. Andrieu E, Darmon N, Drewnowski A. Low-cost diets: more energy, fewer nutrients. Eur J Clin Nutr 2006;60:434–6.
128. Cade J, Upmeier H, Calvert C, et al. Costs of a healthy diet: analysis from the UK Women's Cohort Study. Public Health Nutr 1999;2:505–12.
129. Darmon N, Briend A, Drewnowski A. Energy-dense diets are associated with lower diet costs: a community study of French adults. Public Health Nutr 2004;7:21–7.
130. Drewnowski A, Specter SE. Poverty and obesity: the role of energy density and energy costs. Am J Clin Nutr 2004;79:6–16.
131. Drewnowski A, Darmon N, Briend A. Replacing fats and sweets with vegetables and fruits–a question of cost. Am J Public Health 2004;94:1555–9.
132. Schroder H, Marrugat J, Covas MI. High monetary costs of dietary patterns associated with lower body mass index: a population-based study. Int J Obes (Lond) 2006;30:1574–9.
133. Jetter KM, Cassady DL. The availability and cost of healthier food alternatives. Am J Prev Med 2006;30:38–44.
134. Monro D, Young L, Wilson J, et al. The sodium content of low cost and private label foods: implications for public health. J N Z Dietetic Association 2004;58:4–10.

135. Mhurchu CN, Ogra S. The price of healthy eating: cost and nutrient value of selected regular and healthier supermarket foods in New Zealand. N Z Med J 2007;120:U2388.
136. Wilson N, Mansoor O. Food pricing favours saturated fat consumption: supermarket data. N Z Med J 2005;118:U1338.
137. Lopez-Azpiazu I, Sanchez-Villegas A, Johansson L, et al. Disparities in food habits in Europe: systematic review of educational and occupational differences in the intake of fat. J Hum Nutr Diet 2003;16:349–64.
138. Irala-Estevez JD, Groth M, Johansson L, et al. A systematic review of socio-economic differences in food habits in Europe: consumption of fruit and vegetables. Eur J Clin Nutr 2000;54:706–14.
139. Wright L, Hickson M, Frost G. Eating together is important: using a dining room in an acute elderly medical ward increases energy intake. J Hum Nutr Diet 2006; 19:23–6.
140. Wu A, Ying Z, Gomez-Pinilla F. Docosahexaenoic acid dietary supplementation enhances the effects of exercise on synaptic plasticity and cognition. Neuroscience 2008;155:751–9.
141. Vaynman S, Ying Z, Gomez-Pinilla F. Hippocampal BDNF mediates the efficacy of exercise on synaptic plasticity and cognition. Eur J Neurosci 2004;20: 2580–90.
142. Chan RS, Lok KY, Sea MM, et al. Clients' experiences of a community based life-style modification program: a qualitative study. Int J Environ Res Public Health 2009;6:2608–22.
143. Lok KY, Chan RS, Sea MM, et al. Nutritionist's variation in counseling style and the effect on weight change of patients attending a community based lifestyle modification program. Int J Environ Res Public Health 2010;7:413–26.

Falls, Osteoporosis, and Hip Fractures

Lenise A. Cummings-Vaughn, MD[a,b,]*, Julie K. Gammack, MD[b]

KEYWORDS

• Falls • Osteoporosis • Hip fracture • Risk factors

Although osteoporosis and falls are distinct conditions that are often evaluated and managed separately, they share the potential and serious clinical endpoint of fracture. This article explores the intertwined associations between osteoporosis and falls by examining the epidemiology, risk factors, risk prevention, and treatments. This relationship is shown in **Fig. 1**.

By examining the epidemiology of falls and the associated mortality, the impact of this condition becomes evident. The ability to predict falls and identify osteoporosis early can be challenging, and this in turn affects the opportunity to prevent fractures. This article outlines the evidence on falls prevention, osteoporosis diagnosis, and fracture risk assessment. It includes several studies that challenge the common view on the use of fall prevention tools, dual energy X-ray absorptiometry (DEXA) testing, and postfracture bisphosphonate treatment. By understanding the evidence, it becomes clearer how to target populations at risk, interpret screening methods, and promote disease prevention and treatment.

FALLS
Epidemiology and Risk Factors

Falls contribute to considerable morbidity and mortality in the elderly.[1] According to Rubenstein,[1] about three-fourths of deaths caused by falls in the United States occur in those 65 years of age or older. The multifactorial nature of falls, with a significant risk for functional decline and mortality in this age group, is a primary reason falls are considered a geriatric syndrome. Rubenstein[1] analyzed 12 large studies of falls risk factors. Those risks found in more than 10% of falls included accidents, environmental hazards, gait/balance disorders, weakness, dizziness/vertigo, and other causes

[a] Jefferson Barracks Division, Department of Internal Medicine, Geriatric Research, Education, and Clinical Center, Saint Louis Veterans Affairs Medical Center, #1 Jefferson Barracks Drive, St Louis, MO 63125, USA
[b] Division of Geriatric Medicine, Department of Internal Medicine, Saint Louis University School of Medicine, 1402 South Grand Boulevard, Room 238, St Louis, MO 63104, USA
* Corresponding author. Jefferson Barracks Division, Geriatric Research, Education, and Clinical Center, Saint Louis Veterans Affairs Medical Center, #1 Jefferson Barracks Drive, St Louis, MO 63125.
E-mail address: lenise.cummingsvaughn@va.gov

Med Clin N Am 95 (2011) 495–506
doi:10.1016/j.mcna.2011.03.003
0025-7125/11/$ – see front matter. Published by Elsevier Inc.

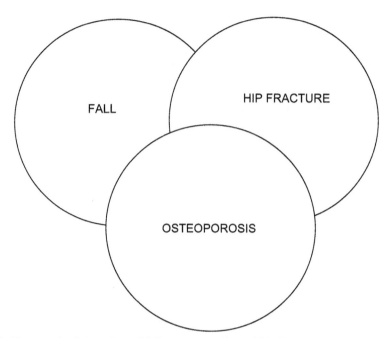

Fig. 1. The complex interaction of falls, osteoporosis, and hip fractures.

including arthritis, acute illness, drugs, alcohol, pain, epilepsy, and falling from bed. Less common risks included drop attack, confusion, postural hypotension, visual disorders, and syncope.

Risk Assessment

Falls occur in various settings including the home, hospital, and nursing home. Fall risk screening tools are needed to identify high-risk individuals in these settings. Screening for fall risk should include a documentation of prior falls, a fear of falling, sensory impairments, and cognitive impairment. Although this type of screening does not quantify risk, it does provide useful clinical information.

Gates and colleagues[2] performed a systematic review assessing the accuracy of 29 different screening instruments for falls. Of these, only 6 were tested more than once. These tools were used in the assessment of the community-dwelling older adult population. The screening tools used included the Tinetti Balance and Gait Assessment Tool (also called the Performance Oriented Mobility Assessment [POMA]), Timed Up and Go (TUG), Mobility Interaction Fall Chart, functional reach, tandem stance, and walking tests (5-minute walk and timed 12-m walk). The POMA was evaluated in 8 studies and the TUG was evaluated in 4 studies. Study heterogeneity, small sample sizes, and lack of methodological standardization (different versions of tests and cutoff values) prevented the quantification of effect sizes via meta-analytical techniques. The review did show that most screening tools possessed a higher specificity than sensitivity. Therefore, Gates and colleagues[2] found insufficient evidence that any screening tool accurately predicted falls. This finding suggests that sole reliance on a single screening tool could mistakenly under-recognize those individuals at risk for falls.

Because existing screening tools do not reliably identify those at risk for falling, or quantify the falls risk, an integrative approach must be used for screening. This means that screening should occur at frequent time intervals and at multiple clinical encounters. Screening should be performed by a variety of observers using a variety of instruments to avoid missing small changes in risk that may accumulate to cause a large likelihood of falling. The skills of multiple disciplines such as physical therapy, occupational therapy, and ophthalmology/optometry are useful in providing this comprehensive risk assessment. In addition, an algorithm similar to the FRAX (fracture risk assessment tool) would be helpful in giving a projected probability of falling.

Risk Reduction/Prevention

Once high-risk individuals are identified, interventions to reduce falls can be implemented. The strongest evidence for falls risk reduction supports strength and balancing training, psychotropic medication limitations, vitamin D and calcium supplementation, and home hazard assessment in high-risk populations.[3] Kam and colleagues[4] performed a systematic review of exercise interventions and found that exercise reduced falls, fall-related fractures, and several risk factors for falls in those with low bone mineral density (BMD). When stratified by type of exercise, most balance studies confirmed the efficacy of balance exercises in the reduction of falls. Not all muscle strengthening exercise studies showed fall reductions, but bone strength was improved with weight-bearing aerobic exercise for at least 1 year regardless of the muscle strengthening program.[4]

In the home care setting, innovative models to reduce falls have been developed. Gombar and colleagues[5] implemented a home health care falls prevention program using a protocol of frequent surveillance similar to that used in the hospital. In this study, caregivers at home were encouraged to check on their care recipient hourly. In addition, all falls and near falls were reported weekly to the clinicians. The investigators showed a trend toward reduction in moderate-severity falls with time. This intervention is time consuming and may be difficult to implement in community nursing homes and those living in their own home; however, the salient feature of Gombar and colleagues' model is frequent reassessment in high-risk individuals.

OSTEOPOROSIS
Epidemiology and Risk Factors

According to the International Osteoporosis Foundation, an estimated 75 million men and women in Europe, the United States, and Japan are affected by osteoporosis. Osteoporosis is not just a disease of women; men experience both osteoporosis and its clinical consequences. One in 3 women and 1 in 5 men more than 50 years of age experience osteoporotic fractures.[6] Of the estimated 9 million osteoporotic fractures in 2000, 1.6 million were of the hip.[6] Thirty-nine percent of these fractures and 30% of hip fractures occur in men. Hasserius and colleagues[7] note that men generally have higher rates of fracture-related mortality. The resulting disability from osteoporosis in Europe is greater than the combined disability of all nonlung cancers.

The risk factors of osteoporosis are many. **Box 1** lists some of the more commonly accepted risk factors. Some of the less common risk factors, and those with a possible contribution to decreased BMD include Parkinson disease (PD), stroke, low vitamin B concentration, depression, and use of selective serotonin reuptake inhibitors.

The decreased BMD observed in PD is likely multifactorial. Causes of decreased BMD have been correlated with immobilization-induced bone resorption, hypovitaminosis D caused by lack of sun exposure, and a compensatory hyperparathyroidism.[8] This low BMD in PD has been observed in the lumbar vertebrae, hip, and second metacarpal bone. Sato and colleagues[8] performed a 2-year, randomized, double-

---

Box 1
Risk factors for osteoporosis

Genetics (parental history of fracture, especially hip fracture)

Physical inactivity/sedentary lifestyle

Impaired neuromuscular function

Smoking

High alcohol intake

Prolonged corticosteroid use

Proton pump inhibitor use. Low body weight

Weight loss

Exercise induced amenorrhea

---

blind, placebo-controlled trial of 121 patients with PD receiving either risedronate 2.5 mg plus vitamin D_2 1000 IU or placebo plus vitamin D_2 1000 IU. The treatment group experienced a significant 2.2% increase in BMD and reduced risk of hip fracture compared with the placebo group.

Pouwels and colleagues[9] noted that stroke can result in a 1.5-fold to fourfold increased risk of hip fracture. Prospective studies suggest that nonuniform patterns in BMD occur rapidly after stroke, especially in patients with the most severe functional deficits. Most significant bone loss occurs on the paretic side.[9]

To investigate the relationship between stroke and fracture, Pouwels and colleagues[9] performed a case-control study 6763 patients with a first-time hip/femur fracture. The odds ratio (OR) for hip/femur fracture was 1.96 (95% confidence interval [CI], 1.65–2.33) any time after stroke occurrence. A higher fracture risk was noted within 3 months of stroke with an OR of 3.34 (95% CI, 1.87–5.97) and female patients with an OR of 2/12 (95% CI, 3.00–8.75). Those at highest risk were patients younger than 71 years and those with a hemorrhagic stroke. These data are useful in identifying previously under-recognized populations at risk for osteoporosis and fracture.

Because increased homocysteine levels have been associated with osteoporotic fracture, McLean and colleagues[10] investigated the association between homocysteine levels and BMD. Homocysteine is believed to impede bone collagen cross-links, causing increased fragility. In addition, the B vitamins, folate, B12, and B6 are cofactors in homocysteine metabolism and are determinants of homocysteine levels in the elderly.[10] In a group of community-dwelling residents from the Framingham Osteoporosis Study, vitamin B, homocysteine, and BMD were followed over time. There was a trend toward increased bone loss with low vitamin B6 levels and a trend toward increased fractures with low vitamin B12 and B6 levels. Those with highest homocysteine levels (more than 14 μmol/L) had higher hip fracture risk despite adjustment for B6 levels. Increased homocysteine levels alone were not associated with greater bone loss.[10]

There have been several studies of the association between major depressive disorder (MDD), selective serotonin reuptake inhibitors (SSRI), and osteoporosis. In a meta-analysis, Yirmiya and colleagues[11] compared BMD and markers of bone turnover between 2327 depressed and 21,141 nondepressed individuals. They found that depressed individuals had lower BMD than nondepressed subjects, in the spine, hip, and forearm. Depressed women were more likely to have lower BMD than depressed men, and premenopausal depressed women were more likely than postmenopausal depressed women. MDD is the second leading cause of years lived with a disability.[11] The association of bone loss and depression may be greater in premenopausal women because the confounding factor in postmenopausal women may be obscured by estrogen depletion, reduced physical activity, nutritional disturbances, and drug treatments. In an animal study, Yirmiya and colleagues[12] showed that chronic mild stress in rodents decreased trabecular bone volume density in the femur and vertebral body. This effect may be induced by an increased in steroid and norepinephrine levels. It is possible that β-adrenergic antagonist treatment could prevent the bone loss in the rodent model, thus showing a brain-to-bone communication pathway.[12] Other possible contributors to bone loss in depression may include inflammatory cytokines, tumor necrosis factor α, endocannabinoid system, and dietary and behavioral patterns (cigarette smoking, alcohol consumption, and decreased consumption of nutrients).

In addition to the effects of glucocorticoids and the adrenergic system, the skeletal serotonergic system is integral to the potential association of SSRIs and osteoporosis. Although increasing serotonin (5-HT) levels is the first-line treatment of depression, the presence of 5-HT receptors and 5-HT transporters in osteoblasts and osteoclasts can cause deleterious skeletal effects. A resulting decreased osteoblastic activity may result in bone loss.[11] Richards and colleagues[13] showed that daily SSRI use also doubled the risk of fragility fractures after adjustment for covariates.

Medication-induced bone loss should be considered when establishing an osteoporosis and fracture risk profile. Allport[14] performed a review of the evidence for medication-induced osteoporosis with the use of corticosteroids, androgen-deprivation therapy, hormone-based therapy, highly-active antiretroviral therapy (HAART), neurologic drugs, and disease-modifying antirheumatic drugs. In comparing 2 cross-sectional studies of osteoporosis, more osteopenia was observed in corticosteroid-naive children versus corticosteroid-treated children. Conversely, greater osteoporosis was found in the corticosteroid-treated group in a study of adolescents and adults. The author identified multiple studies with positive correlations between steroid use and increased incidence and prevalence of fracture alone or fracture and osteoporosis.[14] The data are strongest with oral steroid use in adults. Only 1 study of inhaled steroid treatment in lung disease was noted, and this did not show a significant difference in nonvertebral fractures.

For androgen deficiency, Allport[14] did not find studies comparing the prevalence of osteoporosis in men treated with androgen deprivation versus naive men. However, the incidence of fracture was found to be increased in androgen-deprived men. Hormone therapy with aromatase inhibitors, exemestane, anastrozole, and letrozole for breast cancer has also been studied. These breast cancer treatments have shown an increased risk of bone loss and fracture. HAART therapy with and without protease inhibitors has been shown to increase the prevalence of osteopenia and osteoporosis. Disease-modifying drugs, like methotrexate, did not show a significant difference in osteoporosis and osteopenia prevalence compared with those who were never exposed.

Risk Reduction/Treatment

With so many risk factors associated with osteoporosis, it is important to determine whether knowledge of these risks significantly reduces the prevalence of osteoporosis and the risk of fracture and falls. Burke-Doe and colleagues[15] studied a group of 49 community-dwelling adults older than 50 years and analyzed their knowledge of risk factors, prevalence of risk factors of osteoporosis, falls, and fractures, and the relationship between knowledge and prevalence of osteoporosis risk factors. There was a positive correlation between knowledge of risk factors and increased confidence in performing activities of daily living, greater lower-extremity strength, and lower fall risk. Despite this knowledge, only one-third of respondents scored more than 50% correct on a 20-item Osteoporosis Knowledge Assessment Tool. These results suggest a role for greater individual education in reducing the risk for osteoporosis and falls.

Gardner and colleagues[16] investigated the undertreatment of osteoporosis following hip fracture. A femoral neck fracture is considered an osteoporosis risk equivalent, especially in postmenopausal women and the elderly. Therefore, treatment should be considered or instituted in appropriate patients following acute fracture management. Gardner and colleagues[16] studied the rate of recognition and treatment of osteoporosis in patients with low-energy osteoporotic hip fractures between 1997 and 2000. Less than one-third of the 75 patients with fracture were treated for osteoporosis at the time of discharge. Only 19.3% of the patients received medication management at discharge, 13.3% of the study patients received only calcium, and 6% received an antiresorptive treatment of estrogen, calcitonin, bisphosphonate, or raloxifen.

Treatments focused on preventing osteoporotic fractures or osteopenia, including vitamin D_3, calcium, bisphosphonates, and weight-bearing exercise. These treatments are intended to increase bone strength by supporting bone metabolism. Vitamin D_3 is essential to calcium absorption and low levels of the metabolite 25-hydroxyvitamin D seem to be predictive of low BMD and femoral neck osteoporosis.[17] In a meta-analysis of 8 controlled trials of 12,658 women taking vitamin D_3 or placebo with or without calcium, the use of vitamin D_3 plus calcium resulted in a significantly decreased incidence of nonvertebral fractures (OR, 0.77; 95% CI, 0.6–0.93) and hip fractures (OR, 0.70; 95% CI, 0.53–0.90). The doses in these studies ranged from 400 IU to 800 IU. These doses are generally considered suboptimal because earlier studies note that maximum fracture prevention occurs with vitamin D doses from 700 IU to 1000 IU daily.[17] The dose of vitamin D was not an initial measure in the analysis and the difference in the dose recommendation may reflect this. However, some data suggest that only 4% to 30% of reduced fracture risk that occurs with antiresorptive therapy can be attributed to changes in bone density.[3]

HIP FRACTURE
Epidemiology and Risk Analysis

Most osteoporotic fractures (approximately 61%), occur in women.[6] The International Osteoporosis Foundation projects that by the year 2050, hip fracture incidence in men will increase by 310% and in women by 240%. The measurements of BMD using DEXA are believed to overestimate BMD by 20% to 50%; they are therefore poor predictors of fracture in individuals.

According to Jarvinen and colleagues,[3] falling is more strongly associated with fracture than osteoporosis. Fall height, energy, and direction are important determinants of the type and severity of fracture. Therefore, fall prevention should be included in fracture prevention. Jarvinen and colleagues[3] note that more than 80% of low-trauma fractures occur in people who do not have osteoporosis (defined as a T score of −2.5 or less). Changing the DEXA T score cutoff to −1.5 would only change the figure to 75%. Despite these parameters, many believe that low-trauma fractures, such as hip fractures from a fall, occur because the bone is compromised secondary to osteoporosis.[3,18] In addition, prior fracture is associated with an 86% increased risk of any fracture.[19]

The World Health Organization (WHO) fracture risk assessment tool (FRAX) gives a 10-year hip, clinical spine, humerus, or wrist fracture risk–specific for age, gender, race and clinical profiles. The algorithm is calibrated for geographic variation in risk. Version 3.0 of the FRAX has been shown to give lower probability estimates for major osteoporotic fracture and hip fracture than version 2.0 but has little impact on rank order of risk.[20] Fall risk is not specifically included in the algorithm. This tool bridges the chasm between the parameters for diagnosing osteoporosis and identifying individuals with structurally compromised bone that causes an increase risk of fracture.

Hip fractures are the most significant contributor to osteoporotic morbidity and mortality and a surprising 30% occur in men.[21] The morbidity includes chronic pain, loss of independence, and disability that ultimately results in nursing home placement. An estimated 25% of individuals require long-term care placement after hip fracture, and 60% never return to prefracture levels of independence.[22] These numbers provide a clear picture of the lost independence and disability that a fracture can cause.

Institutionalized elderly represent a high-risk group for hip fracture.[23] Nakamura and colleagues[23] studied 7654 subjects for 1 year who resided in nursing homes and who required moderate or extensive care. Low activities of daily living, dementia, and low weight were independent risk factors for hip fracture–institutionalized elderly. The Japanese women were found to have an incidence of hip fracture of 15 per 1000 person years. This rate is one-third that reported for white women.

Khosla[21] states that osteoporosis in men is an increasingly important public health problem, with an estimated 1 in 5 men more than 50 years old experiencing an osteoporotic fracture in their lifetime. There is a geographic variation in the probability of hip fracture. In 2007, Johnell and colleagues[24] reported a 0.3% increased 10-year probability of hip fracture in men with each 10° increment in latitude.

As with women, there is an increased risk of subsequent fracture after low-trauma fracture. Center and colleagues[25] reported a relative risk of subsequent fracture of 1.95 (95% CI, 1.70–2.25) in women and 3.47 (95% CI, 2.68–4.48) in men. Low-trauma fractures have been associated with an increased mortality risk at 5 to 10 years and were found to be higher in men than women for all ages. The importance of high-trauma falls was also reviewed in this study. Men and women had an increased risk of high-trauma fracture with each 1 standard deviation reduction in total hip BMD. The conclusion from this study states that, as with women, men also need a thorough fracture history and evaluation with imaging.[21]

Both SSRIs and tricyclic antidepressants (TCAs) have been implicated in fracture risk. Ziere and colleagues[26] showed that current SSRI users have a significantly increased risk of nonvertebral fracture, 2.07-fold (95% CI, 1.23–3.50) compared with past TCAs or SSRIs. This increased risk was independent of other potential risk factors such as age, fall history, low BMD, lower-limb disability, and depressive state at baseline and follow-up. The results in this study are limited to only 18 fractures among current users. Ziere and colleagues[26] noted that prior studies have already established that TCAs have been implicated in fracture risk.

Prevention

As previously discussed with osteoporosis, hip fracture can also be associated with specific medication use. There is also an association between hip fracture and polypharmacy. Lai and colleagues[27] investigated the association between polypharmacy and hip fracture. A population-based study using insurance claims data from the Taiwan Bureau of National Health analyzed 2328 elderly patients with newly diagnosed hip fractures from 2005 to 2007. The results indicated that the OR of hip fracture for patients using 10 or more medications was 8.42 (95% CI, 4.73–15) compared with use of 1 or fewer medications. The risk was 23 times greater for those 85 years and older compared with those aged 65 to 74 years. Before this study, the risk of falling was found to be 2 times higher for patients taking 4 drugs a day versus not taking any medications. Therefore, medication management represents an important preventive strategy for falls that becomes critically important for those older than 85 years.

In addition to limiting medications, the use of hip protectors has been identified as a preventive strategy. A Bayesian meta-analysis by Sawka and colleagues[28] concluded that hip protectors decrease the risk of hip fracture in elderly nursing home residents. The analysis was conducted in a nursing home where compliance issues can be monitored. However, hip protector use in community-dwelling adults is significantly complicated by noncompliance. Hip protector compliance was found to be poor, with only 14 of 74 aging adults at risk for hip fracture regularly using the device. Forty-one percent of individuals reported that the hip protector was uncomfortable, and 29% found them difficult to put on.[29] In addition, the most common reason for nonuse appeared to be lack of education on the purpose and benefit of the device. Therefore, hip protectors may represent an underused preventive strategy.

Postfracture Management

Treatment of osteoporosis is often inadequate following fragility fracture despite evidence showing the benefit in decreasing mortality. Reports indicate that the rate of postfracture pharmacotherapy for osteoporosis ranges from 5% to 30%.[18] Miki and colleagues[18] evaluated the use of medication management for osteoporosis at an inpatient unit by orthopedic surgeons in 62 patients with an average age of 79.2 years. The randomized controlled trial consisted of a control group given calcium and vitamin D3 daily and instructed to seek evaluation from their primary physician for osteoporosis. The intervention group was evaluated for osteoporosis in the hospital, started on calcium and vitamin D3, and given a follow-up with an orthopedic osteoporosis clinic. Twenty intervention group participants were started on risedronate at the follow-up clinic visit. One patient in the control group sustained a fragility fracture 6 months after the hip fracture. There was a significant difference in the 6-month post–hip fracture osteoporosis treatment rate (58% vs 29%, $P = .04$). The 6-month difference in fracture was not significant, but this was attributed to the small sample size. This study also reported that only 39% of the control group discussed osteoporosis with their primary physician and none reported speaking with their orthopedic surgeon during the follow-up visit. The intervention group had low 25-hydroxyvitamin D levels and increased parathyroid levels. Miki and colleagues[18] believe that screening for secondary causes of osteoporosis should be encouraged and vitamin D supplementation should be routine after hip fracture. The investigators concluded that an active role by an orthopedic/osteoporosis clinic improves the management of osteoporosis.[18] Additional interventions shown to have success include inpatient protocols,[30] an inpatient metabolic evaluation, and endocrinology consultation.[31]

Some additional barriers to postfracture treatment include physician education, transportation, lack of financial incentives, and the cost of treatment.[18] Some physicians are apprehensive with the use of bisphosphonates after fracture. There is a theoretic concern that bone resorption can be reduced by bisphosphonates and it is used in diseases with excessive osteoclastic activity.[32] The basic mechanism of non–nitrogen containing bisphosphonates (alendronate, pamidronate, risedronate, and zoledronate) is interference with the mevalonate biosynthetic pathway and cellular activity and survival through protein prenylation.[32] Bone resorption can be reduced by bisphosphonates; therefore, they are often used in diseases with excessive osteoclastic activity.[32] The trepidation with bisphosphonate use after fracture stems from the possible inhibition of remodeling during bone healing or repair/bone graft incorporation.[32] **Fig. 2**. shows the steps involved with bone healing after fracture.

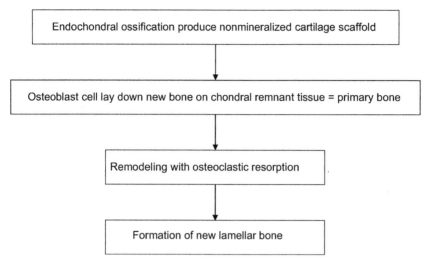

Fig. 2. Bone healing following fracture. (*Data from* Streeten EA, Mohamed A, Gandhi A, et al. The inpatient consultation approach to osteoporosis treatment in patients with a fracture. Is automatic consultation needed? J Bone Joint Surg Am 2006;88:1968–74.)

No studies have been performed in humans to test the hypothesis of impaired bone healing from bisphosphonate use after fracture, but there are multiple animal model studies. These models have supported both positive and negative conclusions about the use of a bisphosphonate after fracture. Matos and colleagues[32] studied 30 immature male albino New Zealand rabbits that received an osteotomy. The experimental group received a single dose of 0.04 mg/kg zoledronic acid, considered the most potent bisphosphonate, via intraperitoneal injection before the osteotomy. The fibulas of a representative sample in both the experimental and control groups were examined at 1, 2, and 4 weeks after osteotomy. There was increased trabecular bone in the experimental group and less periosteal fibrosis in the fourth week of the experimental group compared with the control. The investigators concluded that zoledronic acid did not prevent bone healing and resulted in accentuated stimulation of primary bone production rather than an inhibition of bone remodeling. They noted that bone remodeling is not required for initial fracture repair. The increased woven bone and retention of primary bone suggest an anabolic component to the drug's actions.[15] This might be explained by the potency and biologic actions of zoledronic acid that are most similar to pamidronate. The existing animal study evidence does not suggest that bisphosphonate treatment increases healing time after fracture.

Although surgical correction of the hip fracture is the usual initial treatment, other treatments can be considered but have an associated increased risk of hip displacement, increased pain, and loss of mobility.[33] Neuman and colleagues[33] reported that the most common reasons for nonoperative management of hip fractures are late presentation with an already healing fracture, moribund condition, poor prognosis for recovery of function, or refusal of the procedure. In this study of 165,861 Medicare beneficiaries admitted with a hip fracture between 2002 and 2006, nonoperative management occurred in only 6.2% of patients. Nonoperative patients were generally older, less likely to be female, have more comorbidities (prior myocardial infarction, congestive heart failure, renal failure, chronic obstructive pulmonary disease, Alzheimer disease, paraplegia, or stroke), and be admitted from a skilled nursing facility. Significant differences in nonoperative management in this population included race, with an OR of 1.79 (95%CI, 1.64–1.95) for African Americans versus white people, after controlling for age, sex, comorbidities, and type of hip fracture. Low income was not significantly associated with nonoperative management. Despite the higher odds of nonoperative management in African Americans, when this group did receive operative repair, there was a lower mortality compared with white people (7.96% vs 20.17%, $P<.0001$) at 7 days compared with 30 days (24.14% vs 38.22%, $P<.001$).[33] From this information, the investigators concluded that the difference was not explained by severity of illness and may be explained by inequitable selection for fracture repair. The investigators note that the study does not capture patient and family preferences or difference between physicians and hospitals.

To better identify the factors affecting hip fracture postoperative mortality, the Scottish Hip Fracture Audit database was analyzed for factors associated with early postoperative mortality. Holt and colleagues[34] analyzed data from 18,817 individuals and found a 30-day mortality of 7% and 120-day mortality of 18%. The case mix variables strongly associated with postoperative mortality included age, American Society of Anesthesiologist score (health status before surgery), gender (men greater than women), prefracture residence, prefracture mobility, and type of fracture. Only the management variable of grade of anesthetists showed significance for postoperative mortality.

Functional ability is another important outcome following hip fracture. Hormonal functioning may affect postfracture outcomes because of the regulations of anabolic and catabolic processes, which include bone healing. Insulinlike growth factor-1 (IGF-1) is involved in growth hormone–induced actions and anabolic effects in muscle and bone.[22] Levels in the elderly are noted to be low. Di Monaco and colleagues[22] hypothesized that IGF-1 levels could be associated with functional outcome after hip fracture. They studied 171 women in a rehabilitation hospital. IGF-1 levels were found to be significantly associated with Barthel index scores after adjustment for confounders after rehabilitation and during rehabilitation.

SUMMARY

The relationship between the risks, interventions, and preventive strategies for falls, osteoporosis, and hip fracture is clinically challenging. Continued assessment of risks seems to be a key factor for both falls and osteoporosis. The current research identifies several areas for improvement in the present approaches to assessment and treatment of these conditions. Improving assessment and treatment may have a large impact on the related morbidity and mortality for the elderly and other populations at risk.

REFERENCES

1. Rubenstein LZ. Falls in older people: epidemiology, risk factors and strategies for prevention. Age Ageing 2006;35:37–41.
2. Gates S, Smith LA, Fisher JD, et al. Systematic review of accuracy of screening instruments for predicting fall risk among independently living older adults. J Rehabil Res Dev 2008;45(8):1105–16.
3. Jarvinen TL, Sievanen H, Khan KM, et al. Shifting the focus in fracture prevention osteoporosis to falls. BMJ 2008;336:124–6.
4. Kam D, Smulders E, Weerdesteyn V, et al. Exercise interventions to reduce fall-related fractures and their risk factors in individuals with low bone density: a systematic review of randomized controlled trials. Osteoporos Int 2009;20: 2111–25.

5. Gombar EN, Smith-Stoner M, Mitchell-Mattera SD. 10 Organizational characteristics that may prevent falls in home healthcare and hospice. Home Healthc Nurse 2011;29(1):26–32.
6. Johnell O, Kanis JA. A estimate of the worldwide prevalence and disability associated with osteoporotic fractures. Osteoporos Int 2006;17:1726–33.
7. Hasserius R, Karlsson MK, Nilsson BE, et al. Prevalent vertebral deformities predict increased mortality and increased fracture rate in both men and women: a 10-year population-based study of 598 individuals from the Swedish cohort in the European Vertebral Osteoporosis Study. Osteoporos Int 2003;14:61–8.
8. Sato Y, Honda Y, Iwamoto J. Risedronate and ergocalciferol prevent hip fracture in elderly men with Parkinson disease. Neurology 2007;68:911–5.
9. Pouwels S, Lalmohamed A, Leufkens B, et al. Risk of hip/femur fracture after stroke: a population-based case-control study. Stroke 2009;40:3281–5.
10. McLean RR, Jacques PF, Selhub J, et al. Plasma B vitamins, homocysteine and their relation with bone loss and hip fracture in elderly men and women. J Clin Endocrinol Metab 2008;93:2206–12.
11. Yirmiya R, Bab I. Major depression is a risk factor for low bone mineral density: a meta-analysis. Biol Psychiatry 2009;66:423–32.
12. Yirmiya R, Goshen I, Bajayo A, et al. Depression induces bone loss through stimulation of the sympathetic nervous system. Proc Natl Acad Sci U S A 2006;103:16876–81.
13. Richards JB, Papaioannou A, Adachi JD, et al. Effect of selective serotonin reuptake inhibitors on the risk of fracture. Arch Intern Med 2007;167:188–94.
14. Allport J. Incidence and prevalence of medication-induced osteoporosis: evidence-based review. Curr Opin Rheumatol 2008;20:435–41.
15. Burke-Doe A, Hudson A, Werth H, et al. Knowledge of osteoporosis risk factors and prevalence of risk factors for osteoporosis, falls, and fracture in functionally independent older adults. J Geriatr Phys Ther 2008;31(1):11–7.
16. Gardner MJ, Flik KR, Mooar P, et al. Improvement in the undertreatment of osteoporosis following hip fracture. J Bone Joint Surg Am 2002;84A(8):1342–8.
17. Bergman GJD, Fan T, McFetridge JT, et al. Efficacy of vitamin D3 supplementation in preventing fractures in elderly women: a meta-analysis. Curr Med Res Opin 2010;26:1193–201.
18. Miki RA, Oetgen ME, Kirk J, et al. Orthopaedic management improves the rate of early osteoporosis treatment after hip fracture. J Bone Joint Surg Am 2008;90:2346–53.
19. Kanis JA, Johnell O, De Laet, et al. A meta-analysis of previous fracture and subsequent fracture risk. Bone 2004;35:375.
20. Kanis JA, Johansson H, Oden A, et al. The effects of a FRAX® revision for the USA. Osteoporos Int 2010;21:35–40.
21. Khosla S. Update in male osteoporosis. J Clin Endocrinol Metab 2010;95(1):3–10.
22. Di Monaco M, Vallero F, Di Monaco R, et al. Serum levels of insulin-like growth factor-I are positively associated with functional outcome after hip fracture in elderly women. Am J Phys Med Rehabil 2009;88:119–25.
23. Nakamura K, Takahashi S, Oyama M, et al. Incidence and risk factors associated with hip fracture in institutionalised elderly people in Japan. Age Ageing 2009;38(4):478–82.
24. Johnell O, Borgstrom F, Jonsson B, et al. Latitude, socioeconomic prosperity, mobile phones and hip fracture risk. Osteoporos Int 2007;18:333–7.
25. Center JF, Bliuc D, Nguyen TV, et al. Risk of subsequent fracture after low-trauma fracture in men and women. JAMA 2007;297:387–94.

26. Ziere G, Dieleman JP, van der Cammen TJM, et al. Selective serotonin reuptake inhibiting antidepressants are associated with an increased risk of nonvertebral fractures. J Clin Psychopharmacol 2008;28:411–7.
27. Lai SW, Liao KF, Liao CC, et al. Polypharmacy correlates with increased risk for hip fractures, a population-based study. Medicine 2010;89:295–9.
28. Sawka AM, Boulos P, Beattie K, et al. Hip protectors decrease hip fracture risk in elderly nursing home residents: a Bayesian meta-analysis. J Clin Epidemiol 2007; 60:336–44.
29. Madreka A, Lyons D, O'Connor C, et al. Hip protectors in fracture prevention for aging adults at risk of falling: a study of user compliance. J Geriatr Phys Ther 2009;32:153–8.
30. Kaufman JD, Bolander ME, Bunta AD, et al. Barriers and solutions to osteoporosis care in patients with a hip fracture. J Bone Joint Surg Am 2003;85:1837–42.
31. Streeten EA, Mohamed A, Gandhi A, et al. The inpatient consultation approach to osteoporosis treatment in patients with a fracture. Is automatic consultation needed? J Bone Joint Surg Am 2006;88:1968–74.
32. Matos MA, Tannuri U, Guarniero R. The effect of zolendronate during bone healing. J Orthop Traumatol 2010;11:7–12.
33. Neuman MD, Fleisher A, Evan-Shoshan O, et al. Nonoperative care for hip fracture in the elderly, the influence of race, income and comorbidities. Med Care 2010;48:314–20.
34. Holt G, Smith R, Duncan K, et al. Early mortality after surgical fixation of hip fractures in the elderly: an analysis of data from the Scottish Hip Fracture Audit. J Bone Joint Surg Br 2008;90:1357–63.

Late-Onset Hypogonadism

Nazem Bassil, MD

KEYWORDS

- Hypogonadism • Aging • Testosterone • Muscle mass
- Osteoporosis • Prostate

The percentage of population in the older age group is increasing. With aging, a significant percentage of men have a gradual and moderate decrease in testicular function known as late-onset hypogonadism (LOH), which is a clinical and biochemical syndrome. It is a common disorder in older men, but it is underdiagnosed and often untreated. It has been estimated that only 5% to 35% of hypogonadal males actually receive treatment for their condition. The prevalence of hypogonadism was 3.1% to 7.0% in men aged 30 to 69 years, and 18.4% in men older than 70 years.[1] The most easily recognized clinical signs of relative androgen deficiency in older men are a decrease in muscle mass and strength, a decrease in bone mass and osteoporosis, and an increase in central body fat. None of these symptoms are specific to the low androgen state but may raise suspicion of testosterone deficiency. In addition, symptoms such as a decrease in libido and sexual desire, forgetfulness, loss of memory, difficulty to concentrate, insomnia, and a decreased sense of well-being are more difficult to measure and differentiate from hormone-independent aging. In men, endogenous testosterone concentrations are inversely related to mortality. But this association could not be confirmed in the Massachusetts Male Aging Study (MMAS)[2] or the New Mexico Aging Study.[3]

DECLINE IN SERUM TESTOSTERONE LEVELS

Testosterone levels decline with aging at the rate of 1% per year.[4] In older men, the changes in total testosterone levels are overshadowed by a more significant decline in free testosterone (FT) levels. This overshadowing is a consequence of the age-associated increase of levels of sex hormone–binding globulin (SHBG), which increases gradually as a function of age and binds testosterone with high affinity; less of the total testosterone is free. The rate of age-related decline in serum testosterone levels varies in different individuals and is affected by chronic disease, such as obesity, new illness, serious emotional stress, and medications.[5] There is evidence

Department of Medicine, Saint George Hospital Medical Center, Balamand University, Youssef Sursock Street, PO Box 166378, Achrafieh, Beirut 1100 2807, Lebanon
E-mail address: nbassil@hotmail.com

Med Clin N Am 95 (2011) 507–523
doi:10.1016/j.mcna.2011.03.001
0025-7125/11/$ – see front matter © 2011 Elsevier Inc. All rights reserved.

medical.theclinics.com

that many of these men are not symptomatic. An interesting observation from the MMAS was that half of the men found to have symptomatic androgen deficiency at one stage were found to be eugonadal when retested at a later stage.[6] This observation is probably because there is a subject-to-subject variation in testosterone secretion and the testosterone threshold at which symptoms become manifest. The measurement of low testosterone levels in a patient should be reconfirmed at a later stage before considering treatment.

DIAGNOSIS OF LOH

The diagnosis of LOH requires the presence of symptoms and signs suggesting testosterone deficiency.[1] The symptom most associated with hypogonadism is low libido. Other manifestations of hypogonadism include erectile dysfunction (ED), decreased muscle mass and strength, increased body fat, decreased bone mineral density (BMD) and osteoporosis, mild anemia, breast discomfort and gynecomastia, hot flushes, sleep disturbance, body hair and skin alterations, decreased vitality, and decreased intellectual capacity (poor concentration, depression, fatigue). The problem is that many of the symptoms of late-life hypogonadism are similar to those of other conditions or are physiologically associated with the aging process. Depression, hypothyroidism, and chronic alcoholism should be excluded, as should the use of medications such as corticosteroids, cimetidine, spironolactone, digoxin, opioid analgesics, antidepressants, and antifungal drugs. Diagnosis of LOH should never be undertaken during an acute illness, which is likely to result in temporarily low testosterone levels.

The questionnaires, Androgen Deficiency in Aging Male (ADAM) (**Box 1**) and Aging Male Symptoms Scale (AMS), may be sensitive markers of the low testosterone state (97% and 83%, respectively); they are not tightly correlated with low testosterone state (specificities of ADAM and AMS being 30% and 39%, respectively), particularly in the borderline low serum testosterone range. Therefore, questionnaires are not recommended for screening androgen deficiency in men receiving health care for unrelated reasons. Moreover, healthy ambulatory elderly men older than 70 years,

---

Box 1
The ADAM questionnaire

1. Do you have a decrease in libido or sex drive?

2. Do you have a lack of energy?

3. Do you have a decrease in strength and/or endurance?

4. Have you lost weight?

5. Have you noticed a decreased "enjoyment of life?"

6. Are you sad and/or grumpy?

7. Are your erections less strong?

8. Have you noticed a recent deterioration in your ability to play sports?

9. Are you falling asleep after dinner?

10. Has there been a recent deterioration in your work performance?

A positive ADAM questionnaire result was defined as "yes" for question 1 and 7, and 2–4 for all other items.

assessed by the AMS, had a high perception of sexual symptoms with mild psychological and mild to moderate somatovegetative symptoms.

Hypogonadism in older men may be associated with chronic illnesses such as diabetes mellitus and renal disease. Systemic glucocorticoids can reduce testosterone biosynthesis in the testis and affect the hypothalamic-pituitary-gonadal (HPG) axis by inhibiting the release of luteinizing hormone (LH). Patients being treated with glucocorticoids for chronic conditions such as rheumatoid and osteoarthritic inflammation, skin inflammations, asthma, chronic obstructive pulmonary disease (COPD), and inflammatory bowel disease are at an increased risk of hypogonadism. Patients with COPD have a higher incidence of hypogonadism because of many factors such as steroid treatment, chronic hypoxia, and a systemic inflammatory response. Testosterone therapy can improve lean body mass (LBM) and BMD and strength in hypogonadal men with COPD.[7]

LABORATORY DIAGNOSIS

Diagnosis of late-life hypogonadism requires both symptoms and low testosterone levels. Serum testosterone levels have a diurnal variation; a serum sample should be obtained between 07.00 AM and 11.00 AM. The most widely accepted parameter to establish the presence of hypogonadism is the measurement of serum total testosterone level. The International Society of Andrology/International Society for the Study of Aging Male/European Association of Urology/European Academy of Andrology/ American Society of Andrology guidelines suggest that subjects with total testosterone levels greater than 350 ng/dL do not require substitution. Patients with serum total testosterone levels less than 230 ng/dL usually benefit from testosterone treatment. If the serum total testosterone level ranges between 230 and 350 ng/dL (8–12 nmol/L), patients could benefit from having a repeat measurement of total testosterone levels together with a measurement of SHBG concentrations so as to calculate FT levels, or bioavailable testosterone (BT, free plus albumin bound fractions) levels, particularly if they are obese.[8] The gold standard for BT level measurement is sulfate precipitation and for FT level is equilibrium dialysis. However, both techniques are usually not available in most laboratories so that calculated values seem preferable. The salivary testosterone level, a proxy for unbound testosterone level, has also been shown to be a reliable substitute for FT measurements.[9]

The final step is to determine whether a patient has primary or secondary hypogonadism by measuring the serum LH and follicle-stimulating hormone (FSH) levels. Elevated LH and FSH levels suggest primary hypogonadism, whereas low or low to normal LH and FSH levels suggest secondary hypogonadism. Normal LH or FSH levels with low testosterone levels suggest primary defects in the hypothalamus and/or the pituitary (secondary hypogonadism). However, in elderly men, the increase in serum gonadotropin levels, FSH levels more than LH levels, is not so great as one would expect from the decrease in testosterone levels, suggesting that the decrease in testosterone levels with aging is more due to secondary than primary hypogonadism. Unless fertility is an issue, it is usually not necessary to measure FSH levels, and determining LH levels alone is sufficient. If the total testosterone concentration is less than 150 ng/dL, pituitary imaging studies and prolactin levels are recommended to evaluate for structural lesions in the hypothalamic-pituitary region. Also, in secondary hypogonadism, prolactin levels should be obtained to rule out prolactinoma in addition to screening for hemochromatosis. Karyotyping should be considered in a young teenager or an infertile man with primary hypogonadism to diagnose Klinefelter syndrome.

TREATMENT OF LOH

The principal goal of testosterone therapy is to restore the serum testosterone concentration to the normal range to alleviate the symptoms suggesting hormone deficiency. However, the ultimate goals are to maintain or regain the highest quality of life, reduce disability, compress major illnesses into a narrow age range, and add life to years.

DELIVERY SYSTEMS

Several different methods of testosterone replacement exist including tablets, injections, transdermal systems, oral agents, pellets, and buccal preparations of testosterone. Selective androgen receptor modulators are under development. The selection of the preparation should be a joint decision of an informed patient and the physician. Short-acting preparations may be preferred over long-acting depot preparations in the initial treatment of patients with LOH. The goal of testosterone replacement therapy (TRT) is to increase blood testosterone concentrations to the normal (eugonadal) range and to match the most appropriate treatment to the individual patient. However, older men need higher levels to obtain a therapeutic benefit.

Oral Agents

The modified testosterone 17α-methyl testosterone is an effective oral androgen formulation for hypogonadism; however, it is not recommended because of its hepatotoxic side effects and its potential liver toxicity, including the development of benign and malignant neoplasm in addition to deleterious effects on levels of both low-density-lipoprotein cholesterol (LDL-C) and high-density-lipoprotein-C (HDL-C). Oral testosterone undecanoate (TU), however, bypasses first-pass metabolism through its preferential absorption into the lymphatic system. It is safe because of the lack of adverse liver side effects, but it is available only outside the United States.

Intramuscular Injection

Testosterone cypionate and enanthate were frequently used by intramuscular injection of short-acting testosterone esters that usually produce supraphysiological peaks and hypogonadal troughs in testosterone levels, which in many patients results in fluctuations in energy, mood, and libido corresponding to the fluctuations in serum testosterone levels. These fluctuations are more pronounced as the dosing interval is increased. A long-lasting formulation of TU is available in the European Union and other countries, but not yet in the United States. It consists of injections of 1000 mg of TU at intervals of up to 3 months and offers an excellent alternative for substitution therapy for male hypogonadism; the serum testosterone concentration is maintained within the normal range.[10]

Transdermal Systems

Transdermal testosterone is available in either a scrotal or a nonscrotal skin patch and more recently as a gel preparation, allowing a single application of this formulation to provide continuous transdermal delivery of testosterone for 24 hours, producing circulating testosterone levels that approximate the normal levels. Daily application is required to deliver 5 to 10 mg of testosterone per day.[11] The transdermal gels are colorless hydroalcoholic gels of 1% to 2% testosterone. They are applied once a day to the skin. These gels have a lower incidence of skin irritation compared with the patch, but testosterone can be transferred from the patient to his partner or to children after skin contact. A reservoir-type transdermal delivery system of testosterone was developed using an ethanol/water (70:30) cosolvent system as the vehicle. This device is available in Europe as a body patch without reservoir and applied every 2 days. The advantages include ease of use and maintenance of relatively uniform serum testosterone levels over time, resulting in maintenance of relatively stable energy, mood, and libido in addition to their efficacy in providing adequate TRT.

Sublingual and Buccal

Cyclodextrin-complexed testosterone sublingual formulation is absorbed rapidly into circulation, whereas testosterone is released from the cyclodextrin shell. This formulation has been suggested to have a good therapeutic potential, after adjustment of its kinetics, to produce physiologic levels of testosterone.

A mucoadhesive buccal testosterone sustained-release tablet, delivering 30 mg, applied to the upper gum just above the incisor restores serum testosterone concentrations to the physiologic range within 4 hours of application, with steady-state concentrations achieved within 24 hours of twice-daily dosing, and achieves testosterone levels within the normal range. Studies indicate that Striant is an effective, well-tolerated, convenient, and discreet treatment of male hypogonadism. However, it has had minimal clinical uptake because of the difficulty of maintaining the buccal treatment.[12] The incidence of adverse effects is low, although gum and buccal irritation and alterations in taste have been reported.

Subdermal Implants

Subcutaneous pellets are amongst the earliest effective formulations for administering testosterone. Although not frequently used, they remain available. Six to ten pellets are implanted at one time and they last 4 to 6 months, when a new procedure is required to implant more pellets. At present, testosterone pellets are the only long-acting testosterone treatment option approved for use in the United States.

Subdermal testosterone implants still offer the longest duration of action with prolonged zero-order, steady-state delivery characteristics. The standard dosage is four 200 mg pellets (800 mg) implanted subdermally at intervals of 5 to 7 months.[13] Yet the in vivo testosterone release rate of these pellets and its determinants have not been studied systematically. As a result of their long-lasting effect and the inconvenience of removing them, the risk of infection at the implant site, and extrusion of the pellets, which occurs in 5% to 10% of cases even with the most experienced, their use is limited only in men for whom the beneficial effects and tolerance for TRT have already been established.

Intranasal Testosterone

Testosterone is well absorbed after nasal administration.[14] Application of MPP 10 results in a more pulselike testosterone profile compared with the relatively sustained serum levels attained with transdermal administration. The intranasal drug delivery system represents a mechanism to more closely proximate the normal circadian variation of testosterone levels, in contrast to the abnormal steady-state levels seen with transdermal products or the large fluctuations over longer periods seen with injections. Further studies are necessary to determine the effect of nasal testosterone application in hypogonadal men over prolonged periods.

BENEFITS OF TRT

Restoring testosterone levels in older male patients to within the normal range by using TRT can improve many of the effects of hypogonadism. These benefits are summarized in **Box 2**.

Box 2
Potential benefits of TRT

Improves sexual desire and function

Increases BMD.

Improves mood, energy, and quality of life

Changes body composition and improve muscle mass and strength

Improves cognitive function

Improved Sexual Desire, Function, and Performance

The prevalence of ED increases markedly with age. Men with hypogonadism have a decline in sexual function, as illustrated by an improvement after testosterone treatment. Serum-FT was significantly correlated with erectile and orgasmic function domains of the International Index of Erectile Function questionnaire. Men with greater sexual activity had higher BT levels than men with a lower frequency, and androgen deficiency may contribute to the age-related decline in male sexuality; correspondingly low levels of BT were associated with low sexual activity. Compared with younger men, elderly men require higher levels of circulating testosterone for libido and erectile function. However, ED and/or diminished libido with or without a testosterone deficiency might be related to other comorbidities or medications.

Men with ED and/or diminished libido and documented testosterone deficiency are candidates for testosterone therapy. Randomized controlled clinical trials indicate some benefits of testosterone therapy on sexual health–related outcomes in hypogonadal men.[15] Testosterone replacement has also been shown to enhance libido and the frequency of sexual acts and sleep-related erections.

A short therapeutic trial may be done in the presence of a clinical picture of testosterone deficiency and borderline serum testosterone levels. An inadequate response to testosterone treatment requires reassessment of the causes of the ED. There is evidence that the combined use of testosterone and phosphodiesterase type 5 inhibitors in hypogonadal or borderline eugonadal men have a synergetic effect.[16] The combination treatment should be considered in hypogonadal patients with ED who fail to respond to either treatment alone.

BMD

Osteoporosis is an underrecognized problem in men. Testosterone plays a major role in BMD. Osteopenia, osteoporosis, and fracture prevalence rates are greater in hypogonadal older men. In nursing homes, of elderly men who have experienced hip fractures, 66% are hypogonadal. Patients with prostate cancer treated with androgen deprivation therapy have an increased risk of osteoporotic fracture. Assessment of bone density at 2-year intervals is advisable in hypogonadal men, and serum testosterone measurements should be obtained in all men with osteopenia. All persons with low testosterone levels should have their 25-hydroxyvitamin D levels measured and replaced if low.

Testosterone produces this effect by increasing osteoblastic activity and through aromatization to estrogen reducing osteoclastic activity. In aging men, the role of partial androgen deficiency in bone fracture rate remains to be established.[17,18] The correlation with bioestradiol, the levels of which decline in elderly men, was even stronger, suggesting that part of the androgen effects on bone are at least partially indirect, mediated via their aromatization.[19] An increase in osteocalcin levels, an index of osteoblast activity, was observed, and a decrease of hydroxyproline excretion, an index of bone resorption, was also noted.

Trials of the effects of TRT on BMD yielded mixed results. Increases in spinal bone density have been realized in hypogonadal men, with most treated men maintaining bone density above the fracture threshold. An improvement in both trabecular and cortical BMDs of the spine was seen independent of age and type of hypogonadism; in addition, a significant increase in paraspinal muscle area has been observed, emphasizing the clinical benefit of adequate replacement therapy for the physical fitness of hypogonadal men. The pooled results of a meta-analysis suggest a beneficial effect on lumbar spinal bone density and equivocal findings on femoral neck BMD. Trials of intramuscular testosterone reported significantly larger effects on lumbar bone density than trials of transdermal testosterone, particularly among patients receiving long-term glucocorticoids.[20]

Improved Body Composition and Muscle Mass and Strength

The decrease of testosterone levels with aging in addition to the significant change in body composition, which is characterized by decreased fat free mass and increased and redistributed fat mass in elderly patients, imposes functional limitations and increased morbidity. Lower levels of baseline FT are associated with a greater risk of incident or worsening mobility limitation,[21] by directly affecting muscle cells by testosterone, or by stimulating insulinlike growth factor-1 expression directly and indirectly, leading to increased muscle protein synthesis and growth.[22]

Testosterone replacement may be effective in reversing age-dependent body composition changes and associated morbidity. Testosterone administration improves body composition, decrease of fat mass, and increase of LBM, but the body weight change does not differ significantly.[23] Changes in lower-extremity muscle strength and measures of physical function were inconsistent among studies. Some studies showed a positive correlation between testosterone and muscle strength parameters of upper and lower extremities, as measured by leg extensor strength and isometric hand grip strength, as well as functional parameters, including the doors test, get-up-and-go test, and 5-chair sit/stand test.[24] On the other hand, some reported an increase in LBM but no change in physical function, or an increase in strength of knee extension or flexion.

A recent study showed that as men age the prevalence of frailty increases, whereas the testosterone level decreases, and a low testosterone level may be a risk factor for development of this syndrome.[25] But it is not clear whether testosterone replacement in frail older men with low testosterone levels can improve physical function and other health-related outcomes or reduce the risk of disability, falls, or fractures. A combination of testosterone and a nutritional supplement markedly reduced hospital admissions in older men and women.

Mood and Energy and Quality of Life

The brain has androgen receptors as sites for the androgen activity, and the administration of testosterone to hypogonadal men enhances brain perfusion.[26] Hypogonadal older men commonly complain of loss of libido, dysphoria, fatigue, and irritability. These symptoms overlap with signs and symptoms of major depression. Depression tends to increase as testosterone levels become reduced.[27]

TRT has variable effects on mood, energy, fatigue, irritability, and sense of well-being. The results of placebo-controlled randomized trials on testosterone's effect on quality of life and depressive mood were inconsistent across trials and imprecise.

Testosterone administered to nondepressed eugonadal men at physiologic doses did not have an effect on mood.[28] Administration of supraphysiological doses of testosterone to eugonadal men has been associated with mania in a small proportion of men. Testosterone replacement therapy in hypogonadal men with major depression disorder might be an effective antidepressant or augmentation to partially effective antidepressant.[29] Testosterone gel had significantly greater improvement as augmentation therapy for depressive symptoms in hypogonadal men with selective serotonin reuptake inhibitor partial response than in subjects receiving placebo. These significant correlations with testosterone levels were only observed when testosterone levels were less than the normal range, which suggests that once a minimally adequate testosterone/dihydrotestosterone level was achieved, further increase did not contribute to further improvement of mood. However, the studies reported were of limited size and duration, there is a lack of large-scale trials with extended long-term follow-up. This effect may be a direct effect of testosterone or related to positive effects of testosterone on weight and/or other anthropometric indices.

On the other hand, the testosterone-placebo difference distinguishable with respect to mood was not consistent. No relationship between the testosterone level and depressive symptoms was found in the MMAS. This discrepancy in the results of the effects of TRT on mood may be explained by the genetic polymorphism in the androgen receptor, which defines a vulnerable group in whom depression is expressed when testosterone levels decrease below a particular threshold.

Finally, testosterone treatment must be considered experimental. More controlled studies using exogenous testosterone for depression in elderly men are needed. The best candidates for treatment may be hypogonadal men who are currently taking an existing antidepressant with inadequate response.

Cognitive Function

Dementia is a major problem for older men. The decrease in serum testosterone concentrations that occurs with aging in men may be associated with a decline in verbal and visual memory and visuospatial performance and a faster rate of decline in visual memory.[30] Men with a higher ratio of total testosterone to SHBG predict a reduced incidence of Alzheimer disease, and patients with Alzheimer disease had a lower ratio of total testosterone to SHBG compared with age-matched controls.[31] Low BT is strongly associated with amnestic mild cognitive impairment. Higher BT and FT concentrations have each been associated with better performance in specific aspects of memory and cognitive function, with optimal processing capacity found in men aged 35 to 90 years even after adjustment for potential confounders including age, educational attainment, and cardiovascular morbidity, whereas the total testosterone level was not.[32]

On the other hand, contradictory findings have also been reported between total or FT levels and measures of working memory, speed/attention, or spatial relations in older men. No association was found between lower FT levels and higher performance on spatial visualization tasks and between higher FT and total testosterone levels and poorer verbal memory and executive performance. However, there is a correlation with faster processing speed.[33] A possible source of conflicting results in these studies may be interactions between testosterone levels and other risk factors for cognitive impairment, such as apolipoprotein E IV genotype and systemic illness, which cause low testosterone levels.

In men receiving hormonal therapy for prostate cancer, suppression of endogenous testosterone synthesis and blockade of the androgen receptor resulted in a beneficial effect on verbal memory, but an adverse effect on spatial ability slowed reaction times in several attention domains; plasma amyloid levels increased as testosterone levels decreased. Discontinuation of treatment resulted in improved memory but not visuo-spatial abilities. One of the possible protective mechanisms of action of testosterone would be through its conversion into estradiol (E2), the most potent estrogen that could exert protective effects on the brain structures in the aging patient.

To date, trials of testosterone therapy in men to evaluate the effects of estradiol on measures of cognitive function and memory are relatively small, were of a relatively short duration, and have shown mixed results. Androgen supplementation in elderly hypogonadal men improves spatial cognition and verbal fluency, and in elderly men without dementia, it may reduce working memory errors. Intramuscular testosterone improved verbal and spatial memory and constructional abilities in nonhypogonadal men with mild cognitive impairment and Alzheimer disease. On the other hand, in a patient with Alzheimer disease, testosterone treatment seemed to improve quality of life and verbal memory without imprecise effects on several dimensions of cognition.

Therefore, although the evidence from studies is not uniform, lower FT levels seems to be associated with poorer outcomes on measures of cognitive function, particularly in older men, and testosterone therapy in hypogonadal men may have some benefit for cognitive performance.

EFFECT ON METABOLIC SYNDROME AND CARDIOVASCULAR RISK FACTORS

Testosterone has a positive effect on reducing the risk factors for metabolic syndrome and cardiovascular disease. The increased correlation between low testosterone levels and the severity of coronary artery disease may be related to the fact that low androgen levels are accompanied by an accumulation of abdominal visceral fat, which is known to be associated with increased cardiovascular risk factors[34] such as impaired glucose tolerance and non–insulin-dependent diabetes mellitus (syndrome X). Low endogenous testosterone concentrations are related to mortality due to cardiovascular disease and all causes.

There is a relationship between testosterone levels and body mass index (BMI), waist circumference, waist-hip ratio, serum leptin, LDL-C, triglyceride and fibrinogen levels, hypertension, and diabetes. At the same time, adipose tissue affects testosterone levels by increasing the aromatization of testosterone to estradiol, which provides negative feedback on the HPG axis, and by decreasing testosterone levels via a decrease in SHBG levels. Thus, adiposity potentially leads to hypogonadism, which itself promotes further adiposity.

Low testosterone concentrations are known to occur in association with type 2 diabetes. Prevalence in diabetic men has been estimated at 33% to 50%. There is no relation between the degree of hyperglycemia and testosterone concentration. Prostate-specific antigen (PSA) is significantly lower in type 2 diabetics, and this is related to their lower plasma testosterone concentrations.[35] Low testosterone concentrations predict the development of type 2 diabetes. Testosterone may also suppress insulin resistance independent of its effects on adiposity. In addition, diet and exercise increased testosterone levels in hypogonadal men with metabolic syndrome and newly diagnosed type 2 diabetes.

The effect of androgen replacement in elderly men on LDL-C and HDL-C is controversial. The relationship between testosterone and HDL is confounded by the fact that both HDL and testosterone levels are inversely related to BMI. Data from the MMAS have demonstrated that low total or FT levels correlate with low HDL-C levels. TRT in men with hypogonadism has little effect on serum concentrations of total cholesterol and LDL-C. HDL-C levels decrease in patients on oral testosterone therapy but not when given as a transdermal gel to hypogonadal men. In a meta-analysis of 10 studies of intramuscular testosterone esters and plasma lipids in hypo-gonadal men, a small, dose-dependent decrease was seen in total cholesterol, LDL, and HDL levels.[36] The mechanism of decrease in lipid levels might be related to the decrease in the visceral abdominal fat mass under the influence of androgens, which inhibit lipoprotein lipase activity and increase lipolysis with improvement of insulin sensitivity and mobilization of triglycerides from abdominal fat tissue. Supraphysiolog-ical testosterone levels induce an increase in LDL-C and a decrease of HDL-C levels and may increase the risk of cardiovascular disease.

Testosterone treatment in elderly patients with chronic heart failure might improve insulin sensitivity and various cardiorespiratory and muscular outcomes. The adminis-tration of testosterone in physiologic concentration increases coronary blood flow in patients with coronary heart disease. Transdermal TRT was found to be beneficial for men with chronic stable angina because they had greater angina-free exercise tolerance than placebo-treated controls. However, no consistent relationship between the levels of FT or total testosterone levels and coronary atherosclerosis has been observed in men undergoing coronary angiography.

IMPROVING ANEMIA

Endogenous androgens are known to stimulate erythropoiesis and increase reticulo-cyte count, blood hemoglobin levels, and bone marrow erythropoietic activity.[37] Anemia is a frequent finding in men with hypogonadism and in men on antiandrogenic therapy.[38] Testosterone deficiency results in a 10% to 20% decrease in the blood hemoglobin concentration, which can result in anemia. The main androgen involve-ment in the mechanism of normal hematopoiesis is thought to involve direct stimulation of renal production of erythropoietin by testosterone, which is more pronounced in older men, an effect that may be independent of erythropoietin and transferrin receptor levels.[39] Moreover, the latter may also act directly on erythropoietic stem cells.

RISKS OF TRT

The risks of TRT depend on age, life circumstances, and other medical conditions. Potential risks for TRT in elderly men are summarized in **Box 3**.

THE PROSTATE AND TRT

In aging men with LOH, TRT may normalize serum androgen levels but seems to have little effect on prostate tissue androgen levels and cellular functions and causes no significant adverse effects on the prostate. At present, there is no conclusive evidence that testosterone therapy increases the risk of prostate cancer or benign prostatic hyperplasia (BPH).

BPH

With aging, some men experience an exacerbation of BPH symptoms, predominantly lower urinary tract symptoms (LUTS), because of urinary outflow obstruction. The testosterone dependency of BPH has been known for a long time. Testosterone supplements increase prostate volume with eventually mild increase in PSA levels in old men. Although a meta-analysis showed that the total number of prostate events combined was significantly greater in testosterone-treated men than in placebo-treated men, most events are because of prostate biopsy. At the same time, many

---

Box 3
Potential risks for TRT in elderly men

Stimulate growth of prostate cancer and breast cancer

Worsen symptoms of benign prostatic hypertrophy

Cause liver toxicity and liver tumor

Cause gynecomastia

Cause erythrocytosis

Cause testicular atrophy and infertility

Cause skin diseases

Cause or exacerbate sleep apnea

---

studies have failed to show significant exacerbation of voiding symptoms attributable to BPH during testosterone supplementation. Complications such as urinary retention have not occurred at higher rates than in controls receiving placebo and there has been no difference in the urine flow rates, postvoiding residual urine volumes, and prostate voiding symptoms with patients receiving treatment in these studies. The poor correlation between prostate volume and urinary symptoms explain this illogicality. There are no compelling data to suggest that testosterone treatment exacerbates LUTS or promotes acute urinary retention. However, severe LUTS, because of BPH, represents a relative contraindication, which is no longer applicable after successful treatment of lower urinary tract obstruction. Patients needs to be made aware that there might be increased voiding symptoms during treatment.

PROSTATE CANCER

Prostate cancer is well known to be, in most cases, an androgen-sensitive disease, and androgen replacement therapy in patients with prostate cancer is an absolute contraindication. The prevalence of prostate cancer in many patients receiving TRT was similar to that in the general population.[40] So far, there is no compelling evidence that testosterone has a causative role in prostate cancer. There is, however, unequivocal evidence that testosterone can stimulate growth and aggravate symptoms in men with locally advanced and metastatic prostate cancer. A fuller explanation may be that prostate cancer is very sensitive to changes in serum testosterone levels when at low concentrations but is insensitive at higher concentrations because of saturation of the androgen receptors. Men successfully treated for prostate cancer and diagnosed with hypogonadism are candidates for testosterone replacement after a prudent interval if there is no clinical or laboratory evidence of residual cancer.[41] In addition, no effect was found of TRT on PSA levels, and the change in PSA levels was not influenced by the mode of TRT, patient age, or baseline levels of PSA or testosterone.

In summary, there is no convincing evidence that the normalization of serum testosterone levels in men with prostate problems and low levels is deleterious. TRT can be cautiously considered in selected hypogonadal men treated with curative intent for prostate and without evidence of active disease.

LIVER PROBLEMS

Benign and malignant hepatic tumors, intrahepatic cholestasis, hepatotoxicity, and liver failure have been reported with TRT. These unfavorable hepatic effects do not seem to be associated with transdermal or intramuscular injections. Therefore, use of oral forms of testosterone, with the exception of TU, is discouraged. Other liver abnormalities associated with TRT include peliosis hepatis, hepatocellular adenoma, and carcinoma.

SLEEP APNEA

Sleep apnea was worse in men with hypogonadism treated with testosterone. In contrast, in a recent meta-analysis, the frequency of sleep apnea did not differ between testosterone and placebo-treated men. Physicians should inquire symptoms, such as excessive daytime sleepiness and witnessed apnea during sleep by a partner, and if indicated, polysomnography should be performed.

ERYTHROCYTOSIS

There is a correlation between high testosterone levels and high hemoglobin levels. Erythrocytosis is a common adverse effect of testosterone administration. Testosterone-treated men were almost 4 times more likely to have a hematocrit greater than 50%. Erythrocytosis can develop during testosterone treatment, especially in older men treated with injectable testosterone preparations. The elevation in hemoglobin above certain levels may have a greater overall mortality and cardiovascular mortality, particularly in elderly, because the increase in blood viscosity can exacerbate vascular disease in the coronary, cerebrovascular, or peripheral vascular circulations, especially in people with other diseases that cause secondary polycythemia, such as COPD. Testosterone dosage correlates with the incidence of erythrocytosis, and polycythemia is mostly related to supraphysiological levels.

Periodic hematologic assessment is indicated (ie, before treatment, at 3 to 4 months and 12 months in the first year of treatment, and then annually thereafter). Although it is not yet clear what critical threshold is desirable, dose adjustment and/or periodic phlebotomy may be necessary to keep hematocrit les than 52% to 55%.

OTHER SIDE EFFECTS OF TRT

Supraphysiological doses of androgens may cause decreased testicular size, acne, and azoospermia. The decrease in testicular size and compromised fertility during TRT occur because of the down regulation of gonadotropins. It is related to aromatization of testosterone into estradiol in peripheral fat and muscle tissues. Even the ratio of estradiol to testosterone usually remains normal. It occurs especially with testosterone enanthate or cypionate. Dose adjustment may be necessary. Gynecomastia is another benign complication of testosterone treatment. Testosterone is anabolic, and it causes some nitrogen, sodium, and water retention. Edema may be worsened in patients with preexisting cardiac, renal, or hepatic disease. Hypertension has rarely been reported.

SYMPTOM RELIEF

The time course of the effects of testosterone replacement is variable. Once testosterone levels are restored to a stable normal range, there is an improvement in libido, sexual function, mood and energy levels, insulin resistance, and fat-free mass relatively early in the course of treatment. The reduction in fat body mass and an increase in LBM and an improvement in BMD at the hip and spine started after a period between 6 and 24 months.

MONITORING PATIENTS ON TESTOSTERONE REPLACEMENT

Patients who are treated with testosterone should be monitored to determine that normal serum testosterone concentrations are being achieved. If the patient has primary hypogonadism, normalization of the serum LH concentration should also be used to judge the adequacy of the testosterone dose, no matter which testosterone preparation is used. They should be monitored for both desirable and undesirable effects.

Patients should be monitored for signs of edema, gynecomastia, sleep apnea, LUTS, and low BMD. Laboratory parameters should be monitored before and during treatment. There are clinical practice guidelines from the Endocrine Society for monitoring patients receiving TRT. Testosterone level, digital rectal examination (DRE), PSA levels, hematocrit, BMD, lipids, and liver function tests should be checked at baseline, and the patient should be evaluated at 3 and 6 months after treatment starts and then annually to assess whether symptoms have responded to treatment and whether the patient is suffering from any adverse effects. If hematocrit is more than 54%, therapy should be stopped until hematocrit decreases to a safe level, the patient should be evaluated for hypoxia and sleep apnea, and therapy should be reinitiated with a reduced dose. The BMD of lumbar spine and/or femoral neck should be measured at baseline every 1 to 2 years of testosterone therapy in hypogonadal men with osteoporosis or low-trauma fracture.

Testosterone levels should be monitored 3 months after initiation of testosterone therapy. A midmorning total serum testosterone level should be obtained. A target range of 400 to 500 ng/dL (14.0–17.5 nmol/L) for older men is suggested. However, if there is no symptomatic response, higher levels may be necessary. For injectable testosterone, the serum level can be measured between injections. For men treated with a transdermal testosterone patch, the serum level should be measured 3 to 12 hours after patch application. In patients receiving buccal testosterone tablets, the serum level should be measured immediately before application of a fresh system. Patients on testosterone gel may have levels checked anytime after at least 1 week of therapy.[42] In all cases, BT levels should also be monitored because testosterone therapy lowers SHBG.

For patients with BPH, LUTS should be assessed by the International Prostate Symptom Score (IPSS). For prostate cancer, DRE and measurement of serum PSA levels should be performed before initiating testosterone replacement, 3 months after initiation of treatment, and then in accordance with evidence-based guidelines for prostate cancer screening, depending on the age and race of the patient. All men who present for TRT should undergo prostate biopsy if they have an abnormal PSA level or an abnormal result on DRE with low threshold to do or repeat prostate biopsy if the PSA level or DRE changes. The American Urological Association suggests obtaining urologic consultation for any of the following: an abnormal DRE result, PSA levels exceeding 2.5 ng/mL in men younger than 60 years or 4 ng/mL in men older than 60 years, and a velocity change of 0.75 ng/mL or greater in a year.[43]

The use of testosterone preparations should be discussed with the patients, and the patients should be closely monitored for efficacy and toxicities. Failure to benefit from clinical manifestations should result in discontinuation of treatment for libido and sexual function, muscle function, and improved body fat after 3 months; andfor BMD after a longer interval. Further investigation for other causes of symptoms is then mandatory.[42]

PRECAUTIONS AND CONTRAINDICATIONS TO TRT

Health care providers must rule out contraindications to treatment before starting TRT. The presence of a clinical prostatic carcinoma is an absolute contraindication for hormone replacement therapy (HRT) and should be carefully excluded by PSA levels, rectal examination, and, eventually, biopsy before starting any therapy.[42] There is also no clear recommendation for men successfully treated for prostate cancer who would be potential candidates for testosterone substitution after a prudent interval if there is no clinical or laboratory evidence of residual cancer.[42]

Breast cancer as well as prolactinoma are contraindications for TRT because their growth may be stimulated by HRT. Very high risk of serious adverse outcomes, undiagnosed prostate nodules or indurations, unexplained PSA level elevation, erythrocytosis (hematocrit >50%), severe LUTS with BPH with an IPSS greater than 19, unstable congestive heart failure (class III or IV), and untreated obstructive sleep apnea are considered as moderate to high risk factors for potential adverse outcomes.[44]

SUMMARY AND RECOMMENDATION

LOH is a common condition in the men, but it is still underdiagnosed and undertreated. The diagnosis should be made only in men with consistent symptoms and signs and unequivocally low serum testosterone levels. The symptoms in the elderly have a complex origin. It may be reasonably assumed that the age-associated decrease in testosterone levels is in part responsible for the symptoms of aging. In the absence of known pituitary or testicular disease, the authors suggest testosterone therapy only for older men with low serum testosterone concentrations and clinically important symptoms of androgen deficiency. The benefits and risks of testosterone therapy must be clearly discussed with the patient, and assessment of the major risk factors must be before commencing testosterone treatment. The major contraindication for androgen supplementation is the presence of breast or prostate cancer. Response to testosterone treatment should be assessed. If treatment is undertaken, the patient should be screened before treatment and monitored during treatment for evidence of testosterone-dependent diseases. The target serum testosterone concentration in older men should be lower than that for younger men, for example, 300 to 400 ng/dL, rather than 500 to 600 ng/dL, to minimize the potential risk of testosterone-dependent diseases.[42,45]

If there is no improvement of symptoms and signs, treatment should be discontinued and the patient investigated for other possible causes of the clinical presentations. Many questions in the treatment of hypogonadism remain unanswered, and there is a need for large clinical trials to assess the long-term benefits and risks of TRT in older men with LOH.

REFERENCES

1. Araujo AB, Esche GR, Kupelian V, et al. Prevalence of symptomatic androgen deficiency in men. J Clin Endocrinol Metab 2007;92:4241–7.
2. Araujo A, Kupelian V, Page ST, et al. Sex steroids and all-cause mortality and cause-specific mortality in men. Arch Intern Med 2007;167:1252–60.
3. Morley JE, Kaiser FE, Perry HM, et al. Longitudinal changes in testosterone, luteinizing hormone, and follicle-stimulating hormone in healthy older men. Metabolism 1997;46:410–3.
4. Matsumoto AM. Andropause: clinical implications of the decline in serum testosterone levels with aging in men. J Gerontol A Biol Sci Med Sci 2002;57A:M76–99.
5. Gray A, Feldman HA, McKinlay JB, et al. Age, disease, and changing sex hormone levels in middle-aged men: results of the Massachusetts Male Aging Study. J Clin Endocrinol Metab 1991;73:1016–25.

6. Travison TG, Shackelton R, Araujo AB, et al. The natural history of symptomatic androgen deficiency in men: onset, progression, and spontaneous remission. J Am Geriatr Soc 2008;56:831–9.
7. Morley JE, Melmed S. Gonadal dysfunction in systematic disorders. Metabolism 1979;28:1051–73.
8. Wang C, Nieschlag E, Swerdloff R, et al. Investigation, treatment, and monitoring of late-onset hypogonadism in males: ISA, ISSAM, EAU, EAA, and ASA recommendations. J Androl 2009;30:1–9.
9. Morley JE, Perry HM III, Patrick P, et al. Validation of salivary testosterone as a screening test for male hypogonadism. Aging Male 2006;9:165–9.
10. Schubert M, Minnemann T, Hubler D, et al. Intramuscular testosterone undecanoate: pharmacokinetic aspects of a novel testosterone formulation during long-term treatment of men with hypogonadism. J Clin Endocrinol Metab 2004; 89:5429–34.
11. Dobs AS, Meikle AW, Arver S, et al. Pharmacokinetics, efficacy, and safety of a permeation-enhanced testosterone transdermal system in comparison with bi-weekly injections of testosterone enanthate for the treatment of hypogonadal men. J Clin Endocrinol Metab 1999;84:3469–78.
12. Wang C, Swerdloff R, Kipnes M, et al. New testosterone buccal system (Striant) delivers physiological testosterone levels: pharmacokinetics study in hypogonadal men. J Clin Endocrinol Metab 2004;89:3821–9.
13. Handelsman DJ. Clinical pharmacology of testosterone pellet implants. In: Nieschlag E, Behre HM, editors. Testosterone action deficiency substitution. 2nd edition. Heidelberg: Springer; 1998. p. 349–64.
14. Banks WA, Morley JE, Niehoff ML, et al. Delivery of testosterone to the brain by intranasal administration: comparison to intravenous testosterone. J Drug Target 2009;17:91–7.
15. Hajjar RR, Kaiser FE, Morley JE. Outcomes of long-term testosterone replacement in older hypogonadal males: a retrospective analysis. J Clin Endocrinol Metab 1997;82:3793–6.
16. Greco EA, Spera G, Aversa A. Combining testosterone and PDE5 inhibitors in erectile dysfunction: basic rationale and clinical evidences. Eur Urol 2006;50: 940–7.
17. Tivesten A, Moverare-Skrtic S, Chagin A, et al. Additive protective effects of estrogen and androgen treatment on trabecular bone in ovariectomized rats. J Bone Miner Res 2004;19:1833–9.
18. Davey RA, Morris HA. Effects of estradiol and dihydrotestosterone on osteoblast gene expression in osteopenic ovariectomized rats. J Bone Miner Metab 2005; 23:212–8.
19. Michael H, Härkönen PL, Väänänen HK, et al. Estrogen and testosterone use different cellular pathways to inhibit osteoclastogenesis and bone resorption. J Bone Miner Res 2005;20(12):2224–32.
20. Tracz MJ, Sideras K, Bolon ER. Clinical review: testosterone use in men and its effects on bone health. A systematic review and meta-analysis of randomized placebo-controlled trials. J Clin Endocrinol Metab 2006;91(6):2011–6.
21. Krasnoff JB, Basaria S, Pencina MJ, et al. Free testosterone levels are associated with mobility limitation and physical performance in community-dwelling men: the Framingham Offspring Study. J Clin Endocrinol Metab 2010;95(6):2790–9.
22. Sinha-Hikim I, Cornford M, Gaytan H, et al. Effects of testosterone supplementation on skeletal muscle fibre hypertrophy and satellite cells in community-dwelling older man. J Clin Endocrinol Metab 2006;91:3024–33.

23. Harman SM, Blackman MR. The effects of growth hormone and sex steroid on lean body mass, fat mass, muscle strength, cardiovascular endurance and adverse events in healthy elderly women and men. Horm Res 2003;60:121–4.
24. Breuer B, Trungold S, Martucci C, et al. Relationship of sex hormone levels to dependence of daily living in the frail elderly. Maturitas 2001;39:147–59.
25. Hyde Z, Flicker L, Almeida OP, et al. Low free testosterone predicts frailty in older men: the health in men study. J Clin Endocrinol Metab 2010;95(7):3165–72.
26. Azad N, Pitales S, Barres WE, et al. Testosterone treatment enhances regional brain perfusion in hypogonadal men. J Clin Endocrinol Metab 2003;88:3064–8.
27. Barrett-Connor E, Von Mühlen DG, Kritz-Silverstein D. Bioavailable testosterone and depressed mood in older men: the Rancho Bernardo study. J Clin Endocrinol Metab 1999;84:573–7.
28. Haren MT, Wittert GA, Chapman IM, et al. Effect of oral testosterone undecanoate on visuospatial cognition, mood and quality of life in elderly men with low–normal gonadal status. Maturitas 2005;50:124–33.
29. Seidman SN, Rabkin JG. Testosterone replacement therapy for hypogonadal men with SSRI-refractory depression. J Affect Disord 1998;48:157–61.
30. Greenlee MW. Human cortical areas underlying the perception of optic flow: brain imaging studies. Int Rev Neurobiol 2000;44:269–92.
31. Hogervorst E, Bandelow S, Combrinck M, et al. Low free testosterone is an independent risk factor for Alzheimer's disease. Exp Gerontol 2004;39:1633–9.
32. Thilers PP, Macdonald SW, Herlitz A. The association between endogenous free testosterone and cognitive performance: a population-based study in 35–90 year-old men and women. Psychoneuroendocrinology 2006;31:565–76.
33. Yonker JE, Eriksson E, Nilsson L-G, et al. Negative association of testosterone on spatial visualisation in 35 to 80 year old men. Cortex 2006;42:376–86.
34. Kannell WB, Cupples LA, Ramaswami R, et al. Regional obesity and the risk of coronary disease: the Framingham Study. J Clin Epidemiol 1991;44:183–90.
35. Dhindsa S, Upadhyay M, Viswanathan P, et al. Relationship of prostate-specific antigen to age and testosterone in men with type 2 diabetes mellitus. Endocr Pract 2008;14:1000–5.
36. Whitsel EA, Boyko EJ, Matsumoto AM, et al. Intramuscular testosterone esters and plasma lipids in hypogonadal men: a meta-analysis. Am J Med 2001;111:261–9.
37. Claustres M, Sultan C. Androgen and erythropoiesis: evidence for an androgen receptor in erythroblasts from human bone marrow cultures. Horm Res 1988;29:17.
38. Ferruci L, Maggio M, Bandinelli S, et al. Low testosterone levels and the risk of anemia in older men and women. Arch Intern Med 2006;166:1380–8.
39. Coviello AD, Kaplan B, Lakshman KM, et al. Effects of graded doses of testosterone on erythropoiesis in health young and older men. J Clin Endocrinol Metab 2008;93:914–9.
40. Coward RM, Simhan J, Carson CC 3rd. Prostate-specific antigen changes and prostate cancer in hypogonadal men treated with. testosterone replacement therapy. BJU Int 2009;103(9):1179–83.
41. Khera M, Lipshultz LI. The role of testosterone replacement therapy following radical prostatectomy. Urol Clin North Am 2007;34:549–53.
42. Bhasin S, Cunningham GR, Hayes FJ, et al. Testosterone therapy in men with androgen deficiency syndromes: an Endocrine Society clinical practice guideline. J Clin Endocrinol Metab 2010;95(6):2536–59.

43. Carroll P, Albertsen PC, Babaian RJ, et al. Prostate-specific antigen best practice statement: 2009 update. New York (NY): American Urological Association; 2009.
44. Wang C, Nieschlag E, Swerdloff R, et al. ISA< ISSAM, EAU, EAAS and ASA recommendations: investigation, treatment and monitoring of late-onset hypogonadism in males. Int J Impot Res 2009;21:1–8.
45. Bhasin S, Cunningham GR, Hayes FJ, et al. Testosterone therapy in adult men with androgen deficiency syndromes: an endocrine society clinical practice guideline. J Clin Endocrinol Metab 2006;91:1995–2010.

Hypertension: How Does Management Change with Aging?

Milta O. Little, DO

KEYWORDS

• Hypertension • Aging • Elderly • Orthostatic • Pharmacologic

Age is a question of mind over matter. If you don't mind, it doesn't matter.
– Mark Twain

Aging is an inevitable part of life and brings along two inconvenient events: physiologic decline and disease states.[1] Practitioners who care for elderly patients note a higher incidence of hypertension in this population, in part due to age-related cardiovascular changes. According to the Seventh Report of the Joint National Committee on Prevention, Detection, Evaluation, and Treatment of High Blood Pressure (JNC-7), "Hypertension occurs in more than two-thirds of individuals after age 65. This is also the population with the lowest rates of BP control. Treatment recommendations for older people with hypertension, including those who have isolated systolic hypertension, should follow the same principles outlined for the general care of hypertension."[2] Although the JNC-7 recommendations follow conventional practice, many have questioned the safety and value of aggressive blood pressure control in elderly patients. When does hypertension cause harm in people older than 65 years? What is "ideal blood pressure" in the elderly? When do the risks of lowering blood pressure outweigh the potential benefits? What is the best treatment regimen? This article attempts to answer those questions through a review of aging physiology, the classification of hypertension, the relevance of orthostatic hypotension, nonpharmacologic and pharmacologic management of hypertension, and finally, when to consider secondary hypertension.

AGING PHYSIOLOGY

Before thirty, men seek disease; after thirty, diseases seek men.
– Chinese Proverb

No funding support was used in the writing of this article.

The author has nothing to disclose.

Division of Gerontology and Geriatric Medicine, Department of Internal Medicine, Saint Louis University School of Medicine, 1402 South Grand Boulevard, Room M238, St Louis, MO 63139, USA

E-mail address: mlittle6@slu.edu

Med Clin N Am 95 (2011) 525–537

doi:10.1016/j.mcna.2011.02.002

Age-related anatomic and physiologic changes occur independently of disease; however, these changes predispose the individual to disease. Understanding the cardiovascular changes that occur with aging is the first step to understanding hypertension in the elderly. **Box 1** outlines the relevant cardiovascular changes associated with aging.

Box 1
Effects of aging on cardiovascular structure and function

Cardiac

    Increases with aging:

        Heart weight

        Collagen in cross-linking

        Degeneration of sympathetic nerve supply

        End diastolic filling[a]

        Release of natriuretic peptides

    Decreases with aging:

        Early diastolic filling

        Chronotropic response to β-adrenergic stimuli[a]

        Inotropic response to β-adrenergic stimuli[a]

        Cardiac relaxation

        Peak cardiac output to maximal effort

    No change with aging:

        Ejection fraction

        Stroke volume

        Cardiac output[a]

Vascular

    Increases with aging:

        Artery wall thickness[a]

        Subendothelial collagen

        Total peripheral resistance

        Endothelial permeability

        Inflammatory markers/mediators

    Decreases with aging:

        Elastin

        Artery distensibility[a]

        Endothelial nitric oxide release

        β-Adrenergic-mediated vasodilatation

[a] See additional comments in text for relevance to blood pressure regulation.
Data from Ferrari AU, Radaelli A, Centola M. Invited review: aging and the cardiovascular system. J Appl Physiol 2003;95:2591–7.

With age, cardiac output remains unchanged at rest, due to preserved ejection fraction and stroke volume. Despite the blunting of heart rate and contractile response during exercise, cardiac output is maintained through the Frank-Starling mechanism by increasing end-systolic and end-diastolic volume. The latter compensatory mechanism reflects diastolic changes that often lead to heart failure.[3]

In addition, prolonged ejection time and the age-related vascular changes of hypertrophy and stiffness predispose to increased systolic and pulse pressures (PP), which are often described in older people. Isolated systolic hypertension (ISH) and widened PP lead to increased workload on the heart, decreased coronary perfusion during diastole, and higher pressures to other end organs, predisposing to myocardial infarction, stroke, and renal failure.[4] Although there is an association between age and increase in blood pressure, there is evidence that it does not have to be an essential part of human biology. For example, in industrialized societies systolic pressure rises progressively with age and if individuals live long enough, nearly all develop hypertension.[5] Also, diastolic pressure rises until the age of 50 years and decreases thereafter, producing a progressive increase in pulse pressure.[5] In less industrialized societies where consumption of calories and salt is low, blood pressures remain low and do not increase with age.[6]

Finally, blunted baroreceptor response occurs with aging, which may impair moment-to-moment vascular adjustments, causing postural or postprandial hypotension and excessive blood pressure peaks. Taken together, the age-related changes of predisposition to diastolic heart failure, increased systolic and pulse pressures, and baroreceptor alterations affect the management of hypertension in the elderly.

CLASSIFICATION OF HYPERTENSION

One way to get high blood pressure is to go mountain climbing over molehills.
– Earl Wilson

Hypertension is defined by the JNC-7 as systolic blood pressure (SBP) greater than 140 and diastolic blood pressure (DBP) greater than 90, confirmed with 2 or more readings on at least 2 visits, multiple weeks apart.[2] This definition is derived from epidemiologic and drug trial outcome data.[7] Hypertension has long been recognized as an important treatable risk factor for stroke, myocardial infarction, heart failure, peripheral vascular disease, aortic dissection, atrial fibrillation, and end-stage kidney disease.[6] In the 1950s, DBP was thought to be the most important determinant of cardiovascular risk. Through major trials, such as the Framingham Heart Study and Multiple Risk Factor Intervention Trial (MRFIT), it was concluded that SBP and pulse pressure are better predictors of risk than DBP, particularly in older patients.[5]

Current recommendations by the JNC-7 for achieving blood pressure 140/90 mm Hg or less, or 130/80 mm Hg or less for patients with diabetes or chronic kidney disease[8] are based on prospective observational studies, which taken together demonstrate that for each 20 mm Hg decrease in SBP down to 115 mm Hg or 10 mm Hg decrease in DBP down to 75 mm Hg, there is an associated twofold reduction in vascular mortality risk in people older than 60 years.[9] This difference falls slightly in those older than 80; however, there is still nearly a one-third risk difference. Note that there is little or no evidence for the benefit of lowering blood pressure to below 115/75 in any age group.

A reanalysis of the Framingham all-cause and cardiovascular mortality data, which in the original article reported a direct linear relationship with increasing SBP and death, found no correlation in risk until the SBP reached the 80th percentile (correlating to a value of around 160) (**Fig. 1**). The investigators also note age-dependent

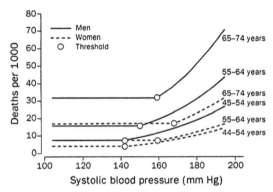

Fig. 1. Horizontal-logistic-spline fits from Framingham data. (*Reprinted from* Port S, Demer L, Jennrick R, et al. Systolic blood pressure and mortality. Lancet 2000;355:177.)

and sex-dependent differences, which indicate that older people and women can have higher SBP than younger people or men, respectively, without increased risk. This analysis challenges the traditional definition of hypertension and suggests that many people, particularly the elderly, are unnecessarily overtreated.[10]

The European Working Party on High Blood Pressure in the Elderly trial, which randomized people older than 60 years to active diuretic treatment or placebo, reported mortality based on blood pressure tertiles. In patients on active treatment, total, cardiovascular, and noncardiovascular mortality was lowest for the middle tertile, revealing a U-shaped mortality curve. In patients on placebo, the mortality curve was linear; however, the lowest SBP tertile was in the same range as the middle tertile of the active treatment group (approximately 150/88).[11]

Other studies, including the Helsinki Ageing Study[12] and the International Verapamil SR/Trandolapril Study (INVEST), also question the appropriateness of aggressive treatment in older people by reporting a J-shaped mortality curve with blood pressure control. The INVEST trial was designed to investigate two hypertension treatment strategies in patients with coronary artery disease. The study included a large number of individuals older than 80 years, and a secondary analysis of this group was performed to assess the effects of strict blood pressure control (**Fig. 2**).[13]

It is unclear whether the U-shaped or J-shaped mortality curves from these studies are attributable to severe end-stage disease alone or whether iatrogenesis plays a significant role. However, the data should cause one to be cautious in lowering blood pressures to below 130/70 in older patients, including those at high risk of adverse cardiovascular outcomes, and to consider changing hypertension goals with age and comorbid state.

SECONDARY HYPERTENSION

The older I get, the better I used to be!
– Lee Trevino

The majority of cases of high blood pressure are due to essential hypertension. However, it is important to consider an identifiable, correctable cause of hypertension, also known as secondary hypertension, especially when the patient requires multiple antihypertensive medications. A simple mnemonic to remember the causes of secondary hypertension was created by Edward Onusko: ABCDE (**Table 1**).

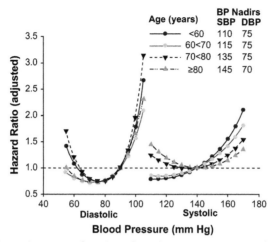

Fig. 2. Adjusted hazard ratio as a function of age (in 10-year increments). Reference systolic and diastolic blood pressure for hazard ratio: 10 and 90 mm Hg, respectively. The quadratic terms for both systolic and diastolic blood pressures were statistically significant in all age groups. (*From* Denardo SJ, Gong Y, Nichols WW, et al. Blood pressure and outcomes in very old hypertensive coronary artery disease patients: an INVEST substudy. Am J Med 2010;123:725.)

Ensuring accurate diagnosis of high blood pressure is very important in all patients, but particularly in patients at high risk of orthostatic hypotension and falls. It is critical to make certain that the blood pressure cuff is the correct size and that the pressure is measured with the patient standing in addition to sitting. Pseudohypertension is common in older people, and is caused by atherosclerotic and other vascular changes associated with aging. While people with pseudohypertension are at higher risk of cardiovascular disease, they are also likely to experience adverse effects of excessive blood pressure lowering. The Osler maneuver should be performed when pseudohypertension is considered, though it has low sensitivity and specificity. Finally, white-coat hypertension is also common in older people, and ambulatory blood pressure measurements are necessary to prevent overtreatment.[14]

Table 1
ABCDE: causes of secondary hypertension, mnemonic by Dr Edward Onusko

A	Accuracy of diagnosis obstructive sleep Apnea Aldosteronism (consider in any patient with low potassium)
B	renal artery Bruits (suggesting renal artery stenosis) Bad kidneys (renal parenchymal disease)
C	excess Catecholamines (pheochromocytoma, extreme stress) Coarctation of the aorta Cushing syndrome
D	Drugs (notably nonsteroidal anti-inflammatories, alcohol, estrogen, and decongestants) Diet
E	excess Erythropoietin Endocrine disorders (thyroid, parathyroid, and growth hormone abnormalities)

Data from Onusko E. Diagnosing secondary hypertension. Am Fam Physician 2003;67(1):67–4.

Evaluation of hypertension begins with a thorough history, including the Epworth Sleepiness Scale to screen for obstructive sleep apnea, a complete review of all prescription and over-the-counter medications, and a quantification of tobacco and alcohol ingestion. The physical examination should emphasize the cardiovascular system and include documentation of peripheral pulses, presence of bruits, and fundoscopic condition. Laboratory evaluations are ordered based on the results of the history and physical examination, but generally include a renal function panel, complete blood count, urinalysis, thyroid-stimulating hormone, and 12-lead electrocardiogram.[15] Treatment of secondary hypertension is primarily aimed at correcting the underlying cause along with the use of antihypertensive medications.

ORTHOSTATIC HYPOTENSION

Age does not diminish the extreme disappointment of having a scoop of ice cream fall from the cone.

– Jim Fiebig

Normal age-related cardiovascular changes and age-associated disease states predispose older adults to orthostatic hypotension (OH). The presence of postprandial and postural hypotension may not be readily apparent, and this is another reason to be cautious when managing hypertension in the elderly. OH is associated with multiple adverse outcomes, including recurrent falls[16] and increased vascular and all-cause mortality.[17] These studies also suggest that frail elderly are at the highest risk for the adverse consequences of OH. Standing blood pressures should be measured in every patient to exclude OH. In patients with hypertension and postural changes, anti-hypertensive should be titrated very slowly over several weeks and home blood pressures should be monitored frequently. Consider discontinuing other medications that may contribute to OH and employ nonpharmacologic interventions, such as avoiding a low sodium diet, straining, or rapid rising.[17]

Postprandial hypotension, caused by an increased release of the vasodilating calcitonin gene-related peptide following a meal, is also associated with falls and decreased survival.[18] In patients with recurrent syncope or falls, particularly in the morning, it is important to screen for postprandial hypotension, as this can be easily treated with α-glucosidase inhibitors, which slow the release of vasodilating hormones.[19]

NONPHARMACOLOGIC MANAGEMENT OF HYPERTENSION IN ELDERLY PATIENTS

I've been trying for some time to develop a lifestyle that doesn't require my presence.

– G.B. Trudeau

The JNC-7 recommends implementing lifestyle modifications when high blood pressures are first detected, regardless of the decision to begin medications. These modifications include weight reduction (results in a 5–20 mm Hg decrease in SBP per 10 kg loss), DASH eating plan (8–14 mm Hg decrease in SBP), dietary sodium reduction (2–8 mm Hg decrease in SBP), physical activity (4–9 mm Hg decrease in SBP), and moderate alcohol consumption (2–4 mm Hg decrease in SBP).[8] Most of the data supporting these recommendations are derived from trials with a paucity of older adults.

A randomized trial was completed in adults aged 60 to 80 years to assess the effects of weight loss and sodium restriction on blood pressure control and cardiovascular outcomes.[20] The Trial of Nonpharmacologic Interventions in the Elderly (TONE) enrolled seniors (mean age 66.5 years) with medication-controlled hypertension and randomized them to usual care versus sodium restriction (>1.8 gm/d) and/or weight loss (≥10 lb [4.5 kg]) with the help of nutritionists and exercise counselors. Whereas a significantly greater percentage of subjects in the intervention group were able to successfully withdraw from antihypertensive medications, there was no difference between groups in the rates of cardiovascular disease events.[20] Moreover, the mean reduction in blood pressure (−4.3/2) experienced in the sodium-restricted group was significantly different from usual care in those aged 60 to 69, but not those in the 70 to 80 age group.[21] Mortality data were not reported, which is important considering the evidence for poor outcomes with weight loss and very low salt intake in older people.[14,22]

Other nonpharmacologic interventions have been shown to be of benefit in lowering blood pressure by reducing arterial stiffness. As stated previously, arterial stiffness is a prominent age-related change that contributes to the development of hypertension in older people. Dietary measures that may ameliorate this arterial change include garlic powder (reported in a group of healthy people aged 50–80 who ingested 3–9 100-mg garlic tablets daily for an average of 7 years),[23] α-linoleic acid (reported with a daily intake of 20 g of flax oil-based margarine products for 4 weeks),[24] fish oil (based on a crossover study of 10 capsules of fish oil vs olive oil daily for 6 weeks),[25] and dietary isoflavins (as shown with regular intake of phytoestrogens).[26]

In older patients with hypertension, it is reasonable to recommend regular aerobic exercise, a diet rich in whole grains, fruits, and vegetables, and moderation of alcohol consumption. Caution must be taken when recommending diet restrictions or weight loss to older patients, especially those at risk for frailty or osteoporosis.[20]

PHARMACOLOGIC MANAGEMENT OF HYPERTENSION IN ELDERLY PATIENTS

If you're a person with a heart condition or hypertension, you're going to want a very good drug benefit.

– Ray Werntz

When lifestyle measures fail to lower blood pressure to goal, pharmacotherapy should be instituted. The choice of medication is affected by multiple factors, including cost, ease of administration (once daily is preferred), tolerability, and the patient's comorbid diseases. Another important consideration is polypharmacy. As more medications are added to the daily regimen, the number of drug interactions increases and adherence decreases. One observational study showed that 82% of patients on 6 or more medicines experienced a drug interaction.[27]

The safety and efficacy of multiple medication classes has been studied in elderly patients over the last 30 years. **Tables 2** and **3** summarize the results of 5 major trials involving older subjects. Note that for most trials, the goal and achieved blood pressures are higher than that recommended by JNC-7, while still showing a significant benefit of treatment.

A 2010 Cochrane review of 15 trials with mean age 63 to 84 years (average across trials 73.8 years) reported mortality and morbidity data based on age groups (≥60 and ≥80 years). The mean duration of the trials was 4.5 years (60 years and older) and 2.2 years (80 years and older). More than 70% of the trials used thiazide diuretics as first-line therapy. Cardiovascular morbidity was significantly reduced in all age groups. Overall, total (relative risk [RR] = 0.9, number needed to treat [NNT] = 84), cardiovascular (absolute risk reduction = 1.5%, NNT = 67), and cerebrovascular (RR = 0.66) mortality were all significantly reduced in the 60 and older group but not for the 80 and older group.[33]

Table 2
Characteristics of the 5 major trials on hypertension in the elderly

Major Hypertension Trials	Mean Age (y)	Mean Starting BP (mm Hg)	Goal BP (mm Hg)	Length of Follow-Up
EWPHE[11,28]	72	183/101	<160/90	7 y
SHEP[29]	72	170.3/76.6	For baseline SBP >180: goal SBP <160 For baseline SBP 160–179: reduction of >20 mm Hg	5 y
STOP-HTN 2[30]	76	Supine 194/98 Standing 187/101	<160/95	60 mo
ALLHAT[31]	67	145/83	<140/90 with lowest possible drug dose	Median 3.3 y
HYVET[32]	84 (range 80–105)	Sitting 173/91 Standing 168/88	<150/80	Median 1.8 y

Abbreviations: ALLHAT, Antihypertensive and Lipid-Lowering Treatment to Prevent Heart Attack Trial; EWPHE, European Working Party on High Blood Pressure in the Elderly; HYVET, Hypertension in the Very Elderly Trial; SHEP, Systolic Hypertension in the Elderly Program; STOP-HTN 2, Swedish Trial in Old Patients with Hypertension-2 Study.

The JNC-7 recommends a thiazide diuretic as initial drug therapy with consideration for angiotensin-converting enzyme inhibitors (ACEI), angiotensin receptor blockers (ARB), β-blockers, calcium channel blockers (CCB), or combination based on compelling indications or to reach goal.[8] Despite these recommendations and convincing evidence, thiazides remain underused.[34]

The evidence for the safety and efficacy of thiazide diuretics in preventing cardiovascular and renal disease is well established for all age groups, particularly the elderly (see **Table 3**).[35] Unfortunately, thiazide treatment is associated with an increase in blood glucose by as much as 5 to 10 mg/dL. This finding caused some concern about diuretic-induced diabetes; however, reanalysis of the ALLHAT (Antihypertensive and Lipid-Lowering Treatment to Prevent Heart Attack Trial) data indicates that new-onset diabetes associated with thiazides do not increase cardiovascular disease. In fact, thiazides remained unsurpassed in all clinical outcomes (cardiovascular and renal) compared with α-blockers, CCB, or ACEI.[36] Only the recent Avoiding Cardiovascular events through COMbination therapy in Patients LIving with Systolic Hypertension (ACCOMPLISH) trial favored the ACEI/CCB combination over the ACEI/thiazide combination. However, the hydrochlorothiazide dose used (12.5–25 mg/d) was half the dose used in other trials, indicating the need to titrate to higher doses.[35] Data support the following dosages of thiazides: hydrochlorothiazide 25 to 50 mg/d, chlorthalidone 12.5 to 25 mg/d, indapamide 2.5 mg/d.[35]

ACEI can also be considered for first-line or combination therapy, especially if another compelling indication is present such as diabetes, heart failure, postmyocardial infarction, or chronic kidney disease.[8] Patients with or at risk of sarcopenia may particularly benefit, as ACEI have been shown to improve muscle strength and walking speed in older hypertensive individuals.[37] Therefore, this group of antihypertensives may be a good first choice for the frail elderly.

Table 3
Summary of results from 5 major trials on hypertension in the elderly

Major Hypertension Trials	Medications Used	Mean Achieved BP (mm Hg)	Primary End Point
EWPHE[11,28]	HCTZ + triamterene or Placebo	Year 1: active 151/88, placebo 172/95 Year 7: active 148/85, placebo 167/90	Cerebrovascular mortality and morbidity 36% reduction in terminating events
SHEP[29]	Step 1: Chlorthalidone vs placebo Step 2: Atenolol or reserpine	Active treatment: 26 mm Hg lower Placebo: 15 mm Hg or lower	Total stroke Absolute 5-year risk reduction of 30 strokes/1000 patients (NNT = 33)
STOP-HTN 2[30]	Conventional (diuretics ± β-blockers) or ACE inhibitors or CCB	Decrease from baseline: Conventional treatment: 34.8/16.6 ACE inhibitor: 34.5/16.2 CCB: 34.5/17.5	Prevention of cardiovascular death No difference between groups
ALLHAT[31]	Chlorthalidone or Doxazosin	Year 1: chlorthalidone 137/79, doxazosin 140/79 Year 4: chlorthalidone 135/76, doxazosin 137/76	Composite of fatal CHD and nonfatal MI No difference between the 2 groups Stopped early due to 25% higher risk of combined CVD outcomes 2× risk of CHF in doxazosin group
HYVET[32]	Indapamide or Placebo	Decrease from baseline at 2 years: Active treatment 29.5/12.9 Placebo 14.5/6.8 Over 5 years, mean blood pressures in active treatment arm ranged from 140–150/75–90	Any stroke (fatal or nonfatal) 30% reduction (equivalent to preventing 1 stroke by treating 94 patients for 2 years) NNT 48 for 2 years

Abbreviations: ACE, angiotensin-converting enzyme; CCB, calcium channel blockers; CHD, coronary heart disease; CHF, congestive heart failure; CVD, cardiovascular disease; HCTZ, hydrochlorothiazide; MI, myocardial infarction; NNT, number needed to treat.

Box 2
Take-home points

Hypertension is a significant risk factor for cardiovascular morbidity and mortality in people older than 60 years

ISH and widened pulse pressure appear to be more important than diastolic hypertension

Very low blood pressure and OH are associated with increased mortality and should be checked for at every visit

Best evidence suggests adjusting hypertension goals with age, starting therapy when blood pressure is >160/90

When facing resistant hypertension, evaluate for a secondary cause using the ABCDE mnemonic

Medication tips:

Start low and go slow

Therapy should start with a thiazide diuretic (best evidence) or an ACEI

Use older medications and combination pills that are taken once a day to improve compliance

---

Beta-Blockers have an important role in patients with heart failure or postmyocardial infarction[27]; however, they should be used with caution in older patients. Multiple studies fail to show the benefit of β-blockers compared with placebo regarding cardiovascular mortality or coronary heart disease morbidity, even showing poorer outcomes when added to diuretics versus diuretics alone in one trial.[38] β-Blockers tend to be poorly tolerated in older people, probably because of their tendency to enhance the hemodynamic changes experienced with aging and to decrease exercise tolerance.[38] For these reasons, β-blockers should not be considered first-line antihypertensives and should be reserved for patients with a compelling reason for use.

CCB have been shown to lower blood pressure and prevent cardiovascular mortality, as have diuretics and ACEI.[30] CCB are typically considered second-line agents because of the increased risk of constipation, edema, and heart failure.[27,30] Data from the ALLHAT trial indicate that alpha-blockers should be avoided unless needed for treatment of benign prostatic hypertrophy.[27,31]

SUMMARY

Based on the current available data, it is reasonable to recommend lifestyle changes and pharmacotherapy for patients older than 60 years, whose blood pressures are greater than 160/90, to achieve a blood pressure goal of 130–150s/70–80s. Secondary hypertension should be considered and evaluated using the ABCDE mnemonic. Exercise is an important component in managing hypertension in the elderly; however, weight loss and sodium restriction should be used with caution and be limited to more robust patients. The medication regimen depends on several factors, but should start with a thiazide diuretic (best evidence) or ACEI. Alpha-blockers and beta-blockers are not recommended as first-line drugs and should be used with caution in the elderly. Electrolytes and renal function should be monitored on drug therapy, and orthostatic blood pressure assessed at each visit. Medications should be started at the lowest dose possible and titrated slowly (the "start low and go slow" principle). It is critically important to remember cost and ease of administration. Whenever possible, generic and combination medications that are taken once daily should be used to improve compliance. Older medications typically tend to be less expensive and have the most efficacy and safety data available, making them more reliable for use in older patients. In conclusion, hypertension is a significant contributor to cardiovascular morbidity and mortality in the elderly and, if appropriately treated, can improve outcomes (**Box 2**). However, best evidence suggests that treatment goals ought to be adjusted with increasing age and disease state.

ACKNOWLEDGMENTS

The author wishes to acknowledge the help of Dr Joshua William Little in commenting on an early draft of the article.

REFERENCES

1. Abrass IB. The biology and physiology of aging. West J Med 1990;153(6):641–5.
2. Hyman DJ, Pavlik VN. Characteristics of patients with uncontrolled hypertension in the United States. N Engl J Med 2001;345(7):479–86.
3. Ferrari AU, Radaelli A, Centola M. Invited review: aging and the cardiovascular system. J Appl Physiol 2003;95(6):2591–7.
4. Lim MA, Townsend RR. Arterial compliance in the elderly: its effect on blood pressure measurement and cardiovascular outcomes. Clin Geriatr Med 2009;25(2): 191–205.
5. Mosley WJ 2nd, Lloyd-Jones DM. Epidemiology of hypertension in the elderly. Clin Geriatr Med 2009;25(2):179–89.
6. Goldman L, editor. Goldman's Cecil medicine. 23rd edition. Philadelphia: Saunders Elsevier; 2007. p. 119–24. Chapter 23.
7. Cushman WC. JNC-7 guidelines: are they still relevant? Curr Hypertens Rep 2007;9(5):380–6.
8. Chobanian AV, Bakris GL, Black HR, et al. The seventh report of the joint national committee on prevention, detection, evaluation, and treatment of high blood pressure: the JNC 7 report. JAMA 2003;289(19):2560–72.
9. Lewington S, Clarke R, Qizilbash N, et al. Age-specific relevance of usual blood pressure to vascular mortality: a meta-analysis of individual data for one million adults in 61 prospective studies. Lancet 2002;360(9349):1903–13.
10. Port S, Demer L, Jennrich R, et al. Systolic blood pressure and mortality. Lancet 2000;355(9199):175–80.
11. Staessen J, Bulpitt C, Clement D, et al. Relation between mortality and treated blood pressure in elderly patients with hypertension: report of the European Working Party on High Blood Pressure in the Elderly. BMJ 1989;298(6687): 1552–6.
12. Hakala SM, Tilvis RS, Strandberg TE. Blood pressure and mortality in an older population. A 5-year follow-up of the Helsinki Ageing Study. Eur Heart J 1997; 18(6):1019–23.
13. Denardo SJ, Gong Y, Nichols WW, et al. Blood pressure and outcomes in very old hypertensive coronary artery disease patients: an INVEST substudy. Am J Med 2010;123(8):719–26.
14. Morley JE. Hypertension: is it overtreated in the elderly? J Am Med Dir Assoc 2010;11(3):147–52.
15. Onusko E. Diagnosing secondary hypertension. Am Fam Physician 2003;67(1): 67–74.
16. Ooi WL, Hossain M, Lipsitz LA. The association between orthostatic hypotension and recurrent falls in nursing home residents. Am J Med 2000;108(2):106–11.

17. Mukai S, Lipsitz LA. Orthostatic hypotension. Clin Geriatr Med 2002;18(2): 253–68.
18. Fisher AA, Davis MW, Srikusalanukul W, et al. Postprandial hypotension predicts all-cause mortality in older, low-level care residents. J Am Geriatr Soc 2005;53(8): 1313–20.
19. Shibao C, Gamboa A, Diedrich A, et al. Acarbose, an alpha-glucosidase inhibitor, attenuates postprandial hypotension in autonomic failure. Hypertension 2007; 50(1):54–61.
20. Whelton PK, Appel LJ, Espeland MA, et al. Sodium reduction and weight loss in the treatment of hypertension in older persons: a randomized controlled trial of nonpharmacologic interventions in the elderly (TONE). TONE Collaborative Research Group. JAMA 1998;279(11):839–46.
21. Appel LJ, Espeland MA, Easter L, et al. Effects of reduced sodium intake on hypertension control in older individuals: results from the Trial of Nonpharmacologic Interventions in the Elderly (TONE). Arch Intern Med 2001;161(5):685–93.
22. Cohen HW, Hailpern SM, Alderman MH. Sodium intake and mortality follow-up in the Third National Health and Nutrition Examination Survey (NHANES III). J Gen Intern Med 2008;23(9):1297–302.
23. Breithaupt-Grogler K, Ling M, Boudoulas H, et al. Protective effect of chronic garlic intake on elastic properties of aorta in the elderly. Circulation 1997;96(8): 2649–55.
24. Nestel PJ, Pomeroy SE, Sasahara T, et al. Arterial compliance in obese subjects is improved with dietary plant n-3 fatty acid from flaxseed oil despite increased LDL oxidizability. Arterioscler Thromb Vasc Biol 1997;17(6):1163–70.
25. McVeigh GE, Brennan GM, Cohn JN, et al. Fish oil improves arterial compliance in non-insulin-dependent diabetes mellitus. Arterioscler Thromb 1994;14(9): 1425–9.
26. van der Schouw YT, Pijpe A, Lebrun CE, et al. Higher usual dietary intake of phytoestrogens is associated with lower aortic stiffness in postmenopausal women. Arterioscler Thromb Vasc Biol 2002;22(8):1316–22.
27. Cooney D, Pascuzzi K. Polypharmacy in the elderly: focus on drug interactions and adherence in hypertension. Clin Geriatr Med 2009;25(2):221–33.
28. Amery A, Birkenhager W, Brixko P, et al. Mortality and morbidity results from the European Working Party on High Blood Pressure in the Elderly trial. Lancet 1985; 1(8442):1349–54.
29. Prevention of stroke by antihypertensive drug treatment in older persons with isolated systolic hypertension. Final results of the Systolic Hypertension in the Elderly Program (SHEP). SHEP Cooperative Research Group. JAMA 1991; 265(24):3255–64.
30. Hansson L, Lindholm LH, Ekbom T, et al. Randomised trial of old and new antihypertensive drugs in elderly patients: cardiovascular mortality and morbidity the Swedish Trial in Old Patients with Hypertension-2 study. Lancet 1999; 354(9192):1751–6.
31. Major cardiovascular events in hypertensive patients randomized to doxazosin vs chlorthalidone: the antihypertensive and lipid-lowering treatment to prevent heart attack trial (ALLHAT). ALLHAT Collaborative Research Group. JAMA 2000; 283(15):1967–75.
32. Beckett NS, Peters R, Fletcher AE, et al. Treatment of hypertension in patients 80 years of age or older. N Engl J Med 2008;358(18):1887–98.
33. Musini VM, Tejani AM, Bassett K, et al. Pharmacotherapy for hypertension in the elderly. Cochrane Database Syst Rev 2009;4:CD000028.

34. Moser M. From JNC I to JNC 7—what have we learned? Prog Cardiovasc Dis 2006;48(5):303–15.
35. Rashidi A, Wright JT Jr. Drug treatment of hypertension in older hypertensives. Clin Geriatr Med 2009;25(2):235–44.
36. Wright JT Jr, Probstfield JL, Cushman WC, et al. ALLHAT findings revisited in the context of subsequent analyses, other trials, and meta-analyses. Arch Intern Med 2009;169(9):832–42.
37. Burton LA, Sumukadas D. Optimal management of sarcopenia. Clin Interv Aging 2010;5:217–28.
38. Messerli FH, Grossman E, Goldbourt U. Are beta-blockers efficacious as first-line therapy for hypertension in the elderly? a systematic review. JAMA 1998;279(23):1903–7.

Incontinence

Alayne D. Markland, DO, MSc[a], Camille P. Vaughan, MD, MS[b],
Theodore M. Johnson II, MD, MPH[b], Kathryn L. Burgio, PhD[a],
Patricia S. Goode, MSN, MD[a],*

KEYWORDS

- Urinary incontinence • Urinary tract disorders
- Benign prostatic enlargement • Geriatric

EPIDEMIOLOGY AND IMPACT OF URINARY INCONTINENCE

Urinary incontinence (UI), the complaint of any involuntary leakage of urine, is a common geriatric syndrome that affects between 30% and 60% of older women and between 10% and 35% of older men in the community, and up to 80% of nursing home residents.[1,2]

The most common types of UI are stress, urge or urgency, and mixed (stress and urgency) incontinence. Stress incontinence is the involuntary leakage of urine on effort or exertion, with activities that increase intra-abdominal pressure, such as coughing, sneezing, or lifting.[3] Urgency incontinence is the involuntary leakage of urine accompanied by or immediately preceded by a sensation of urgency, or the sudden compelling desire to pass urine which is difficult to defer.[3] In older women, mixed incontinence (stress and urgency incontinence) is the most common type, accounting for about half of all cases, with urgency incontinence alone less common, and stress incontinence alone the least common.[4] In older men, urgency incontinence is the most common type, followed by mixed incontinence, stress incontinence being the least common type.

Incontinence is not a normal part of aging, but age-related conditions and changes in bladder and pelvic floor function[5,6] contribute to the loss of bladder control in older adults. In addition to age, risk factors for men and women include cognitive

---

The authors have the following disclosures: Patricia Goode: Pfizer (research grant). Kathryn Burgio: Astellas (advisory board), GlaxoSmithKline (consultant), Johnson & Johnson (consultant), Pfizer (consultant, research grants). Theodore Johnson II: Boehringer-Ingelheim (consultant), Ferring (consultant), Johnson & Johnson (consultant), Pfizer (consultant and research grants), Vantia (consultant and research grant). Camille Vaughan: Astellas Pharmaceuticals (grant support). Alayne Markland: Pfizer (nonpaid consultant).
[a] Department of Medicine, University of Alabama at Birmingham, and Birmingham/Atlanta Geriatric Research, Education, and Clinical Center, Veterans Affairs Medical Center, GRECC/11G, 700 19th Street South, Birmingham, AL 35233, USA
[b] Department of Medicine, Emory University, and Birmingham/Atlanta Geriatric Research, Education, and Clinical Center, Atlanta Veterans Affairs Medical Center, Mailstop 508/11B, 1670 Clairmont Road, Decatur, GA 30033, USA
* Corresponding author.
E-mail address: pgoode@aging.uab.edu

impairment, mobility impairment, diabetes, neurologic conditions, and other lower urinary tract symptoms. Factors increasing the risk for UI in woman include white race, increased parity, oral hormone therapy, higher body mass index, and menopause. In men, despite advances in surgical technique, radical prostatectomy remains strongly associated with transient or persistent incontinence.

Although UI is not a life-threatening condition, it can greatly diminish quality of life. In fact, its impact exceeds that of many comorbid diseases (such as diabetes mellitus, stroke, and arthritis in the hands and wrists).[7,8] Incontinence can contribute to social isolation, anxiety, and depression, and is associated with an increased risk of falls and fractures (urgency UI) and admission to long-term care facilities.[9-14]

DETECTION AND EVALUATION OF URINARY INCONTINENCE

The first step in evaluation of older adults with incontinence is detection. However, community-based studies in the United States indicate that only 30% to 45% of older adults with incontinence seek care.[15] Because of the high prevalence of undiagnosed incontinence, it should be included in the *Review of Systems*. Older adults reporting infrequent incontinence should be alerted that occasional incontinence is a risk factor for more frequent incontinence.[16] Also, evidence exists that behavioral intervention is effective in preventing new incontinence or reducing the progression of infrequent incontinence.[17]

The basic evaluation for UI should include a focused history, paying close attention to the severity, duration, and burden of incontinence, clues to the type of UI, and any potentially modifiable contributing factors; a physical examination; and a urinalysis (**Tables 1** and **2**).

Urinalysis should be interpreted with caution to avoid overtreatment of asymptomatic bacteriuria, which is found in at least 20% of older women. Diagnosis of symptomatic urinary tract infection requires relevant symptoms (urgency, frequency, dysuria, suprapubic tenderness, or costovertebral angle pain or tenderness) and a positive urine culture of 10^5 CFU/mL or greater with no more than 2 species of microorganisms.[18] Having a positive leukocyte esterase or urinary nitrite in addition to pyuria or a positive Gram stain is contributory, but not sufficient for the diagnosis.

Postvoid residual volume (PVR) should be determined in patients with acute UI or suspected retention. There are no evidence-based criteria for an "abnormal" PVR; in general, PVR greater than 150 to 200 mL is considered clinically significant in men. Women may tolerate PVRs in this range without symptoms or morbidity; thus, PVR interpretation should be individualized.

A brief cognitive assessment should be considered for patients who give a history that is inconsistent or unclear, or who have no response to initial treatments (see section on special considerations for patients with cognitive impairment).

URINARY INCONTINENCE TREATMENTS
Behavioral Treatments

Behavioral treatments have been well studied and have been shown to be effective in older adults, reducing leakage by 50% to 80%, with 10% to 30% of patients achieving continence.[19-23] Behavioral treatments are recommended by most treatment guidelines as initial management for UI and related symptoms (**Fig. 1**).[24] These interventions improve incontinence by teaching skills and assisting the patient to change behavior. Behavioral treatment programs usually comprise multiple individualized components, which may include pelvic floor muscle training and exercise, bladder control strategies, self-monitoring (bladder diary), scheduled or prompted voiding, delayed voiding, caffeine reduction, fluid management, weight loss, and/or other lifestyle changes.

Table 1
Modifiable contributors to urinary incontinence

Condition	Mechanism	Treatment
Medical Conditions		
Urinary tract infection	Cystitis with resulting urgency and frequency may precipitate urgency incontinence	Consider treatment of bacteriuria when incontinence is of new onset, suddenly worsens, or with altered mental status Caveat: Asymptomatic bacteriuria is common in the elderly patient and does not need treatment
Constipation	Rectal distension may cause detrusor instability with mass effect	Manage with increased dietary fruit, fiber, and fluids, stool softeners, and laxatives as needed
Diabetes mellitus	Diuresis associated with glycosuria precipitates urgency incontinence Diabetic neuropathic bladder can result in a chronically full bladder with precipitation of frequency, urgency, and stress incontinence	Improve diabetic control or diagnose and treat undetected diabetes
Mobility impairment	Postponed voiding to avoid pain related to degenerative joint disease or other conditions can result in urgency incontinence Slowed mobility from any cause can precipitate urgency incontinence	Improve pain management (pharmacologic or nonpharmacologic) and education concerning regular toileting, which helps decrease stiffness and improves incontinence Improve mobility with physical therapy, assistive devices, or other interventions
Obesity	Pressure on the bladder from central obesity may worsen urgency incontinence and chronic stress on the pelvic floor muscles may lead to stress incontinence	Consider a weight loss program in younger obese geriatric patients. Caution with frail older patients
Obstructive sleep apnea	Nocturnal diuresis due to production of atrial natriuretic peptide may precipitate urgency incontinence or nocturia	Screen for sleep apnea (snoring, daytime sleepiness, witnessed apnea) and consider sleep study. Continuous positive airway pressure treatment decreases nocturnal diuresis and decreases nocturia
Diet		
Caffeine	Caffeine is a mild diuretic and a bladder irritant	Eliminating or reducing caffeine can improve incontinence
Medications		
Diuretics	Rapid increases in bladder volume may precipitate urgency incontinence	Consider discontinuing diuretic. Loop diuretics can be changed to mid to late afternoon to allow useful daytime hours without frequency with diuresis ending before bedtime

(continued on next page)

Table 1 (continued)		
Condition	**Mechanism**	**Treatment**
Angiotensin-converting enzyme inhibitors	Cough, a common side effect in the elderly, precipitates stress incontinence	Change to other agents such as angiotensin II receptor blockers
Anticholinergics, sedatives, and hypnotics	Sedation may cause cognitive impairment that interferes with ability to sense and respond to the need to void, particularly at night, resulting in enuresis Anticholinergics may cause incomplete bladder emptying and constipation, and thus contribute to frequency, urgency, and urinary incontinence	Discontinue or reduce dose when possible

Adapted from Goode PS, Burgio KL, Richter HE, et al. Incontinence in older women. JAMA 2010;303(21):2172–81; with permission.

The purpose of pelvic floor muscle exercises (also known as Kegel exercises) is to strengthen the pelvic floor muscles so they can be used more effectively to prevent urine leakage. Multiple methods have been effectively used to help patients contract their pelvic floor muscles, including self-help books,[25] biofeedback,[20,23] verbal feedback based on vaginal or anal palpation,[20] and electrical stimulation.[21] Careful training with coaching through verbal feedback during physical examination (during the vaginal examination for women or during the rectal examination for men or women) can be as effective as biofeedback and electrical stimulation.[20,23] A reasonable initial approach in a busy primary care practice may be a verbal explanation of the technique reinforced with written materials available through the National Association For Continence (www.nafc.org) and the Simon Foundation (http://www.simonfoundation.org/About_Incontinence_Treatment_Options_Pelvic_Floor_Exercises.html). One of the most effective verbal explanations of a proper contraction of the pelvic floor muscles is to tell the patient to tighten up the muscles that they use to hold in gas (flatus). One of the benefits of pelvic floor muscle strengthening includes better control of flatus, the involuntary loss of which is common and embarrassing for many older adults.

A reasonable and effective exercise prescription for older adults is to contract and relax their pelvic floor muscles for 2 seconds with 15 repetitions 3 times a day.[19–21,23] Patients should gradually increase the duration of squeeze/relaxations by about 1 second each week, until they achieve 10-second contractions and relaxations. At this point they can begin a maintenance prescription of 10-second contractions and relaxations with 10 repetitions once a day. It is essential to continue the maintenance program to maintain strength and effectiveness.

The strategic use of the pelvic floor muscles to prevent leakage is an essential component of behavioral therapy. Effective strategies are shown in **Table 3**.[25] The urge suppression skills outlined in **Table 3** are also effective in reduction of urinary urgency, frequency, and nocturia.[26,27] These symptoms as well as fear of leakage can have a major impact on quality of life. Bladder training, incremental voiding schedules supplemented with techniques to resist the sensation of urgency such as relaxation, distraction, or pelvic floor muscle contraction, or simply delaying voiding for increasing intervals can be added to a behavioral treatment program to help reduce urgency and frequency.[22]

Table 2
Evaluation of urinary incontinence

Evaluation Type	Components
Focused history	Review of chronic conditions and medications Onset, duration, previous history/treatments Characteristics of symptoms and impact on quality of life Frequency/severity Fluid status Concomitant symptoms—ie, constipation, fecal incontinence, dysuria, nocturia, vaginal dryness/vaginal bulging (in women) Cognitive assessment (if indicated, see section on special considerations for patients with cognitive impairment)

Physical examination	General
	    Volume status
	    Abdominal examination (masses, suprapubic tenderness, palpable bladder)
	    Neurologic examination (tremor, cogwheeling, reflexes, sensation)
	    Musculoskeletal (strength, balance, gait)
	    Cognition (delirium)
	Vaginal examination (cough stress test, prolapse evaluation, muscular strength—circumferential squeeze around examining finger(s), internal and anterior displacement—scarring in perineal body, anal wink, vaginal atrophy)
	Rectal in women and men (resting and squeezing sphincter tone, sphincter asymmetry with squeeze, impaction, prostate size/contour/tenderness in men)
	Perineal skin evaluation (contact dermatitis, skin tags, scars, perineal warts)

Laboratory	Urinalysis/culture (rule out infection or hematuria) Fluid status (metabolic panel) Other for consideration: thyroid studies, vitamin B12 levels as indicated, vitamin D levels (25-OH vitamin D)
Radiology (not always indicated)	Postvoid residual volume: bladder ultrasonography, if available Abdominal kidney/ureter/bladder radiograph for constipation, hematuria, or abdominal pain

Adapted from Gibbs CF, Johnson TM 2nd, Ouslander JG. Office-based management of geriatric urinary incontinence. Am J Med 2007;120:211–20; with permission.

Sometimes the pattern of leakage is unclear. A bladder diary (http://kidney.niddk.nih.gov/kudiseases/pubs/pdf/diary.pdf), in which the patient writes down the times they void and the time and circumstances of any leakage, may help identify a pattern that can be treated with a behavioral strategy. Diaries are also helpful for identifying times when a strategy might have prevented leakage, planning for the next time, and monitoring progress of behavioral interventions.

Behavioral lifestyle changes are generally used in addition to other behavioral interventions such as pelvic floor muscle exercises and bladder control strategies, but evidence shows that they can be sufficient treatments alone. Reducing caffeine intake may reduce both stress and urgency incontinence.[28] To avoid withdrawal symptoms, caffeine reduction should be gradual, and may include mixing caffeinated and decaffeinated beverages incrementally.

To evaluate fluid intake, an intake diary or patient's recall of types and amounts of fluid consumed in a usual day can provide very helpful information. Although reducing excess fluid intake can decrease incontinence,[29] many older women attempt to control

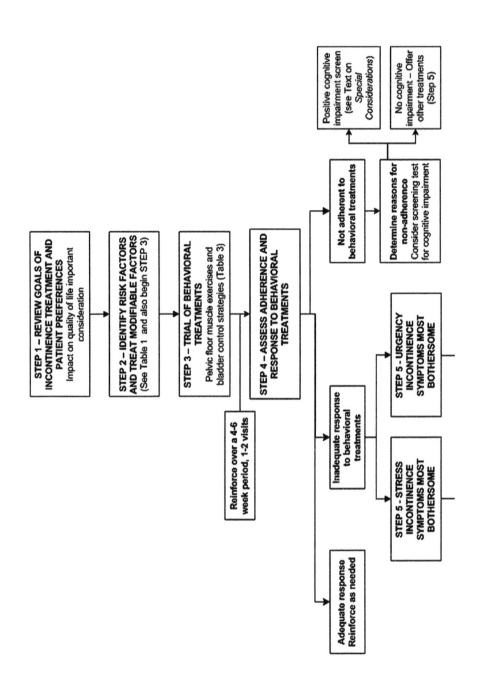

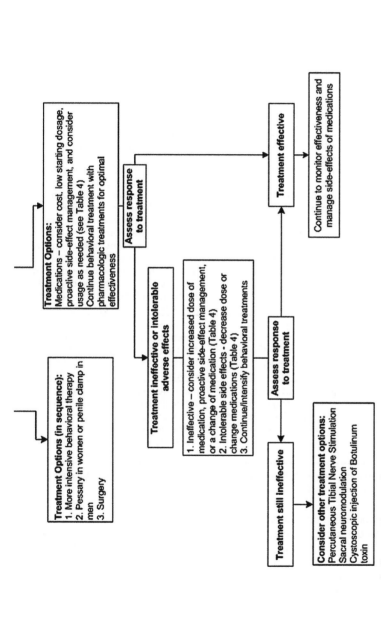

Fig. 1. Stepwise approach to treatment of urinary incontinence in older adults. (*Modified from* Goode PS, Burgio KL, Richter HE, et al. Incontinence in older women. JAMA 2010;303(21):2172–81. Copyright 2010, American Medical Association. All rights reserved; with permission.)

Table 3
Behavioral strategies to prevent urine leakage

Type of Leakage	Patient Complaint	Strategy
Stress incontinence	Urine loss during sneezing, coughing, or lifting Urine loss during exercise	Squeeze and hold the pelvic floor muscles just before and during these activities (Squeeze before you sneeze!). If it happens too suddenly, squeeze anyway, it will be too late that time, but will help establish the habit When possible, squeeze for certain components of exercise, but also know that as strength increases with continued exercise, leakage with exercise will decrease
Urge or urgency incontinence	Urine loss following an urge to urinate—can't get to the bathroom in time Urine leakage starts with sudden urgency when running water, pumping gas, driving up to the house, or putting the key in the front door	Instead of rushing to the bathroom, stay still and repeatedly tighten the pelvic floor muscles without relaxing them until the urgency is gone (Freeze and squeeze!). Then walk to the bathroom at a normal pace. Repeat the Freeze and squeeze if urgency reoccurs on the way to the bathroom Anticipate and prevent urgency. Squeeze and hold the pelvic floor muscles before turning on the water, pumping gas, getting out of the car, or opening the front door. Also, consider voiding before doing dishes or pumping gas
Leakage without warning	Urine starts flowing when the person stands up from a chair or the bed, without urgency	Squeeze and hold the pelvic floor muscles before standing and hold them as you stand up. This helps prevent the sudden detrusor contraction that causes the leakage
Post-void dribbling	Urine drips on the floor after standing up from voiding. Urine seeps out in the underwear after voiding	Tighten the pelvic floor muscles before the final wiping or shaking. If the person sits to void, tighten the pelvic floor muscles as they stand up to prevent leakage. Men may "milk" the penis to empty the urethra

Adapted from Burgio KL, Pearce KL, Lucco AJ. Staying dry: a practical guide to bladder control. Baltimore (MD): Johns Hopkins University Press; 1989; with permission.

incontinence by restricting fluid intake. Although fluid restriction can be helpful at certain times, such as before social activities, restricting overall fluid intake is not recommended because of the risk of dehydration. Though it may seem counterintuitive, it is beneficial to encourage older patients to consume at least 6 8-ounce glasses of fluid each day.[30]

Weight loss studies have shown significant improvement in incontinence for younger women following bariatric surgery[31] and with 5% weight reduction in a more traditional weight loss program.[32] However, more evidence is needed to evaluate the effectiveness of weight loss as an incontinence treatment for older women or for men.

Behavioral interventions are safe, and result in significant reduction in symptoms and improved quality of life. Such interventions do require the active participation of a motivated patient or caregiver and a knowledgable clinician. Behavioral interventions are commonly implemented by advanced practice nurses (http://www.wocncenter.com/public/member_directory.cfm), physical therapists with special training (http://www.apta.org), or other professionals who have developed the appropriate expertise (www.nafc.org). Behavioral treatments usually work gradually at first and rely on patient self-management; therefore, it is important to follow patients regularly to sustain behavioral changes over time.

Pharmacologic Therapy

Various drug therapies (**Table 4**) are available to treat UI depending on the underlying etiology. Anticholinergic antimuscarinic drugs, which target bladder smooth muscle leading to relaxation, are most often used to treat urgency or mixed incontinence.[33,34] These drugs can be used in men and women, and all have similar efficacy.[35] Anticholinergic side effects such as dry mouth and constipation are common,[35,36] and long-term adherence is often limited.[37] Older adults with evidence of incomplete bladder emptying should be monitored for worsening urinary retention while taking antimuscarinic agents. Further, there is potential for negative effects on cognition, particularly when using antimuscarinic drugs which are less selective for the bladder or more likely to cross the blood-brain barrier.[38]

Antimuscarinic agents may be used alone in men for symptoms of urgency incontinence, but are often paired with drug treatments targeting benign prostatic enlargement (BPE).[39] α-Adrenergic antagonists and 5α-reductase inhibitors are effective for symptoms associated with BPE, which may include urgency incontinence.[40,41] The use of a selective α-adrenergic antagonist is associated with less risk of orthostatic hypotension compared with nonselective agents. 5α-Reductase inhibitors, alone or in combination with an α-adrenergic antagonist, have been shown to reduce urinary symptoms, the risk of acute urinary retention, and the need for future invasive surgical therapy.[40]

Fewer pharmacologic treatments have been studied for stress UI, and only among women. Duloxetine, a serotonin and norepinephrine reuptake inhibitor, has been evaluated in several randomized controlled trials, and a recent systematic review suggests it may be beneficial for stress incontinence in women,[42] but is not approved for this indication in the United States.

Low-dose, topical vaginal estrogen therapy can be effective in older women for the reduction of symptoms associated with overactive bladder syndrome, including urgency incontinence.[43] Systemic absorption while using dosages typical for treating urogenital atrophy (0.5 g of estrogen cream 3 times a week) is low,[44] although such treatment should be used with caution among women with a history of breast cancer. The estradiol ring, which is placed vaginally every 90 days, may be a convenient method of treatment for many older women.

Devices

For women with stress incontinence or mixed incontinence with stress predominance, intravaginal mechanical devices can reduce episodes of UI. Both tampons and pessaries have been studied in a randomized controlled trial, and have demonstrated decreased volumes of incontinence compared with no treatment.[45] A large randomized controlled trial showed that the use of a pessary was as effective as pelvic floor muscle exercise–based behavioral therapy in reducing episodes of stress incontinence and leading to satisfaction with treatment at 12 months.[46] Pessaries must be fitted in a clinic setting to optimize comfort and performance. Further, their use requires regular cleaning and reinsertion of the device, which may be difficult for some older women, thus necessitating frequent visits to their clinician for proper maintenance of the device.

For men with stress UI or continuous leakage, penile clamps or collection devices such as condom catheters can offer self-management options. One small study

Table 4
Drugs commonly used to treat different types of incontinence

Drugs	Usual Adult Dose	Comments
Drugs with Predominantly Anticholinergic or Antimuscarinic Effects		
Darifenacin	7.5–15.0 mg daily orally	The drug is selective for the bladder M3 muscarinic receptor, and may have fewer cognitive side effects than other anticholinergic agents
Fesoterodine	4–8 mg daily orally	This prodrug is easily converted to an active metabolite chemically identical to the active metabolite of tolterodine
Oxybutynin[a]	2.5–5.0 mg 1–3 times daily orally (short-acting) 5–30 mg daily orally (long-acting) 3.9 mg over a 96-h period (transdermal) 10% topical gel 0.5–1 g daily	Long-acting and transdermal preparations have fewer side effects than short-acting preparations The transdermal patch can cause local skin irritation in some patients
Solifenacin	5–10 mg daily orally	The drug has some selectivity for the bladder M3 muscarinic receptor over other muscarinic receptors
Tolterodine[a]	2–4 mg daily orally	The drug has relatively low lipophilicity with limited ability to penetrate the central nervous system
Trospium	20 mg twice daily orally 60 mg daily orally (long-acting)	The agent is a quaternary ammonium compound, which is less likely to cross the blood-brain barrier and may have fewer cognitive side effects than other anticholinergic agents
Estrogen (for Women)		
	Approximately 0.5 g cream applied topically nightly for 2 weeks, then twice per week Estradiol ring, replaced every 90 days Estradiol, 1 vaginal tablet daily for 2 weeks, then 1 tablet twice a week	Local vaginal preparations are probably more effective for urgency related to local irritation than oral estrogen, but definitive data on effectiveness are lacking
Serotonin and Noradrenaline Reuptake Inhibitor		
Duloxetine	20–80 mg daily	Not approved for this indication in the USA; however, a systematic review of clinical trial data suggests improvement in stress UI Transient nausea is a common side effect
α-Adrenergic Antagonists (for Men)		
Alfuzosin (selective)	10 mg daily orally	Postural hypotension can be a serious side effect Doses of nonselective agents must be increased gradually to facilitate tolerance

(continued on next page)

Table 4 (continued)		
Drugs	**Usual Adult Dose**	**Comments**
α-adrenergic Antagonists (for Men)		
Doxazosin (nonselective)[a]	1–8 mg daily orally at bedtime	
Prazosin (nonselective)	1–5 mg twice daily orally	Also used for posttraumatic stress disorder in men
Silodosin (selective)	4–8 mg daily orally	
Tamsulosin (selective)[a]	0.4–0.8 mg daily orally	
Terazosin (nonselective)[a]	1–10 mg daily orally at bedtime	
5α-Reductase Inhibitors (for Men)		
Dutasteride	0.5 mg daily orally	
Finasteride[a]	5 mg daily orally	

[a] Available as a generic.

Data from Ouslander JG. Management of overactive bladder. N Engl J Med 2004;350:786–99; and Gibbs CF, Johnson TM 2nd, Ouslander JG. Office-based management of geriatric urinary incontinence. Am J Med 2007;120:211–20.

assessed different types of penile clamps and found the Cunningham clamp (a rigid metal and foam clamp) to be the most comfortable and effective but, even at the loosest setting, penile artery Doppler ultrasonography revealed decreased systolic blood flow.[47] Penile clamps must be removed at least every 4 hours to prevent penile erosion. Before they recommend a penile clamp, clinicians should confirm that men are cognitively intact and have the manual dexterity to open and close the device. Collection devices provide a method for containment of incontinence. Condom catheters were studied in one randomized study[48] and were shown to reduce the risk of bacteriuria, symptomatic urinary tract infection, and death compared with indwelling catheters in a group of hospitalized older men, particularly in those without dementia, but likely result in a higher infection rate than diapering.[49] Newer types of collection devices are becoming available and can be explored using consumer advocacy Web sites such as the National Association for Continence (www.nafc.org) and the Simon Foundation (www.simonfoundation.org).

Absorptive undergarments may be a preferred method of containment for some patients,[50] but generally should not be the first response to incontinence as a treatment option. In addition, these products are costly and are not covered by Medicare or most insurance plans. If continence products are preferred, proper fit for comfort and use are essential. Assessment of self-care practices to prevent skin breakdown (changing undergarments when wet, use of barrier creams or treatment of fungal infections if necessary) is important in those who use absorptive products.

Surgical Treatment

Minimally invasive surgeries for UI include midurethral slings for stress incontinence in women and men and artificial urinary sphincters in men.[51–53] Midurethral sling surgeries are often done in the outpatient setting for women and men with stress urinary incontinence.[51–53] In men, less evidence regarding the different types of sling surgeries exists in comparison with women.[53] Men with stress urinary incontinence also have the option of surgical implantation of an artificial urinary sphincter.[53]

For refractory urgency incontinence, minimally invasive procedures and surgeries include implantation of a sacral neuromodulation device, percutaneous tibial nerve stimulation, and botulinum toxin A bladder injections (off-label usage). Sacral neuro-modulation therapy involves an outpatient surgical implantation of an electronic device approved by the Food and Drug Administration (FDA) that stimulates the S3 sacral nerve.[54] Neuromodulation also occurs through projections from the posterior tibial nerve to the sacral nerve plexus at the S2-S4 junction. Electrical stimulation of the posterior tibial nerve can be performed via a fine-needle electrode inserted percu-taneously near the ankle.[55] Treatments last 30 minutes and are done in clinic once a week for 12 weeks, then repeated as needed. Although not currently FDA-approved, botulinum toxin A injected cystoscopically into the detrusor muscle is increasingly being used for patients who are refractory to other treatments for urgency, frequency, and urgency incontinence.[56,57]

SPECIAL CONSIDERATIONS FOR TREATMENT OF PATIENTS WITH COGNITIVE IMPAIRMENT

Patients with cognitive impairment and incontinence need modified evaluation and treatment approaches. Symptoms of urinary tract infection can be nonspecific in cognitively impaired older adults, and can include worsening incontinence as well as decreased cognitive status. Although it is important not to treat asymptomatic bacteriuria, if a functional decline occurs in conjunction with worsening or new incon-tinence, a urinalysis and culture are indicated.

In identifying factors that may have precipitated or worsened incontinence, medica-tions may play a role (see **Table 1**). Cholinesterase inhibitors used to treat dementia work to increase acetylcholine levels and therefore may precipitate incontinence.[58] The benefits of the cholinesterase inhibitor need to be balanced with the burden of incontinence in deciding whether the medication should be withdrawn or changed.

During the physical examination, an abdominal and a digital rectal examination are necessary to rule out constipation as a precipitating factor in patients unable to monitor their frequency of bowel movements.[59] Also, perineal skin should be inspected and any perineal irritation treated with an antifungal cream if indicated, and with a moisture barrier ointment.

For patients with mild to moderate cognitive impairment, a behavioral program limited to caffeine reduction and timed voiding can reduce incontinence. For patients with a caregiver, the active involvement of the caregiver is usually essential for optimal outcomes with behavioral treatment. Prompted voiding works very well in reducing incontinence in community-dwelling older persons.[60] A 3-day trial of prompted void-ing can determine if quality of life improves for the caregiver and patient.[61] If there is no improvement after 3 days, a "check and change" management strategy, using appro-priate absorbent garments, can contain incontinence and preserve dignity. Substituting pull-ups for the patient's usual underwear can provide considerable relief for the caregiver without being bothersome to the patient.

Antimuscarinic medications can worsen cognitive function, and should be used with caution in older patients with preexisting cognitive impairment.[38] Careful monitoring for worsening mental status should be part of the instructions given to the caregiver. If improvement is not noted within a month or if the patient has a functional decline sooner, the medication should be discontinued.

Although surgical procedures may be indicated, such as in cases of severe pelvic organ prolapse and incontinence, in general, patients with dementia may sustain cognitive and functional decline with surgical interventions.

> **Box 1**
> **Reasons for referral of older adults with urinary incontinence for specialty evaluation**
>
> Surgery or pelvic floor radiation within the past 6 months and not responding to a behavioral treatment plan
>
> Recurrent urinary tract infections (2 or more urinary tract infections in a 12-month period)
>
> Postvoid residual volume >200 mL
>
> Asymptomatic microscopic or macroscopic hematuria (as per guidelines)[18]
>
> Incontinence with new-onset neurologic symptoms and/or muscular weakness
>
> Persistent bothersome symptoms after trials with behavioral and/or drug treatment
>
> Failure to isolate pelvic floor muscles in a patient desiring to try behavioral therapy
>
> No longer able to tolerate or lack of response to a pessary or other adjunctive treatment
>
> Pelvic pain associated with incontinence
>
> In women: pelvic organ prolapse past the introitus or less severe prolapse with discomfort
>
> In men: abnormal prostate examination on digital rectal examination

REFRACTORY SYMPTOMS/REFERRAL

Many older patients with UI are referred to specialists for further evaluation and treatment. Common reasons for referral are listed in **Box 1**. However, most UI can be evaluated and treated in the primary care setting.

REFERENCES

1. Hunskaar S, Arnold EP, Burgio KL, et al. Epidemiology and natural history of urinary incontinence. Int Urogynecol J Pelvic Floor Dysfunct 2000;11:301–19.
2. Abrams P, Cardozo L, Khoury S, Wein A, editors. 4th International Consultation on Incontinence. Recommendations of the international scientific committee: epidemiology of urinary and fecal incontinence and pelvic organ prolapse. 4th edition. Paris (France): Health Publication Ltd; 2009.
3. Abrams P, Cardozo L, Fall M, et al. The standardization of terminology of lower urinary tract function: report from the standardization subcommittee of the international continence society. Neurourol Urodyn 2002;21:167–78.
4. Minassian VA, Stewart WF, Wood GC. Urinary incontinence in women: variation in prevalence estimates and risk factors. Obstet Gynecol 2008;111:324–31.
5. Diokno AC, Brown MB, Brock BM, et al. Clinical and cystometric characteristics of continent and incontinent noninstitutionalized elderly. J Urol 1988;140:567–71.
6. Staskin DR. Age-related physiologic and pathologic changes affecting lower urinary tract function. Clin Geriatr Med 1986;2:701–10.
7. Lin SJ, Salmon JW, Bron MS. The impact of urinary incontinence on quality of life of the elderly. Am J Manag Care 2005;11(Suppl 4):S103–11.
8. Huang AJ, Brown JS, Kanaya AM, et al. Quality-of-life impact and treatment of urinary incontinence in ethnically diverse older women. Arch Intern Med 2006; 166(18):2000–6.
9. Brown JS, Vittinghoff E, Wyman JF, et al. Urinary incontinence: does it increase risk for falls and fractures? Study of osteoporotic fractures research group. J Am Geriatr Soc 2000;48(7):721–5.

10. Chiarelli PE, Mackenzie LA, Osmotherly PG. Urinary incontinence is associated with an increase in falls: a systematic review. Aust J Physiother 2009;55(2):89–95.

11. Thom D, Haan M, Van Den Eeden S. Medically recognized urinary incontinence and risks of hospitalization, nursing home admission and mortality. Age Ageing 1997;26(5):367–74.

12. Holroyd-Leduc JM, Mehta KM, Covinsky KE. Urinary incontinence and its association with death, nursing home admission, and functional decline. J Am Geriatr Soc 2004;52(5):712–8.

13. Johnson TM II, Bernard SL, Kincade JE, et al. Urinary incontinence and risk of death among community-living elderly people: results from the national survey on self-care and aging. J Aging Health 2000;12(1):25–46.

14. Nakanishi N, Tatara K, Shinsho F, et al. Mortality in relation to urinary and faecal incontinence in elderly people living at home. Age Ageing 1999;28(3):301–6.

15. Burgio KL, Ives DG, Locher JL, et al. Treatment seeking for urinary incontinence in older adults. J Am Geriatr Soc 1994;42(2):208–12.

16. Goode PS, Burgio K, Redden D, et al. Population-based study of incidence and predictors of urinary incontinence in African American and white older adults. J Urol 2008;179(4):1449–53.

17. Diokno AC, Sampselle CM, Herzog AG, et al. Prevention of urinary incontinence by behavioral modification program: a randomized controlled trial among older women in the community. J Urol 2004;171(3):1165–71.

18. Centers for disease control and prevention: guidelines for prevention of catheter-associated urinary tract infections. 2009. Available at: http://www.cdc.gov/HAI/ca_uti/uti.html. Accessed March 15, 2011.

19. Burgio KL, Locher JL, Goode PS, et al. Behavioral versus drug treatment for urge incontinence in older women: a randomized clinical trial. JAMA 1998;23:1995–2000.

20. Burgio KL, Goode PS, Locher JL, et al. Behavioral training with and without biofeedback in the treatment of urge incontinence in older women: a randomized controlled trial. JAMA 2002;288:2293–9.

21. Goode PS, Burgio KL, Locher JL, et al. Effect of behavioral training with or without pelvic floor electrical stimulation on stress incontinence in women: a randomized controlled trial. JAMA 2003;290:345–52.

22. Fantl JA, Wyman JF, McClish DK, et al. Efficacy of bladder training in older women with urinary incontinence. JAMA 1991;265:609–13.

23. Goode PS, Burgio KL, Johnson TM, et al. Behavioral therapy with or without biofeedback and pelvic floor electrical stimulation for persistent postprostatectomy incontinence—a randomized controlled trial. JAMA 2011;305(2):151–9.

24. Abrams P, Andersson K, Birder L, et al. Fourth International Consultation on Incontinence recommendations of the International Scientific Committee: evaluation and treatment of urinary incontinence, pelvic organ prolapse, and fecal incontinence. Neurourol Urodyn 2010;29:213–40.

25. Burgio KL, Pearce KL, Lucco AJ. Staying dry: a practical guide to bladder control. Baltimore (MD): Johns Hopkins University Press; 1989.

26. Burgio KL, Kraus SR, Borello-France D, et al, Urinary Incontinence Treatment Network. The effects of drug and behavioral therapy on urgency and voiding frequency. Int Urogynecol J Pelvic Floor Dysfunct 2010;21(6):711–9.

27. Johnson TM, Burgio KL, Redden DT, et al. Effects of behavioral and drug therapy on nocturia in older incontinent women. J Am Geriatr Soc 2005;53(5):846–50.

28. Bryant CM, Dowell CJ, Fairbrother G. Caffeine reduction education to improve urinary symptoms. Br J Nurs 2002;11:560–5.

29. Swithinbank L, Hashim H, Abrams P. The effect of fluid intake on urinary symptoms in women. J Urol 2005;174:187–9.
30. Kincade JE, Dougherty MC, Carlson JR, et al. Randomized clinical trial of efficacy of self-monitoring techniques to treat urinary incontinence in women. Neurourol Urodyn 2007;26:507–11.
31. Burgio KB, Richter HE, Clements RH, et al. Changes in urinary and fecal incontinence symptoms with weight loss surgery in morbidly obese women. Obstet Gynecol 2007;110(5):1034–40.
32. Subak LL, Wing R, West DS, et al, Program to Reduce Incontinence by Diet and Exercise (PRIDE). Weight loss to treat urinary incontinence in overweight and obese women. N Engl J Med 2009;360:481–90.
33. Ouslander JG. Management of overactive bladder. N Engl J Med 2004;350:786–99.
34. Nabi G, Cody JD, Ellis G, et al. Anticholinergic drugs versus placebo for overactive bladder syndrome in adults. Cochrane Database Syst Rev 2006;4:CD003781 [online].
35. Hay-Smith J, Herbison P, Ellis G, et al. Which anticholinergic drug for overactive bladder symptoms in adults. Cochrane Database Syst Rev 2005;3:CD005429 [online].
36. Goode PS, Burgio KL, Richter HE, et al. Incontinence in older women. JAMA 2010;303:2172–81.
37. Gopal M, Haynes K, Bellamy SL, et al. Discontinuation rates of anticholinergic medications used for the treatment of lower urinary tract symptoms. Obstet Gynecol 2008;112:1311–8.
38. Kay GG, Abou-Donia MB, Messer WS Jr, et al. Antimuscarinic drugs for overactive bladder and their potential effects on cognitive function in older patients. J Am Geriatr Soc 2005;53:2195–201.
39. Kaplan SA, Roehrborn CG, Rovner ES, et al. Tolterodine and tamsulosin for treatment of men with lower urinary tract symptoms and overactive bladder: a randomized controlled trial. JAMA 2006;296:2319–28 [erratum JAMA 2007;297(11):1195].
40. McConnell JD, Roehrborn CG, Bautista OM, et al. The long-term effect of doxazosin, finasteride, and combination therapy on the clinical progression of benign prostatic hyperplasia. N Engl J Med 2003;349:2387–98.
41. Lepor H, Williford WO, Barry MJ, et al. The efficacy of terazosin, finasteride, or both in benign prostatic hyperplasia. Veterans affairs cooperative studies benign prostatic hyperplasia study group. N Engl J Med 1996;335:533–9.
42. Mariappan P, Alhasso A, Ballantyne Z, et al. Duloxetine, a serotonin and noradrenaline reuptake inhibitor (SNRI) for the treatment of stress urinary incontinence: a systematic review. Eur Urol 2007;51:67–74.
43. Cardozo L, Bachmann G, McClish D, et al. Meta-analysis of estrogen therapy in the management of urogenital atrophy in postmenopausal women: second report of the hormones and urogenital therapy committee. Obstet Gynecol 1998;92:722–7.
44. Ponzone R, Biglia N, Jacomuzzi ME, et al. Vaginal oestrogen therapy after breast cancer: is it safe? Eur J Cancer 2005;41:2673–81.
45. Nygaard I. Prevention of exercise incontinence with mechanical devices. J Reprod Med 1995;40:89–94.
46. Richter HE, Burgio KL, Brubaker L, et al. Continence pessary compared with behavioral therapy or combined therapy for stress incontinence: a randomized controlled trial. Obstet Gynecol 2010;115:609–17.
47. Moore KN, Schieman S, Ackerman T, et al. Assessing comfort, safety, and patient satisfaction with three commonly used penile compression devices. Urology 2004;63:150–4.

48. Saint S, Kaufman SR, Rogers MA, et al. Condom versus indwelling urinary catheters: a randomized trial. J Am Geriatr Soc 2006;54:1055–61.

49. Ouslander JG, Greengold B, Chen S. External catheter use and urinary tract infections among incontinent male nursing home patients. J Am Geriatr Soc 1987;35:1063–70.

50. Johnson TM, Ouslander JG, Uman GC, et al. Urinary incontinence treatment preferences in long-term care. J Am Geriatr Soc 2001;49:710–8.

51. Bemelman BC, Chapple CR. Are slings now the gold standard treatment for the management of female urinary stress incontinence and if so, which technique? Curr Opin Urol 2003;13:301–7.

52. Novara G, Ficarra V, Boscolo-Berto R, et al. Tension-free midurethral slings in the treatment of female stress urinary incontinence: a systematic review and meta-analysis of randomized controlled trials of effectiveness. Eur Urol 2007;52:663–78.

53. Herschorn S, Bruschini H, Comiter C, et al. Surgical treatment of stress incontinence in men. Neurourol Urodyn 2010;29:179–90.

54. Herbison GP, Arnold EP. Sacral neuromodulation with implanted devices for urinary storage and voiding dysfunction in adults. Cochrane Database Syst Rev 2009;2:CD004202.

55. MacDiarmid SA, Peters KM, Shobeiri A, et al. Long-term durability of percutaneous tibial nerve stimulation for the treatment of overactive bladder. J Urol 2010;183:234–40.

56. Brubaker L, Richter HE, Visco AG, et al. Refractory idiopathic urge incontinence and Botulinum A injection. J Urol 2008;180:217–22.

57. Flynn M, Amundsen CL, Perevich M, et al. Short term outcomes of a randomized, double blind placebo controlled trial of botulinum A toxin for the management of idiopathic detrusor overactivity incontinence. J Urol 2009;181(6):2608–15.

58. Gill SS, Mamdani M, Naglie G, et al. A prescribing cascade involving cholinesterase inhibitors and anticholinergic drugs. Arch Intern Med 2005;165:808–13.

59. DuBeau C, Kuchel G, Johnson T II, et al. Incontinence in the frail elderly. In: Abrams P, Cardozo L, Khoury S, editors. 4th International Consultation on Incontinence. Recommendations of the International scientific committee: evaluation and treatment of urinary incontinence, pelvic organ prolapse and faecal incontinence. 4th edition. Paris (France): Health Publication Ltd; 2009. p. 961–1024.

60. Ostaszkiewicz J, Johnston L, Roe B. Timed voiding for the management of urinary incontinence in adults. Cochrane Database Syst Rev 2004;1:CD002802.

61. Ouslander JG, Schnelle JF, Uman G, et al. Predictors of successful prompted voiding among incontinent nursing home residents. JAMA 1995;273:1366–70.

The Evaluation and Management of Delirium Among Older Persons

Joseph H. Flaherty, MD[a,b,*]

KEYWORDS

- Evaluation • Management • Delirium • Older persons

OVERVIEW

Delirium can be a devastating diagnosis for older persons. For health care professionals, delirium represents one of the most challenging situations in terms of making an accurate and timely diagnosis, identifying all the underlying causes, trying to prevent its occurrence, and managing the symptoms that often are associated with it.

Although references to patients with delirium date as far back as the time of Hippocrates, delirium has received the clinical, research, and public attention it deserves only in the past 3 decades. The first textbook dedicated solely to this topic described delirium as "a ubiquitous and thus clinically important sign of cerebral functional decompensation caused by physical illness."[1] The diagnostic criteria have continued to evolve. The *Diagnostic and Statistical Manual of Mental Disorders (Fifth edition)* (DSM-V) (due out in 2011–2012) will likely define delirium as a disturbance in level of awareness or attention (rather than consciousness as in the previous edition), marked by the acute or subacute onset of cognitive changes attributable to a general medical condition; and it tends to have a fluctuating course. DSM-V will also likely add supportive features and subtypes, such as hypoactive, hyperactive, and mixed.[2]

PATHOPHYSIOLOGY

There are numerous proposed neuropathophysiologic mechanisms of delirium, most of which are related to imbalances of the release, degradation, and synthesis of neurotransmitters in the brain. Perhaps the strongest neurotransmitter change occurs

[a] Geriatric Research, Education and Clinical Center, St Louis Veterans Affairs Medical Center, #1 Jefferson Barracks Road, St Louis, MO 63125, USA
[b] Division of Geriatrics, Department of Internal Medicine, Saint Louis University School of Medicine, 1402 South Grand Boulevard, Room M238, St Louis, MO 63104, USA
* Geriatric Research, Education and Clinical Center, St Louis Veterans Affairs Medical Center, #1 Jefferson Barracks Road, St Louis, MO 63125.
E-mail address: Flaherty@slu.edu

Med Clin N Am 95 (2011) 555–577
doi:10.1016/j.mcna.2011.02.005
0025-7125/11/$ – see front matter. Published by Elsevier Inc.

medical.theclinics.com

within the dopaminergic system, but other neurotransmitters such as serotonin, acetylcholine, γ-aminobutyric acid, glutamine, and norepinephrine may also be involved, whether in combination with the dopaminergic system, or as the primary system.[3] Hypoxia and hypoxic ischemic injury are also proposed mechanisms.[4] There may also be a genetic predisposition for development of delirium.[5]

The pathophysiology of delirium is not well elucidated, which poses trouble for the treating clinician. Currently, it is impossible for the clinician to determine which neuro-transmitter(s) is/are predominately involved in any particular case. By keeping the complex systems and mechanisms in mind when trying to diagnose or manage a patient with delirium, clinicians are better able to understand the challenges in making an accurate diagnosis (especially in the face of dementia) and the significant limitations that medications have in the treatment of delirium.

PREVALENCE AND INCIDENCE FOR VARIOUS SITES AND SITUATIONS

Delirium is one of the most common illnesses older patients can develop and one that clinicians should not miss at the reported rate of 32% to 66%.[6] The prevalence of delirium on admission to medical units among well-performed studies (delirium assessment within 24 hours of admission) ranged from 10% to 31%. (The low of 10% was believed to be an underestimate because this study had strict selection criteria.) In the same systematic review, the incidence during hospitalization was 3% to 29%.[7]

In general, surgical patients have been found to have higher rates of delirium than medical patients. Rates are highest postoperatively among patients with coronary artery bypass graft, ranging from 17% to 74% (>50% in 5 of the 14 studies reviewed), rates among orthopedic surgical patients ranged from 28% to 53% (>40% in 5 of the 6 studies), and rates among urological patients (2 studies) ranged from 4.5% to 6.8%.[8] Past biases have blamed anesthesia agents for most cases, which have wrongly kept alive the belief, like that found in the intensive care unit (ICU), that delirium is unpreventable. Several studies that have evaluated the association between routes of anesthesia (general, epidural, spinal, regional) and the risk of postoperative delirium have found that the route of anesthesia was not associated with the development of delirium.[9]

One of the sites with the highest rates of delirium is the ICU. Rates as low as 19% and as high as 80% have been found.[10,11] It is more evident from the recent studies that the higher rates are more accurate.[12]

Data from postacute care facilities (under such names as subacute care facilities, skilled nursing facilities, rehabilitation centers, and long-term care facilities) reveal 2 major issues: patients are discharged from acute hospitals with unresolved delirium, and delirium at these sites persists for an extended period. In 1 study, 72% of 214 patients in nursing homes who were hospitalized for delirium still had delirium at the time of discharge back to the nursing home. The delirium persisted for 55% of the patients at 1 month and 25% at 3 months after discharge.[13] Another study found that 39% of 52 patients with hip fractures were discharged with delirium, which persisted for 32% of the patients at 1 month and 6% at 6 months after discharge.[14] In a study of more than 80 postacute care facilities using the Minimum Data Set (MDS) to identify patients with any symptoms of delirium, a prevalence rate of 23% was found on admission. Among these patients, 52% still had the symptoms at 1-week follow-up.[15]

Two studies found point prevalence within nursing facilities to be 14% using the MDS[16] and 33% using a validated instrument.[17] Although neither study could determine whether the delirium was persistent after a hospital stay, or was an incident (new episode of) delirium, it is evident that delirium is common among nursing home residents.

Home care is an understudied site concerning delirium. However, 2 studies showed lower rates of delirium among ill, older persons cared for at home compared with similarly ill, older persons cared for in the hospital. It is unclear whether something positive is being done in the home that prevents delirium or whether something negative is occurring in the hospital that contributes to the development of delirium.[18,19]

CONSEQUENCES OF DELIRIUM

Data about the adverse outcomes associated with delirium among older persons have typically compared patients with delirium with patients without delirium. In the hospital setting, most studies have found that delirium is associated with hospital complications, loss of physical function, increased length of stay (LOS) in the hospital, increased instances of discharge to long-term care facilities, and higher mortality.[20–33] **Table 1** details some of these differences among medical inpatients.

Associated adverse outcomes among delirious patients in the ICU have shown prolonged ICU stay, prolonged hospital stay, and increased mortality compared with patients in the ICU without delirium.[10,11] Data from postacute facilities and nursing homes have also shown associated adverse outcomes related to loss of physical function and mortality.[13,15,17]

A recently identified consequence of delirium, particularly delirium in the ICU, has been termed long-term cognitive impairment (LTCI). Although the final term for this syndrome has not been decided, the relationship seems real based on reviews of several studies.[34,35] The proposed mechanisms include delirium as a marker of an underlying progressive disease, acute brain damage causing delirium that in turn causes LTCI, delirium as a cause of LTCI, and drug treatment of delirium as a cause of LTCI.

Table 1
Studies comparing LOS and mortality among hospitalized medical patients with and without delirium

References	Year	No Delirium	Delirium	No Delirium	Delirium
		LOS (days)		Mortality (% who died)	
Thomas et al[20]	1988	11	21[a]	—	—
Rockwood[21]	1989	14	20	—	—
Francis et al[22]	1990	7	12[a]	5	16
Ramsay[23]	1991	—	—	14	62[a]
Jitapunkul et al[24]	1992	16	20	—	—
Kolbeinsson and Jonsson[25]	1993	17	20	—	—
Rockwood[26]	1993	28	32	—	—
O'Keeffe and Lavan[27]	1997	11	21[a]	—	—
Inouye[6,28]	1998	6	7	3	9
Zanocchi et al[29]	1998	—	—	9.9	24.6[a]
Vazquez et al[30]	2000	7	10[a]	—	—
Villalpando-Berumen et al[31]	2003	10	13[a]	2.3	6.1
Adamis et al[32]	2006	14	28[a]	—	—
Edlund et al[33]	2006	10	15[a]	1.8	8.8[a]

[a] Significant difference P<.05

EVALUATION

For the most comprehensive approach, health care providers need to be able to evaluate older people who are at risk of developing delirium and who have already developed delirium. Another key player in the comprehensive approach is the health care system, which needs to be set up to allow the best approaches, depending on the site where older people receive their care.

Components of the evaluation may be considered in a stepwise fashion or along a spectrum. They include:

- Awareness and screening
- Differentiating delirium from dementia
- Identifying and treating the underlying causes of the delirium.

Awareness and Screening

Awareness of delirium means knowing how commonly it occurs, how frequently it is missed, that it is often mislabeled (as a normal part of aging or the hospitalization, or as dementia), where it occurs, and the consequences of having it. Delirium should become part of the medical jargon for all who care for older persons, and terms such as mental status change or acute confusional state should be avoided. A search using Ovid (a medical search engine) from 1996 to 2010 found more than 2000 citations for delirium, but just more than 200 for both mental status change or acute confusional state combined.

There are at least 2 approaches to screening for delirium. One method is to identify predisposing or precipitating factors for developing delirium, and then implement screening and preventive interventions targeted at those with more risk factors than others. One example of this graded risk includes the following predisposing factors among patients: vision impairment, severe illness, cognitive impairment, blood urea nitrogen/creatinine ratio greater than 18. Patients with the following number of factors have the following respective risk (rate) of developing delirium: no factor (low risk: 3%–9% rate), 1 to 2 factors (intermediate risk: 16%–23% rate), 3 to 4 factors (high risk: 32%–83% rate).[6]

Although this approach is useful to target resources (preventive interventions) toward those most at risk, a second approach is to use a validated screening instrument on all older patients who interface with the health care system. The frequency of use of the screening instruments depends on the site. For example, because patients in the ICU are at particularly high risk, screening could be performed on a daily basis or every nursing shift change.[11] In postacute care or nursing facilities, screening could be performed on admission from the hospital and then weekly.[15] There is even a case to be made, given the frequency with which delirium is seen and the seriousness of this diagnosis, that a vital sign for mental status should be instituted across all health care sites for older people.[36]

A large number of validated delirium scales exist. When choosing which one to use, the following should be kept in mind: (1) there is no unanimity about which scale is best; (2) scales differ according to whether they screen for delirium or measure the severity of the symptoms of delirium; (3) they differ by length of time to administer; (4) some scales are designed for health care professionals with knowledge of the full range of constructs associated with delirium and some are designed for those without this depth of knowledge; (5) some scales are better in certain sites compared with others; and (6) some may have better sensitivity but lower specificity, and vice versa. It is beyond the scope of this article to discuss any of the scales in detail, but good reviews and comparison studies that cover these points are available.[37-39]

Differentiating Delirium from Dementia

A mislabeling, or lack of differentiation between these 2 diagnoses, is believed to be the reason why delirium is missed by physicians and nurses. Misdiagnosis or late diagnosis may also partly explain why delirium is associated with so many negative consequences.[22,40] **Table 2** details some of the differentiating characteristics between delirium and dementia. Note that one of the criteria not in **Table 2** is that delirium occurs in the context of a medical illness, metabolic derangement, drug toxicity, or withdrawal.

Altered level of consciousness (LOC) is an excellent clue in differentiating delirium and dementia because it is not always possible to know the patient's baseline mental status. Without ever having seen the patient before, one can determine whether the patient's LOC lies toward the agitated or vigilant side of the spectrum of LOC, or toward the lethargic, drowsy, or stuporous side of the spectrum.

One can ask orientation questions, but because disorientation and problems with memory are present in both delirium and dementia, the key in determining delirium from dementia is how the patient answers. The delirious patient often gives disorganized answers, which can be described as rambling or even incoherent.

The classic identifiers of delirium are acute onset and fluctuating course, both of which are usually obtained by close caregivers (family or nurses). Although acute implies 24 hours, the term subacute is used to emphasize that subtle mental status changes can be overlooked by caregivers. Over a period of many days, the patient may slowly decline mentally, and health care professionals may contribute this to the underlying dementia. If left unchecked, this subacute delirium may impair other necessary functions, leading to further medical problems, such as dehydration and malnutrition. This snowball effect explains in part why the cause of delirium is typically multifactorial. Thus, if it is unclear how long the change has been occurring, patients should be put in the category of delirium and an evaluation should be performed.

Attention is also one of the classic identifiers of delirium, which may often be helpful if the patient's baseline mental status is not known. It can be tested by having a conversation. Patients may have difficulty maintaining or following the conversation,

Table 2
Differentiating delirium from dementia

	Delirium	Dementia
Consciousness	Decreased alertness or hyperalert, clouded	Alert
Orientation	Disorganized	Disoriented
Course	Fluctuating	Steady slow decline
Onset	Acute or subacute	Chronic
Attention	Impaired	Usually normal
Psychomotor	Agitated or lethargic	Usually normal
Hallucinations	Perceptual disturbances May have hallucinations	Usually not present
Sleep-wake cycle	Abnormal	Usually normal
Speech	Slow, incoherent	Aphasic, anomic Difficulty finding words

perseverate on the previous question, or become easily distracted. Attention can also be tested with cognitive tasks such as days of the week backward or months of the year backward.

Psychomotor agitation or lethargy, hallucinations, sleep-wake cycle abnormalities, and slow or incoherent speech can all be seen in patients with delirium, but these features are not necessary for the diagnosis.

Identifying and Treating the Underlying Causes of the Delirium

General guidelines are to consider all possible causes, proceed cautiously with appropriate testing, and keep in mind that delirium is usually caused by a combination of underlying causes. The mnemonic D-E-L-I-R-I-U-M-S can be used as a checklist to cover most causes of delirium (**Box 1**).

Drugs are one of the most common causes of delirium. According to most investigators in this area, "virtually any" and "practically every" drug can be considered deliriogenic.[41,42] Several drugs have been found in vitro to have varying amounts of anticholinergic properties. However, because the pathophysiologic and neurotransmitter mechanisms of delirium go beyond anticholinergic mechanisms, a more practical approach is to remember certain medications and categories of medications that have been reported to cause or are associated with delirium.[43] Some are more common offenders than others, and thus considered high risk, as opposed to moderate to low risk. However, determining risk depends on the vulnerability (frailty) of the person taking the medications as much as it depends on the medication itself (**Table 3**). Also, many older reports did not use delirium criteria, but described psychiatric side effects that might indicate the presence of delirium, such as hallucinosis, paranoia, delusions, psychosis, general confusion, aggressiveness, restlessness, and drowsiness.[44]

A few caveats are worth noting. Tricyclic antidepressants (TCAs) can cause delirium, with an overall incidence ranging from 1.5% to 20%. The highest rates seem to be among older, previously cognitively impaired, and medically ill patients. Serotonin selective reuptake inhibitor (SSRI) antidepressants have a safer side effect profile compared with the TCAs as far as delirium is concerned. However, one of the main side effects of SSRIs, hyponatremia, can present as delirium in older persons.[43] This finding has been reported with fluoxetine, fluvoxamine, paroxetine, and sertraline. Although frank delirium caused by SSRIs is rare, most reported cases seem to point toward drug interactions as a plausible cause. However, to emphasize that no

---

Box 1
Causes of delirium

D Drugs

E Eyes, ears

L Low oxygen states or insults (myocardial infarction, stroke, pulmonary embolus)

I Infection

R Retention (of urine or stool)

I Ictal (ie, postictal states)

U Uncontrolled pain

M Metabolic

(S) Subdural

Table 3
Medications or categories of medications that can cause or be associated with delirium[a]

High Risk	Moderate to Low Risk
Benzodiazepines	Acetylcholinesterase inhibitors
Diphenhydramine	Anticonvulsants
Dopamine agonists	Antidepressants
Meperidine	Antispasmodics
Muscle relaxants	β-Blockers
Neuroleptics	Clonidine
Scopolamine	Corticosteroids
	Digoxin
	H_2 blockers
	Meclizine
	Memantine
	Metoclopramide
	Narcotics, other than meperidine
	Nonsteroidal antiinflammatory agents
	Sedative-hypnotics
	Some antibiotics
	Some antivirals

[a] Diphenhydramine is the most common agent found in over-the-counter sleeping pills. Meperidine is a narcotic, but because of its high risk for delirium, it is listed separately. Neuroleptics are also known as antipsychotics. Antispasmodics refer to drugs used for overactive bladder or urinary incontinence. Long-acting agents are less deliriogenic than short-acting ones. H_2 blockers are most risky in patients with chronic kidney disease because they are renally excreted. Some of the reported antiviral and antibiotics reported to cause delirium include acyclovir, antimalarials, fluoroquinolones, isoniazid, linezolid, macrolides, and interferon.

centrally acting drug is completely safe, in a study of 10 healthy volunteers, paroxetine increased ratings of confusion and fatigue.[45] There are also case reports of confusion caused by antidepressants such as mirtazapine and venlafaxine.[46,47]

Narcotics can be used safely in older persons with little risk of developing delirium, but a few important details need to be remembered. Meperidine is particularly risky in older persons, likely because of the anticholinergic activity of its active metabolite normeperidine. The main problems associated with the use of narcotics are probably related to toxicity, overuse, or overdosage in patients with impaired hepatic or renal function.[42]

Muscle relaxant is a misnomer because these medications act centrally in the brain, not locally at the muscles. Some of the commonly used muscle relaxants include cyclobenzaprine, methocarbamol, and carisoprodol, and have been reported to cause delirium.

Seizure medications have been reported to cause varying types of cognitive impairment, including drowsiness, agitation, depression, psychosis, and delirium. The cognitive impairment is believed to be related to serum levels, but clinicians should keep in mind that most anticonvulsants are protein bound and if the patient's nutritional status is poor then there is potential that the amount of free drug is higher than what is measured by the serum level.

The E in the D-E-L-I-R-I-U-M mnemonic stands for emotions and reminds the clinician that depression can have psychotic features and may present similar to patients with delirium. Depression can also affect attention and thought process. Although depression has classically been considered the masquerader of dementia, given some of the criteria for delirium such as disorganized thinking, psychomotor lethargy and inattention, depression should be considered a reversible cause of delirium.

Low oxygen states or insults in the mnemonic should highlight to the clinician that older patients with acute cardiovascular or pulmonary illnesses can present with delirium. It could be said that delirium is as serious as a heart attack because older delirious patients can have myocardial infarctions that are commonly missed or present atypically. It is unclear whether patients, because of the delirium, cannot either describe or tell clinicians about chest pain, or whether there exists a cardiocerebral syndrome in which the stress of the myocardial infarction affects the adrenergic system, causing a stress on the balance in the central nervous system, that is, in cognition.[48] Not only are patients with stroke at risk of developing delirium as a complication of the stroke or the underlying comorbidities associated with the stroke but also delirium may be the presenting feature of some patients with stroke.[49]

Infections are one of the most common underlying causes of delirium among older people. The most common types of infections that cause delirium are urinary tract infections and respiratory infections. However, with the recent increase in antibiotic-associated diarrhea caused by *Clostridium difficile* bacteria, some clinicians have urged caution not to overdiagnose urinary tract infections that may be asymptomatic bacteriuria. Subtle infections such as cholecystitis and diverticulitis should be in the differential diagnosis.[50] Although meningitis is on the differential, cerebrospinal fluid analysis is probably not warranted in the initial workup of delirious patients without other symptoms that point toward a central nervous system infection.[51]

Retention of urine and feces can both cause delirium, although typically the presentations differ. Urinary retention causing delirium has been well reported in the literature under the term cystocerebral syndrome. The original report was of 3 cases, all were older men who became acutely agitated and nearly mute. All 3 patients had large volumes of urine in their bladder and in all 3 patients, the agitated delirium resolved within a short time after emptying the bladder.[52] A proposed explanation is that the adrenergic tension related to the urinary retention might increase in the central nervous system and the consequent increase in catecholamines might produce delirium.[53] Although this pathophysiologic explanation has not been proved, clinicians should be aware of this syndrome. One of the best ways to quickly evaluate for urinary retention is with a hand-held bladder ultrasound scanner. Although these scanners have a high initial cost, cost savings from the reduction in use of straight catheterizations may help balance this issue.[54]

Fecal retention as a cause of delirium has not been reported in the literature. However, because older patients for multiple reasons are at risk for fecal impactions, clinicians should be suspicious of this problem when the delirium is of the hypoactive type.

Ictal states are a rare cause of delirium and are not difficult to diagnose clinically for patients with tonic clonic seizures. However, patients who experience absence seizures or partial seizures may go unnoticed by caregivers and may seem to have only fluctuating mental status changes. Although an electroencephalogram is not indicated in the initial medical evaluation of delirium, it should be considered when pertinent history is obtained.

Uncontrolled pain can be a cause of delirium. The patient may present with agitation presumably attributed to an underlying dementia, especially if there is a significant aphasia associated with the dementia. Empiric treatment with at least routine acetaminophen and possibly a low-dose narcotic is justified in some circumstances.[55] Postoperative pain has been found to be associated with delirium risk.[56]

Metabolic abnormalities that cause delirium are not difficult to identify because of the availability of commonly used laboratory tests. A complete metabolic panel usually identifies hyponatremia, hypernatremia, hypocalcemia, hypercalcemia, and abnormalities of liver function or renal function. Thyroid function tests and vitamin B_{12} are typically put in this category, but mild changes, if present, are not likely to be the main cause.

Although delirium is not spelled with an "s" at the end, using the mnemonic DELIRIUMS emphasizes to the clinician that delirium usually has more than 1 cause. The "s" also reminds the clinician that a subdural hematoma can cause a mental status change. Although the mortality of subdural hematomas among younger people is high, the prognosis for older people is good as long as the diagnosis is not missed.[57] The other difference between older and younger patients with subdural hematomas is that older patients may develop the subdural hematoma over a period of a few hours or days. Although there could be some debate as to whether or not all older patients presenting to a hospital with delirium should have some sort of brain imaging, most agree that because this is a reversible problem that may cease to be reversible if the diagnosis is delayed, imaging should be considered if there has been a history of head trauma or falls or any suspicion of an unwitnessed fall.

Management of Delirium

Similar to the comprehensive approach for evaluation, comprehensive management interventions need to be targeted toward patients at risk of developing delirium (and thus prevention of delirium) and patients who have already developed delirium. **Table 4** describes several studies, some of which do both (prevention and management),[14,58–60] and some of which focus on just one.[61–67]

Some of the key components in these studies include: (1) staff education; (2) systematic screening for delirium; (3) use of multiple disciplines; (4) use of multiple components; (5) use of geriatric principles (primarily avoidance of iatrogenic causes of delirium); and (6) a focus on nonpharmacologic interventions.

Based on these studies, it is evident that prevention of delirium, and decrease in the severity of delirium, is possible. Improving function among delirious patients is also possible, but may be more difficult to achieve.

Other outcomes such as LOS and mortality seem difficult to affect, but not impossible. The study by Lundstrom and colleagues[60] was able to show this finding. One of the explanations for the negative studies in this area is the low implementation rates of all the components of an intervention or the consult recommendations.[63,65]

Although a review of studies from other sites (home care, nursing homes, postacute care, ICU) are beyond the scope of this article, it is worth noting that interventions in the ICU such as wake-up-and-breathe protocols, less sedation, early mobilization even while patients are intubated, and use of mental exercises have shown positive results.[68–71]

Prevention of delirium through pharmacologic means has been studied, but no strong evidence exists to support it. One study of an acetylcholinesterase inhibitor among patients in the ICU was stopped early because of increased mortality in the drug group compared with the placebo.[72] Another study among patients undergoing hip surgery (most elective) found that haloperidol compared with placebo did not reduce the incidence of delirium but did decrease the severity when it occurred.[73]

Table 4
Delirium prevention and management studies

References	Focus; Type of Patients	Type of Study (N)	Intervention	Outcome
Wanich et al,[58] 1992	Prevention and management; medical	Nonrandomized: intervention unit vs 2 standard care units (235)	Multidisciplinary nursing, especially geriatric clinical specialist (educate nursing staff, mobilize patients, monitor medications, environmental and sensory modifications)	More likely to improve function if on the intervention unit (adjusted odds ratio, 3.29 [95% confidence interval, 1.26–8.17]). No difference in delirium incidence, LOS, discharge location, mortality
Milisen et al,[59] 2001	Prevention and management; hip fracture	Randomized (120)	Education of nurses, systematic screening, consult by nurse specialist, scheduled pain protocol	Mortality inconclusive, no difference in LOS or function. Decrease in delirium duration and severity, but not incidence
Marcantonio et al,[14] 2001	Prevention and management; hip fracture	Randomized (126)	Geriatrician consultation (61% done pre-operatively, the rest within 24 hours)	No difference in mortality, LOS. Decreased incidence of delirium (32% vs 50%) and incidence of severe delirium (12% vs 29%).
Lundstrom et al,[60] 2005	Prevention and management; medical	Randomized (400)	Multicomponent staff education, assessment, prevention and treatment of delirium and caregiver intervention	Decrease in mortality (2 deaths vs 9 deaths, $P = .03$), decrease in LOS (10.8 days vs 20.5 days), decrease in percent with delirium at day 7 (30% vs 60%).
Inouye et al,[61] 1999	Prevention; medical	Randomized (426)	Multicomponent intervention targeted at patients with certain risk factors to develop delirium	No change in mortality and LOS of patients with delirium. Decreased incidence of delirium (9.9% vs 15%; odds ratio, 0.6; 95% confidence interval, 0.39–0.92), and number of days with delirium

Study	Design (n)	Type	Intervention	Outcomes
Naughton et al,[62] 2005	Observational; preintervention/postintervention (374)	Prevention; medical	Education in the emergency department and admission to an acute geriatric unit	Preintervention vs 4-month postintervention vs 9-month postintervention: delirium incidence decreased from 41% to 22.7% to 19.1%
Cole et al,[63] 1994	Randomized (88)	Management; medical	Systematic detection of delirium, geriatrician consult, geriatric nurse specialist does follow-up	No difference in mortality, LOS, function. Minor difference in delirium severity
Lundstrom,[64] 1999	Randomized (49)	Management; hip fracture	Multicomponent recognition, staff education, cooperation between orthopedics and geriatrics, treat delirium and complications	Improved function, decrease in duration and incidence of delirium
Cole et al,[65] 2002	Randomized (227)	Management; medical	Systematic detection of delirium, geriatrician consult, geriatric nurse specialist does follow-up	No difference in mortality, LOS, function, discharge location, delirium duration
Pitkala et al,[66] 2006	Randomized (174)	Management; medical	Intensified multicomponent geriatric directed management	No difference in mortality, LOS, or rate of institutionalization. Delirium was alleviated better in the intervention group
Flaherty et al,[67] 2010	Observational (148)	Management; medical	Use of a delirium room (specialized restraint-free room with 24-hour nursing) within an Acute Care for the Elderly Unit	Delirious patients compared with nondelirious patients had improved function; equal LOS and mortality

PHYSICAL RESTRAINTS

Physical restraints should not be used for patients who are at risk of developing delirium or who have already developed delirium. Physical restraints are associated with developing delirium and are significantly related to severity of delirium. The proposed reason for their use, to prevent injury primarily related to falls, is misconceived. Of 3 studies of restraint reduction programs in long-term care institutions, 2 showed no change in fall rate and 1 showed an increase in fall rate. However, all 3 studies showed a decrease in fall injury rates.[74–76]

Of 2 studies in the hospital setting, restraint reduction was not associated with an increase in falls.[77,78] The rate of restraint use in the study by Powell and colleagues[77] went from 52 per 1000 patient-days to just 0.3 per 1000 patient-days. Although neither study reported injury rates before and after restraint reduction, the study by Mion and colleagues reported that injury rates after the restraint reduction program were low. Restraint reduction programs were modestly successful ($\geq$20% reduction) in 2 of 6 ICUs and no deaths were reported to have occurred as a result of a fall or disruption in therapy, including in patients in the ICU on mechanical ventilators.[77,78] Furthermore, the fact that restraint-free environments can be achieved, as in some geriatric departments in European hospitals,[79] Acute Care of the Elderly Units in United States hospitals,[80] and some nursing facilities,[81,82] adds to the evidence that restraint-free care should be the standard of care.

USE OF PHARMACOLOGIC AGENTS

No antipsychotic or other pharmacologic agent is approved by the US Food and Drug Administration (FDA) for the treatment of delirium. **Table 5** describes several studies that focus on use of antipsychotics among medical/surgical patients or psychiatric consults of medical/surgical patients, and have at least 10 patients in the study.[83–100] A discussion of antipsychotics in the ICU is beyond the scope of this article, but this area is receiving more attention.[101]

Most of the studies in **Table 5** used a prospective open-label method, and most of these evaluated a single drug. Eight studies compared 2 drugs. One study used a prospective double-blind, randomized method,[91] 1 study used a prospective blinded-rater method,[99] and 1 study had a nonplacebo control group.[94] Only 1 study used a placebo group.[100]

This placebo-controlled trial, performed among non-ICU medical-surgical patients, was a well-designed study with a goal of enrolling 34 patients in each group. However, according to the investigators, the trial was stopped early at the request of the manufacturer because of the FDA's concern about the use of antipsychotic medication in elderly patients. There was no difference in adverse events between the 2 groups, but this study should be considered a pilot study. On subscale analyses, there was a suggestion that the quetiapine group's severity scores improved significantly more quickly than the placebo group's.[100]

Of the 5 studies reporting time-to-peak responses, 3 studies found the average time was more than 6 days, 1 study 5.1 days, and 1 study 3.8 days. The average time for resolution ranged from 4.2 to 7.4 days. Of 4 studies reporting resolution rates, 3 reported high rates (76%–100%). Nine of 10 studies showed that more than 70% of patients had a 50% or more reduction in one of the delirium rating scales (see **Table 5**).

In analyzing these studies, it seems that these medications led to improvement or resolution in delirium. However, without a placebo group, one cannot say for sure if the drug is causing the intended effect or if some of the cases of delirium are improving

Table 5
Review of studies of antipsychotics in delirium among medical/surgical patients or psychiatric consults of medical/surgical patients

References	Methods	N Mean age ± Standard Deviation (Age Range)[a]	Type of Patients	Drugs (n)	Placebo?	Assessment Method[b]	Outcome and Time Frame (If Reported)
Nakamura et al,[83] 1997	Prospective, open-label, randomized	66 68 ± 15 vs 64 ± 13 (40–92 vs 23–86)	Medical and surgical patients	Haloperidol (17) Mianserin (49)	No	DRS	>50% reduction in DRS: 71% haloperidol, 69% mianserin
Sipahimalani and Masand,[84] 1998	Retrospective	22 65 ± 18 vs 64±23 (19–89)	Psychiatric consults on mostly medical, some surgical patients	Haloperidol (11) Olanzapine (11)	No	DRS	Peak response[c]: 6.8 days haloperidol, 7.2 days olanzapine >50% reduction in DRS: 45% haloperidol group 55% olanzapine group
Schwartz and Masand,[85] 2000	Retrospective	22 54 ± 19 vs 58 ± 21 (21–74 vs 19–91)	Psychiatric consults on medical patients	Haloperidol (11) Quetiapine (11)	No	DRS	Peak response: 6.5 days haloperidol, 7.6 days quetiapine >50% reduction in DRS: 91% in both groups
Kim et al,[86] 2001	Prospective, open-label	20 46 ± 18 (19–74)	Psychiatry consults on neurosurgical, neurologic and oncology patients	Olanzapine	No	DRS	Peak response: 3.8 ± 1.7 days >50% decrease in DRS: 70%
Breitbart et al,[87] 2002	Prospective, open-label	79 61 ± 17 (range 19–89)	Oncology patients	Olanzapine	No	MDAS	Resolution rates (MDAS <10): 45% by time 2 (day 2–3) 76% by time 3 (day 4–7)
Sasaki et al,[88] 2003	Prospective, open-label	12 67 ± 15 (37–84)	Psychiatric consults on medical and surgical patients	Quetiapine	No	DRS-J (Japanese version)	Average time to resolution (DRS-J <12): 4.8 ± 3.5 days Resolution rate: 100%

(continued on next page)

Table 5
(continued)

References	Methods	N Mean age ± Standard Deviation (Age Range)[a]	Type of Patients	Drugs (n)	Placebo?	Assessment Method[b]	Outcome and Time Frame (If Reported)
Kim et al,[89] 2003	Prospective, open-label	12 74 ± 4 (64–88)	Psychiatry consults on medical patients	Quetiapine	No	Attending psychiatrist	Average time to stabilization (determined by attending psychiatrist): 5.9 ± 2 days
Parellada et al,[90] 2004	Prospective, open-label	64 67 ± 11	Medical patients	Risperidone	No	DRS	Resolution rate (DRS <13 by day 3): 91%
Han and Kim,[91] 2004	Prospective, double-blind, randomized	24 66 ± 8 vs 67 ± 16	Psychiatry consults on mostly medical, some fractures	Risperidone (12) Haloperidol (12)	No	MDAS	Average time to resolution (MDAS <13): 4.2 ± 2.1 days risperidone 4.2 ± 2.5 days haloperidol Resolution rates: 42% risperidone. 75% haloperidol (P = .11)
Liu et al,[92] 2004	Retrospective	77 68 ± 10 vs 50 ± 15 (40–85 vs 15–77)	Psychiatric consults on mostly medical, some surgical	Risperidone (41) Haloperidol (36)	No	DSM-IV by psychiatrist	Average time to recovery (did not meet DSM-IV delirium criteria for 2 consecutive days according to a psychiatrist): 7 ± 4 days risperidone 8 ± 5 days haloperidol
Pae et al,[93] 2004	Retrospective	22 69 ± 10 (48–85)	Psychiatry consults on medical, neurosurgical, orthopedic, oncology patients	Quetiapine	No	DRS-R-98	Average time to resolution: (DRS-R-98 <15): 7 ± 4 days >50% reduction in DRS-R-98: 86%
Hu et al,[94] 2004	Prospective, open-label controlled study	175 74 ± 8 (65–99)	Mostly medical, some surgical	Olanzapine (74) Haloperidol (72) Control (29)	No	DRS	Reduced DRS scores: 72% olanzapine, 70% haloperidol, 25% control

Study	Design	N / Age[a]	Setting	Drugs (n)	Placebo-controlled	Assessment[b]	Results
Lee et al,[95] 2005	Prospective, open-label, randomized	31; 61 ± 18 vs 63 ± 15	Psychiatry consults on medical, neurosurgical, orthopedic, oncology patients	Amisulpride (16) Quetiapine (15)	No	DRS-R-98	Average time to stabilization (not well defined): 6.3 days amisulpride, 7.4 days quetiapine, >50% reduction in DRS-R-98: 81% vs 80%
Straker et al,[96] 2006	Prospective, open-label	14; 70 ± 11 (18–85)	Psychiatric consults on medical and surgical patients	Aripiprazole	No	DRS-R-98	Peak response: 6.2 ± 3.8 days >50% reduction in DRS-R-98: 50% by day 5 86% by day 7
Takeuchi et al,[97] 2007	Prospective, open-label	38; 69 ± 10	Psychiatric consults on medical and surgical patients	Perisperone	No	DRS-R-98	Peak response: 5.1 ± 4.9 days >50% reduction in DRS-R-98: 71%
Maneeton et al,[98] 2007	Prospective, open-label	17; 56 ± 19	Psychiatric consults on mostly medical and some orthopedic patients	Quetiapine	No	DRS-R-98	Average time to >50% reduction in DRS-R-98: 3.9 ± 2.1 days >50% reduction in DRS-R-98: 88.2%
Kim et al,[99] 2010	Prospective randomized, rater-blinded (1 of the investigators)	32; 67 ± 12 vs 68 ± 11 (36–82)	Psychiatric consults on mostly oncology, some medical and some orthopedic patients	Risperidone (17) Olanzapine (15)	No	DRS-R-98	Median number of days to achieve >50% reduction in DRS-R-98: 5 days risperidone, 3 days olanzapine ($P = .298$) >50% reduction in DRS-R-98: 65% risperidone, 73% olanzapine
Tahir et al,[100] 2010	Prospective randomized, placebo-controlled	84 ± 9 vs 84 ± 7 (58–95 vs 71–98)	Medical and surgical	Quetiapine (21) Placebo (20)	Yes	DRS-R-98	No difference in total DRS-R-98 scores at all time points (days 2, 3, 4, 7, 10)

[a] Age ranges not always available.

[b] Assessment methods: DRS, Delirium Rating Scale. A 10-item scale integrating DSM-III criteria for delirium. Maximum score is 32. Score of more than 13 consistent with delirium[105]; MDAS, Memorial Delirium Rating Scale. A 10-item scale integrating DSM-III criteria for delirium. Maximum score = 30. Score of more than 13 consistent with delirium (more stringent score of <10 was used in Breitbart study for resolution)[106]; DRS-R-98, Delirium Rating Scale-Revised-98 is a 16-item scale with maximum score of 39. It is a revision of the original DRS by Trzepacz and colleagues.[107] Cutoff score of 15.25 had best sensitivity for diagnosis of delirium in original study.

[c] Peak response: number of days receiving antipsychotic before achieving maximum response.

or resolving because of other reasons (eg, the natural course of the syndrome or identifying the underlying causes).

Furthermore, it is not clear how long a typical case of delirium should last.[102] Indirect evidence can be found from nonpharmacologic intervention studies. One study of general medical patients focusing on staff education and system reorganization found that for delirious patients in the intervention group, 70% of delirium resolved by day 7. Only 10% received an antipsychotic drug.[60] Another study of a nurse-led interdisciplinary intervention focusing on older patients with hip fractures found that of the patients with delirium in the intervention group, 92% had resolution of delirium by day 3, and 100% by day 6. Even in the control group, 71% had resolution by day 5.[59]

One of the overlooked problems with using antipsychotic medications is that the mechanisms of action of these agents are not pure.[103] Each of these medications binds to 4 or 5 different parent neurotransmitter systems (dopaminergic, serotonergic, adrenergic, histaminic, and muscarinic) in varying degrees. All of the antipsychotics act as antagonists at their respective neurotransmitter receptor. For example, although risperidone binds tightly to the serotonergic (5-HT$_{2A}$) receptors, it also binds to the dopaminergic, α_1, and histaminergic receptors. Haloperidol has a high binding affinity to the dopamine-2 (D$_2$) receptor. This is in contrast to quetiapine, which has a relatively low binding affinity for the D$_2$ receptor. Olanzapine has strong binding to the muscarinic receptors and, similar to risperidone, binds to the 5-HT$_{2A}$ receptors. However, the sedation properties of olanzapine are probably because of its binding affinity for the histaminic receptors.

The exception to this issue of nonselectivity is for older patients who are experiencing hallucinations. The cause of hallucinations is believed to be through the dopaminergic neurotransmitter system. Dopamine antagonists (as used in schizophrenia) can reduce this symptom. Based on positron emission tomography studies, binding to 60% to 80% of the D$_2$ receptors correlates with antipsychotic efficacy. However, higher binding to a greater percentage of the D$_2$ receptors may be associated with increased adverse drug reactions (extrapyramidal symptoms and hyperprolactinemia).[104]

Based on this discussion, 2 conclusions can be made: (1) because of the complexities of the pathophysiology, the nonselective nature of antipsychotics and the lack of placebo-controlled trials, there is no role for general use of antipsychotics in the treatment of delirium; and (2) there may be a limited role for use among a targeted group of patients with delirium who experience hallucinations or delusions associated with the delirium.

If antipsychotics are used, the goal should be an awake patient who is manageable, not a sedated patient, and the drug should be tapered and discontinued as soon as possible.

NONPHARMACOLOGIC METHODS

Having a philosophy of a restraint-free environment and nonuse of antipsychotics is not possible without a wide array of practical options and educational interventions. The TADA approach, which stands for tolerate, anticipate, and don't agitate, can be used for patients at risk of developing delirium (eg, patients with dementia, one of the highest risk factors) and for patients who have already developed delirium. Two videos depicting scenarios of health care providers using the TADA approach (called *Managing Agitated Behaviors in the Nursing Home* and *Managing Agitated Behaviors in the Hospital*) can be found at the following Web site: http://www.stlouis.va.gov/GRECC/Education.asp.

Tolerating behaviors that may seem to be potentially dangerous is contrary to our nature as health care providers. For example, when patients try to get out of bed by themselves or pull on oxygen tubing or telemetry monitoring systems, a health care provider's first response is to prevent them from doing these things either because we believe that patients are about to harm themselves or the oxygen/telemetry is a necessary part of their care. However, allowing patients to respond naturally to their situation while under close observation (which often means standing or sitting close by), gives the patient some semblance of control in their confused state. Tolerating behaviors also allows the health care provider to get clues about what might be bothering the patient. For example, with a patient who is so delirious that he cannot communicate his need to empty his bladder, his getting out of bed might be the first signal to the nurse that he needs to be toileted right now, not at the 2-hour mark.

Anticipating behaviors, so that the health care provider can either prepare for what the patient might do or avoid the inciting agent, is an important part of the approach. Certain behaviors, actions, and reactions of patients with delirium seem logical once they are described and seen on a regular basis. A few of the most common ones with some options for management include: (1) pulling on anything that is not normally present; hiding these unnatural attachments can help, as can using a decoy (eg, taping a false intravenous [IV] attachment on [not in] the patient's nondominant arm); (2) when an attachment is needed, try to use it briefly, then get rid of it or hide it (eg, give IV fluids as boluses, instead of a continuous rate; cover up the precious IV attachment in between the boluses); (3) getting rid of attachments that are not completely necessary and being flexible with attachments that do seem necessary; the seemingly standard telemetry monitor and oxygen tubing that most patients receive are 2 overused attachments; in today's hospital environment of multiple physicians per patient and fear of not doing enough for a patient, it is not easy for nurses to encourage physicians to discontinue certain attachments; (4) when attachments are necessary, staying flexible in their use can help (eg, it might seem imperative that we have minute-by-minute recordings of heart rate and rhythm for a patient with uncontrolled atrial fibrillation, but having the patient wear the monitor an average of 30 minutes per hour might be better than agitating the patient); (5) getting out of bed is as natural as eating and toileting; this action is so anticipated and encouraged that standby observation is more the culture than standby assistance.

Don't agitate is one of the golden rules of this approach. There are numerous agitators in the hospital environment, some of which agitate certain delirious patients and calm others. Some agitators are predictable; many are not. Reorientation is one of the unpredictable ones. One option is to attempt reorientation, but not to use it if it does not seem to help. When reorientation does not work, use distraction techniques (change the subject) or go along with the disorientation, as long as it is safe.

SUMMARY

Delirium is defined as a disturbance in level of awareness or attention, marked by an acute or subacute onset of cognitive changes attributable to a general medical condition, and it tends to have a fluctuating course. The proposed pathophysiology of delirium involves imbalances in several neurotransmitters systems in the brain. However, it is not well elucidated, making it is impossible for the clinician to determine which neurotransmitter(s) is/are predominately involved in any particular case. Delirium among older persons is near ubiquitous in health care (10%–31% among hospitalized medical patients, as high as 74% among patients with coronary artery bypass graft, and 80% in the ICU). It is also found among patients receiving postacute care and nursing home residents receiving long-term care, and to a lesser extent, home care patients. Delirium is associated with hospital complications, loss of physical function, increased LOS in the hospital and within the ICU, increased risk of discharge to long-term care facilities, and higher mortality. Delirium among some patients, particularly from the ICU, may be associated with long-term cognitive impairment. Evaluation includes awareness and screening, differentiating delirium from dementia, and identifying and treating the underlying causes of the delirium. Models of care in the prevention of patients at risk of delirium and management of patients for whom delirium is not preventable exist and typically include (1) staff education; (2) systematic screening for delirium; (3) use of multiple disciplines; (4) use of multiple components; (5) use of geriatric principles (primarily avoidance of iatrogenic causes of delirium); and (6) a focus on nonpharmacologic interventions. The evidence for use of physical restraints is negative and thus they should not be used for patients at risk of developing delirium or who have already developed delirium. Because of the complexities of the pathophysiology, the nonselective nature of antipsychotics and the lack of placebo-controlled trials, there is no role for general use of antipsychotics in the treatment of delirium. An example of a restraint-free, nonpharmacologic management intervention is the TADA approach: tolerate, anticipate, and don't agitate.

REFERENCES

1. Lipowski ZJ. Delirium. Acute brain failure in man. Springfield (IL): Charles C Thomas; 1980.
2. Meagher D, Trzepacz PT. Phenomenological distinctions needed in DSM-V: delirium, subsyndromal delirium, and dementias. J Neuropsychiatry Clin Neurosci 2007;19(4):468–70.
3. Maldonado JR. Pathoetiological model of delirium: a comprehensive understanding of the neurobiology of delirium and an evidence-based approach to prevention and treatment. Crit Care Clin 2008;24(4):789–856.
4. Janz DR, Abel TW, Jackson JC, et al. Brain autopsy findings in intensive care unit patients previously suffering from delirium: a pilot study. J Crit Care 2010; 25(3):538 e7–12.
5. van Munster BC, de Rooij SE, Yazdanpanah M, et al. The association of the dopamine transporter gene and the dopamine receptor 2 gene with delirium, a meta-analysis. Am J Med Genet B Neuropsychiatr Genet Br 2010;153(2): 648–55.
6. Inouye SK. Delirium in hospitalized older patients: recognition and risk factors. J Geriatr Psychiatry Neurol 1998;11:118–25.
7. Siddiqi N, House A. Delirium: an update on diagnosis, treatment and prevention. Clin Med 2006;6(6):540–3.
8. Dyer CB, Ashton CM, Teasdale TA. Postoperative delirium. A review of 80 primary data-collection studies. Arch Intern Med 1995;155:461–5.
9. Marcantonio ER, Goldman L, Orav EJ, et al. The association of intraoperative factors with the development of postoperative delirium. Am J Med 1998; 105(5):380–4.
10. Ely EW, Shintani A, Truman B, et al. Delirium as a predictor of mortality in mechanically ventilated patients in the intensive care unit. JAMA 2004;291: 1753–62.
11. Pisani MA. Considerations in caring for the critically ill older patient. J Intensive Care Med 2009;24(2):83–95.

12. Vasilevskis EE, Ely EW, Speroff T, et al. Reducing iatrogenic risks: ICU-acquired delirium and weakness–crossing the quality chasm. Chest 2010;138(5): 1224–33.

13. Kelly KG, Zisselman M, Cutillo-Schmitter T, et al. Severity and course of delirium in medically hospitalized nursing facility residents. Am J Geriatr Psychiatry 2001;9:72–7.

14. Marcantonio ER, Flacker JM, Wright RJ, et al. Reducing delirium after hip fracture: a randomized trial. J Am Geriatr Soc 2001;49:516–22.

15. Marcantonio ER, Simon SE, Bergmann MA, et al. Delirium symptoms in post-acute care: prevalent, persistent, and associated with poor functional recovery. J Am Geriatr Soc 2003;51:4–9.

16. Mentes J, Culp K, Maas M, et al. Acute confusion indicators: risk factors and prevalence using MDS data. Res Nurs Health 1999;22:95–105.

17. Cacchione PZ, Culp K, Laing J, et al. Clinical profile of acute confusion in the long-term care setting. Clin Nurs Res 2003;12:145–58.

18. Caplan GA, Ward JA, Brennan NJ, et al. Hospital in the home: a randomized controlled trial. Med J Aust 1999;170:156–60.

19. Leff B, Burton L, Guido S, et al. Home hospital: a feasible and efficacious approach to care for acutely ill older persons. J Am Geriatr Soc 2004; 52:S194.

20. Thomas RI, Cameron DJ, Fahs MC. A prospective study of delirium and prolonged hospital stay. Exploratory study. Arch Gen Psychiatry 1988;45(10): 937–40.

21. Rockwood K. Acute confusion in elderly medical patients. J Am Geriatr Soc 1989;37(2):150–4.

22. Francis J, Martin D, Kapoor WN. A prospective study of delirium in hospitalized elderly. JAMA 1990;263:1097–101.

23. Ramsay R, Wright P, Katz A, et al. The detection of psychiatric morbidity and its effects on outcome in acute elderly medical admissions. Int J Geriatr Psychiatry 1991;6(12):861–6.

24. Jitapunkul S, Pillay I, Ebrahim S. Delirium in newly admitted elderly patients: a prospective study. Q J Med 1992;83(300):307–14.

25. Kolbeinsson H, Jonsson A. Delirium and dementia in acute medical admissions of elderly patients in Iceland. Acta Psychiatr Scand 1993;87(2):123–7.

26. Rockwood K. The occurrence and duration of symptoms in elderly patients with delirium. J Gerontol 1993;48(4):M162–6.

27. O'Keeffe S, Lavan J. The prognostic significance of delirium in older hospital patients. J Am Geriatr Soc 1997;45(2):174–8.

28. Inouye SK, Rushing JT, Foreman MD, et al. Does delirium contribute to poor hospital outcomes? A three-site epidemiologic study. J Gen Intern Med 1998; 13(4):234–42.

29. Zanocchi M, Vallero F, Norelli L, et al. [Acute confusion in the geriatric patient]. Recenti Prog Med 1998;89(5):229–34 [in Italian].

30. Vazquez F, O'Flaherty M, Michelangelo H, et al. [Epidemiology of delirium in elderly inpatients]. Medicina (B Aires) 2000;60(5 Pt 1):555–60 [in Spanish].

31. Villalpando-Berumen JM, Pineda-Colorado AM, Palacios P, et al. Incidence of delirium, risk factors, and long-term survival of elderly patients hospitalized in a medical specialty teaching hospital in Mexico City. Int Psychogeriatr 2003; 15(4):325–36.

32. Adamis D, Treloar A, Martin FC, et al. Recovery and outcome of delirium in elderly medical inpatients. Arch Gerontol Geriatr 2006;43(2):289–98.

33. Edlund A, Lundstrom M, Karlsson S, et al. Delirium in older patients admitted to general internal medicine. J Geriatr Psychiatry Neurol 2006;19(2):83–90.
34. Jackson JC, Gordon SM, Hart RP, et al. The association between delirium and cognitive decline: a review of the empirical literature. Neuropsychol Rev 2004; 4(2):87–98.
35. MacLullich AM, Beaglehole A, Hall RJ, et al. Delirium and long-term cognitive impairment. Int Rev Psychiatry 2009;21(1):30–42.
36. Flaherty JH, Rudolph J, Shay K, et al. Delirium is a serious and under-recognized problem: why assessment of mental status should be the 6th vital sign. J Am Med Dir Assoc 2007;8(6):273–5.
37. Adamis D, Sharma N, Whelan PJ, et al. Delirium scales: a review of current evidence. Aging Ment Health 2010;14(5):543–55.
38. van Eijk MM, van Marum RJ, Klijn IA, et al. Comparison of delirium assessment tools in a mixed intensive care unit. Crit Care Med 2009;37(6):1881–5.
39. Kean J, Ryan K. Delirium detection in clinical practice and research: critique of current tools and suggestions for future development. J Psychosom Res 2008; 65(3):255–9.
40. Lyness JM. Delirium: masquerades and misdiagnosis in elderly inpatients. J Am Geriatr Soc 1990;38:1235–8.
41. Carter GL, Dawson AH, Lopert R. Drug-induced delirium. Incidence, management and prevention. Drug Saf 1996;15:291–301.
42. Lipowski ZJ. Delirium in the elderly patient. N Engl J Med 1989;320:578–82.
43. Flaherty JH. Psychotherapeutic agents in older adults. Commonly prescribed and over-the-counter remedies: causes of confusion. Clin Geriatr Med 1998; 14:101–27.
44. Francis J. Drug-induced delirium: diagnosis and treatment. CNS Drugs 1996;5: 103.
45. Brauer LH, Rukstalis MR, deWit H. Acute subjective responses to paroxetine in normal volunteers. Drug Alcohol Depend 1995;39:223–30.
46. Bailer U, Fischer P, Kufferle B, et al. Occurrence of mirtazapine-induced delirium in organic brain disorder. Int Clin Psychopharmacol 2000;15:239–43.
47. Howe C, Ravasia S. Venlafaxine-induced delirium. Can J Psychiatry 2003;48: 129 Revue Canadienne de Psychiatrie.
48. Malone ML, Rosen LB, Goodwin JS. Complications of acute myocardial infarction in patients > or = 90 years of age. Am J Cardiol 1998;81(5):638–41.
49. Ferro JM, Caeiro L, Verdelho A. Delirium in acute stroke. Curr Opin Neurol 2002; 15:51–5.
50. Freeman NJ, Kirdar JA. An unusual manifestation of a common illness in the elderly. Hosp Pract 1990;25:91–4.
51. Warshaw G, Tanzer F. The effectiveness of lumbar puncture in the evaluation of delirium and fever in the hospitalized elderly. Arch Fam Med 1993;2:293–7.
52. Blackburn T, Dunn M. Cystocerebral syndrome. Acute urinary retention presenting as confusion in elderly patients. Arch Intern Med 1990;150:2577–8.
53. Liem PH, Carter WJ. Cystocerebral syndrome: a possible explanation. Arch Intern Med 1991;151:1884–6.
54. Frederickson M, Neitzel JJ, Miller EH, et al. The implementation of bedside bladder ultrasound technology: effects on patient and cost postoperative outcomes in tertiary care. Orthop Nurs 2000;19:79–87.
55. Chibnall JT, Tait RC, Harman B, et al. Effect of acetaminophen on behavior, well-being, and psychotropic medication use in nursing home residents with moderate-to-severe dementia. J Am Geriatr Soc 2005;53(11):1921–9.

56. Lynch EP, Lazor MA, Gellis JE, et al. The impact of postoperative pain on the development of postoperative delirium. Anesth Analg 1998;86:781–5.
57. Tagle P, Mery F, Torrealba G, et al. [Chronic subdural hematoma: a disease of elderly people]. Rev Med Chil 2003;131:177–82 [in Spanish].
58. Wanich CK, Sullivan-Marx EM, Gottlieb GL, et al. Functional status outcomes of a nursing intervention in hospitalized elderly. Image J Nurs Sch 1992;24(3): 201–7.
59. Milisen K, Foreman MD, Abraham IL, et al. A nurse-led interdisciplinary intervention program for delirium in elderly hip-fracture patients. J Am Geriatr Soc 2001; 49(5):523–32.
60. Lundstrom M, Edlund A, Karlsson S, et al. A multifactorial intervention program reduces the duration of delirium, length of hospitalization, and mortality in delirious patients. J Am Geriatr Soc 2005;53(4):622–8.
61. Inouye SK, Bogardus ST, Charpentier PA, et al. A multicomponent intervention to prevent delirium in hospitalized older patients. N Engl J Med 1999;340:669–76.
62. Naughton BJ, Saltzman S, Ramadan F, et al. A multifactorial intervention to reduce prevalence of delirium and shorten hospital length of stay. J Am Geriatr Soc 2005;53(1):18–23.
63. Cole MG, Primeau FJ, Bailey RF, et al. Systematic intervention for elderly inpatients with delirium: a randomized trial. CMAJ 1994;151(7):965–70.
64. Lundström M, Edlund A, Lundström G, et al. Reorganization of nursing and medical care to reduce the incidence of postoperative delirium and improve rehabilitation outcome in elderly patients treated for femoral neck fractures. Scand J Caring Sci 1999;13(3):193–200.
65. Cole MG, McCusker J, Bellavance F, et al. Systematic detection and multidisciplinary care of delirium in older medical inpatients: a randomized trial. CMAJ 2002;167:753–9.
66. Pitkälä KH, Laurila JV, Strandberg TE, et al. Multicomponent geriatric intervention for elderly inpatients with delirium: a randomized, controlled trial. J Gerontol A Biol Sci Med Sci 2006;61(2):176–81.
67. Flaherty JH, Steele DK, Chibnall JT, et al. An ACE unit with a delirium room may improve function and equalize length of stay among older delirious medical inpatients. J Gerontol A Biol Sci Med Sci 2010;65(12):1387–92.
68. Morandi A, Brummel NE, Ely EW. Sedation, delirium and mechanical ventilation: the 'ABCDE' approach. Curr Opin Crit Care 2011;17(1):43–9.
69. Shehabi Y, Riker RR, Bokesch PM, et al. Delirium duration and mortality in lightly sedated, mechanically ventilated intensive care patients. Crit Care Med 2010; 38(12):2311–8.
70. Schweickert WD, Pohlman MC, Pohlman AS, et al. Early physical and occupational therapy in mechanically ventilated, critically ill patients: a randomised controlled trial. Lancet 2009;373(9678):1874–82.
71. Pandharipande P, Banerjee A, McGrane S, et al. Liberation and animation for ventilated ICU patients: the ABCDE bundle for the back-end of critical care. Crit Care 2010;14(3):157.
72. van Eijk MM, Roes KC, Honing ML, et al. Effect of rivastigmine as an adjunct to usual care with haloperidol on duration of delirium and mortality in critically ill patients: a multicentre, double-blind, placebo-controlled randomised trial. Lancet 2010;376(9755):1829–37.
73. Kalisvaart KJ, de Jonghe JF, Bogaards MJ, et al. Haloperidol prophylaxis for elderly hip-surgery patients at risk for delirium: a randomized placebo-controlled study. J Am Geriatr Soc 2005;53(10):1658–66.

74. Neufeld RR, Libow LS, Foley WJ, et al. Restraint reduction reduces serious injuries among nursing home residents. J Am Geriatr Soc 1999;47:1202–7.
75. Capezuti E, Strumpf NE, Evans LK, et al. The relationship between physical restraint removal and falls and injuries among nursing home residents. J Gerontol A Biol Sci Med Sci 1998;53:M47–52.
76. Dunn KS. The effect of physical restraints on fall rates in older adults who are institutionalized. J Gerontol Nurs 2001;27:40–8.
77. Powell C, Mitchell-Pedersen L, Fingerote E, et al. Freedom from restraint: consequences of reducing physical restraints in the management of the elderly. CMAJ 1989;141:561–4.
78. Mion LC, Fogel J, Sandhu S, et al. Outcomes following physical restraint reduction programs in two acute care hospitals. Jt Comm J Qual Improv 2001;27:605–18.
79. de Vries OJ, Ligthart GJ, Nikolaus T, et al. Differences in period prevalence of the use of physical restraints in elderly inpatients of European hospitals and nursing homes. J Gerontol A Biol Sci Med Sci 2004;59(9):M922–3.
80. Flaherty JH, Tariq SH, Raghavan S, et al. A model for managing delirious older inpatients. J Am Geriatr Soc 2003;51:1031–5.
81. Gatz D. Moving to a restraint-free environment. Balance 2000;4:12–5.
82. Makowski TR, Maggard W, Morley JE. The Life Care Center of St. Louis experience with subacute care. Clin Geriatr Med 2000;16:701–24.
83. Nakamura J, Uchimura N, Yamada S, et al. Does plasma free-3-methoxy-4-hydroxyphenyl(ethylene)glycol increase in the delirious state? A comparison of the effects of mianserin and haloperidol on delirium. Int Clin Psychopharmacol 1997;12:147–52.
84. Sipahimalani A, Masand PS. Olanzapine in the treatment of delirium. Psychosomatics 1998;39:422–30.
85. Schwartz TL, Masand PS. Treatment of delirium with quetiapine. Prim Care Companion J Clin Psychiatry 2000;2(1):10–2.
86. Kim KS, Pae CU, Chae JH, et al. An open pilot trial of olanzapine for delirium in the Korean population. Psychiatry Clin Neurosci 2001;55(5):515–9.
87. Breitbart W, Tremblay A, Gibson C. An open trial of olanzapine for the treatment of delirium in hospitalized cancer patients. Psychosomatics 2002;43(3):175–82.
88. Sasaki Y, Matsuyama T, Inoue S, et al. A prospective, open-label, flexible-dose study of quetiapine in the treatment of delirium. J Clin Psychiatry 2003;64(11):1316–21.
89. Kim KY, Bader GM, Kotlyar V, et al. Treatment of delirium in older adults with quetiapine. J Geriatr Psychiatry Neurol 2003;16(1):29–31.
90. Parellada E, Baeza I, de Pablo J, et al. Risperidone in the treatment of patients with delirium. J Clin Psychiatry 2004;65:348–53.
91. Han CS, Kim YK. A double-blind trial of risperidone and haloperidol for the treatment of delirium. Psychosomatics 2004;45(4):297–301.
92. Liu CY, Juang YY, Liang HY, et al. Efficacy of risperidone in treating the hyperactive symptoms of delirium. Int Clin Psychopharmacol 2004;19(3):165–8.
93. Pae CU, Lee SJ, Lee CU, et al. A pilot trial of quetiapine for the treatment of patients with delirium. Hum Psychopharmacol 2004;19(2):125–7.
94. Hu H, Deng W, Yang H. A prospective random control study comparison of olanzapine and haloperidol in senile delirium. Chongging Med J 2004;8:1234–7.
95. Lee KU, Won WY, Lee HK, et al. Amisulpride versus quetiapine for the treatment of delirium: a randomized, open prospective study. Int Clin Psychopharmacol 2005;20(6):311–4.

96. Straker DA, Shapiro PA, Muskin PR. Aripiprazole in the treatment of delirium. Psychosomatics 2006;47(5):385–91.

97. Takeuchi T, Furuta K, Hirasawa T. Perospirone in the treatment of patients with delirium. Psychiatry Clin Neurosci 2007;61(1):67–70.

98. Maneeton B, Maneeton N, Srisurapanont M. An open-label study of quetiapine for delirium. J Med Assoc Thai 2007;90(10):2158–63.

99. Kim SW, Yoo JA, Lee SY, et al. Risperidone versus olanzapine for the treatment of delirium. Hum Psychopharmacol 2010;25(4):298–302.

100. Tahir TA, Eeles E, Karapareddy V, et al. A randomized controlled trial of quetiapine versus placebo in the treatment of delirium. J Psychosom Res 2010;69(5): 485–90.

101. Skrobik Y. Delirium prevention and treatment. Crit Care Clin 2009;25(3):585–91.

102. Dasgupta M, Hillier LM. Factors associated with prolonged delirium: a systematic review. Int Psychogeriatr 2010;22(3):373–94.

103. Gardner DM, Baldessarini RJ, Waraich P. Modern antipsychotic drugs: a critical overview. CMAJ 2005;172:1703–11.

104. Kapur S, Zipursky R, Jones C, et al. Relationship between dopamine D(2) occupancy, clinical response, and side effects: a double-blind PET study of first-episode schizophrenia. Am J Psychiatry 2000;157(4):514–20.

105. Trzepacz PT, Baker RW, Greenhouse J. A symptom rating scale for delirium. Psychiatry Res 1988;23(1):89–97.

106. Breitbart W, Rosenfeld B, Roth A, et al. The Memorial Delirium Assessment Scale. J Pain Symptom Manage 1997;13(3):128–37.

107. Trzepacz PT, Mittal D, Torres R, et al. Validation of the Delirium Rating Scale-revised-98: comparison with the delirium rating scale and the cognitive test for delirium. J Neuropsychiatry Clin Neurosci 2001;13(2):229–42.

Weight Loss in Older Persons

Ian M. Chapman, MBBS, PhD, FRACP

KEYWORDS

• Weight loss • Anorexia • Aging • Under nutrition

This article focuses on the epidemiology, causes, and associated consequences of weight loss in older people.

CHANGES IN BODY WEIGHT AND BODY COMPOSITION WITH INCREASING AGE
Changes in Body Weight

On average, people in developed countries gain weight until they are about 50 to 60 years old, stay fairly weight stable for a while, then lose weight.[1] The weight loss in elderly people has been demonstrated in numerous cross-sectional and prospective studies.[2] In the large American Cancer Prevention Study, women older than 85 years had body mass indexes (BMIs) 1.8 kg/m^2 less than women aged 55 to 64 years, and men older than 85 years had BMIs 2.6 kg/m^2 lower than men aged 45 to 64 years, corresponding to body weights approximately 4.0 kg (9 lb) and 5.5 kg (12 lb) lower in the older adults than the young women and men, respectively.[3] Although some of the reduced body weight in older people found in cross-sectional studies is caused by the premature death of obese people, declining body weight among older people has also been detected consistently in longitudinal studies; in one American study, community-dwelling men older than 65 years lost on average 0.5% of their body weight per year.[4] As a result of this weight loss and the premature death of obese people at younger ages, the prevalence of overweight and obesity as defined by standard criteria peaks around 55 to 65 years of age and decreases after about 70 to 75 years of age. In the 1997 to 1998 US National Health Interview Survey of 68,556 adults, 4 times as many people aged 75 years and older than those aged 45 to 64 years were underweight (BMI <18.5; 5.0% vs 1.2%) and substantially fewer were overweight (BMI >25; 47.2% vs 63.5%).[2]

The author has received research funding support from the Australian National Health and Medical Research Council.
The author has nothing to disclose.
Division of Medicine, Royal Adelaide Hospital, University of Adelaide, Level 6, Eleanor Harrald Building, North Terrace, Adelaide 5000, Australia
E-mail address: ian.chapman@adelaide.edu.au

Med Clin N Am 95 (2011) 579–593
doi:10.1016/j.mcna.2011.02.004
0025-7125/11/$ – see front matter © 2011 Elsevier Inc. All rights reserved.

Changes in Body Composition

Enlargement and redistribution of fat stores

With increasing age there is an overall increase in fat stores and decrease in fat-free mass, the latter mainly caused by loss of skeletal muscle. At any given weight, older people have, on average, much more body fat than young adults. In one study, the mean body fat percentage of 75-year-old men weighing 80 kg was 29% compared with 15% in weight-matched 20-year-old men.[5] The increase in body fat with aging is multifactorial in origin, with decreased physical activity a cause and contributions from reduced anabolic hormone action and reduced resting metabolic rate and thermic effect of food.

Body fat is also distributed differently in older adults compared with younger adults. A greater proportion of body fat in older people is intrahepatic, intramuscular, and intra-abdominal (vs subcutaneous).[6,7] Intramuscular fat stores are as much as 50% greater, intrahepatic stores 4 times greater, and insulin resistance 2 times greater in older adults than in young adults.[7] Given that the body weight compatible with longest survival increases with increasing age (see later discussion), and much if not all of the increase in body weight is caused by increased fat stores, it may be that advancing age blunts in some way the harmful effects of increasing body fat.

Loss of skeletal muscle (sarcopenia)

Aging is associated with a decrease in muscle mass and strength, with loss of up to 3 kg of lean body mass per decade after 50 years of age. After 60 years of age loss of body weight is disproportionately of lean body tissue, predominantly skeletal muscle. The causes of age-related skeletal muscle loss are multiple and not fully understood, but probably similar to those leading to fat gain. When excessive, this loss of skeletal muscle leads to sarcopenia (from the Greek meaning "poverty of flesh"). Sarcopenia is associated with poor gait and balance, frailty, falls, and fractures.[8] Sarcopenia and its management are considered in more detail in an article by Rolland and colleagues elsewhere in this issue for further exploration of this topic.

In older people, in contrast to the usual situation in young adults, increased body fat commonly coexists with muscle loss. The combination of an excess of fat tissue and a deficiency of muscle tissue (sarcopenic obesity) is associated independently with adverse effects,[9,10] such as disabilities in activities of daily living.[11] This finding helps to explain the demonstrated benefits of exercise programs in elderly people, particularly those that increase muscle mass and function.

CONSEQUENCES OF WEIGHT LOSS IN OLDER PEOPLE

As previously indicated, weight loss is more common that weight gain among the elderly. Additionally, (1) weight loss among the elderly is often associated with adverse effects, particularly if the weight loss is unintentional; (2) ideal weight ranges for survival are higher in older adults than in young adults; and (3) undernutrition, most obviously manifesting as both low body weight and weight loss, is common in older people and is associated with significant adverse effects.

Adverse Effects of Weight Loss in Older People

Numerous studies have shown that weight loss in the elderly is associated with reduced survival, certainly if the weight loss is involuntary but possibly even when deliberate. In the prospective Cardiovascular Health Study,[12] for example, of subjects older than 65 years, those who lost 5% or more of their initial body weight in the 3 years after study entry had twice the death rate (2.09 × ↑[95% confidence interval

(CI) 1.67–2.62]) over the following 4 years compared with the stable-weight group. Mortality was increased with weight loss regardless of starting weight and whether or not the weight loss was intentional. Similarly, among people aged 60 years followed for an average of 4.5 years in the Systolic Hypertension in the Elderly Program (SHEP),[13] those who lost 1.6 kg per year or more weight had a 4.9 times greater death rate (95% CI 3.5–6.8) than those without significant weight change. The adverse association of weight loss with mortality was present even in the subjects who were heaviest at baseline (BMI $\geq$31 kg/m^2) and was independent of baseline weight.

The combination of initially low body weight and weight loss is associated with particularly bad survival outcomes in older people. In the SHEP study, subjects with a baseline BMI less than 23.6 kg/m^2 who lost more than 1.6 kg per year had a mortality rate almost 20 times greater than the mortality rate of those with a baseline BMI of 23.6 to 28.0 kg/m^2 whose weight remained stable.[13] This finding is a concern because the tendency for older people to lose weight is variable, with lean individuals probably most likely to lose weight.[14] In an older person, unintentional weight loss of 5% or more over 6 to 12 months is associated with an increased risk of adverse effects; whereas, a loss of 10% or more likely means protein-energy malnutrition.

Not surprisingly, unintentional weight loss in older people is associated with more adverse effects than intentional weight loss. Although some study results have been interpreted to show increased mortality after even intentional weight loss in older people,[12] it is difficult to determine what proportion of weight loss labeled intentional was instead unintentional. In a meta-analysis of 26 studies examining the connection between weight loss and mortality,[15] weight loss that was unintentional or ill defined was associated with a significant (22%–39%) increase in mortality; whereas, intentional weight loss had no significant effect on mortality. This is topic is discussed later.

An important question is whether the increased death rate in older people who lose weight is caused by the weight loss itself or whether the weight loss is merely a marker of underlying conditions that increase mortality. It is often difficult to know and both are likely to be true to varying degrees in different people. In some cases weight loss is caused by an illness, such as a malignancy, that is mainly responsible for the reduced survival and the weight loss is partly an innocent bystander. There are numerous causes of pathologic anorexia and weight loss in older people (**Box 1**). Nevertheless, the older person or their caregivers do not often appreciate the weight loss, and when it is appreciated it can trigger a search for underlying, often treatable, causes. The weight loss and associated undernutrition is itself often a significant problem because weight lost in older persons is disproportionately composed of lean tissue, with its associated adverse effects. Consistent with this, a reduction of mortality has been described in some groups of older people receiving nutritional supplements.[16]

Ideal Body Weight in Older People

Studies consistently show that the body weight associated with the greatest life expectancy is higher for older adults than for young adults. For example, among subjects older than 60 years in the Systolic Hypertension in the Elderly Program,[13] those whose baseline BMI was in the lowest quintile (<23.6 kg/m^2) had the highest subsequent mortality; whereas, those within the highest BMI quintile ($\geq$31 kgm^2), corresponding to the conventional criteria of obesity, had the lowest mortality. BMI values lower than approximately 22 kgm^2 in people older than 70 years are associated with higher mortality rates than higher weights, and BMIs lower than 18.5 kgm^2 particularly so. The optimum BMI for survival in people older than 70 years is probably in the range of 25 to 30 kg/m^2, and there is recent evidence that higher than so-called normal BMIs may be somewhat more protective in women than in men.[17]

Box 1
Nonphysiologic causes of anorexia in older persons

Social factors

　　Poverty

　　Inability to shop

　　Inability to prepare and cook meals

　　Inability to feed oneself

　　Living alone/social isolation/lack of social support network

　　Failure to cater to ethnic food preferences in institutionalized individuals

Psychological factors

　　Depression

　　Dementia/Alzheimer's disease

　　Alcoholism

　　Bereavement

　　Cholesterol phobia

Medical factors

　　Cardiac failure

　　Chronic obstructive pulmonary disease

　　Infection

　　Cancer

　　Alcoholism

　　Dysphagia

　　Rheumatoid arthritis

　　Malabsorption syndromes

　　Hypermetabolism (eg, hyperthyroidism)

Gastrointestinal symptoms

　　Helicobacter pylori infection/atrophic gastritis

　　Vomiting/diarrhea/constipation

　　Parkinson's disease

Medications

　　Antiinfectives

　　Antineoplastics

　　Antirheumatics

　　Nutritional supplements

　　Pulmonary agents

　　Cardiovascular agents

　　Central nervous system agents

　　Gastrointestinal agents

Undernutrition in Older People

Protein-energy malnutrition is common in the elderly. Reported rates vary, in part because of differing diagnostic methods used, but studies in developed countries have found that up to 15% of community-dwelling and homebound elderly, between 23% and 62% of hospitalized patients, and up to 85% of nursing home residents suffer from the condition.[18]

Protein-energy malnutrition is associated with numerous adverse effects (**Box 2**), and is a strong independent predictor of mortality in elderly people, regardless of whether they live in the community or in a nursing home or other institution.[19] The mortality rate is further increased in the presence of other medical diseases, such as renal failure, cardiac failure, and cerebrovascular disease. For example, the 9-month mortality rate of 205 subjects older than 70 years without cancer, admitted to a medical ward in Sweden, was doubled by both coexistent malnutrition and cardiac failure with a greater than 4-fold increase in subjects with both (80% vs 18%).[19]

CAUSES OF WEIGHT LOSS IN OLDER PEOPLE

Weight loss occurs when energy expenditure exceeds intake. The reasons why older people lose weight are multiple and interacting. Some reasons are discussed later.

Box 2
Effects of weight loss and protein-energy malnutrition on function in the elderly

↓ Muscle relaxation

↓ Muscle mass and strength

↑ Risk of fracture

↓ Bone mass

↑ Incidence of falls

↓ Functional status

↑ Risk of infection

Delayed skin hypersensitivity

T-cell lymphocytopenia

↓ Synthesis of interleukin-2

↓ Cytolytic cell activity

↓ Response to influenza vaccination

↑ Anemia, pneumonia

Poor wound healing

Fatigue

Delayed recovery from surgery

↓ Cognitive function

↓ Cardiac output

↓ Intravascular fluid (dehydration)

↑ Incidence of pressure sores

↑ Hospital admission and length of stay

↑ Mortality

Aging is associated with a physiologic anorexia upon which pathologic anorexia is often superimposed. Energy expenditure may be increased by medical conditions, such as malignancies and increased respiratory effort in chronic airways disease. Weight loss is often unintentional. Deliberate diet-induced weight loss by older people who are overweight or think they are overweight is also common.

The Physiologic Anorexia of Aging

There is an age-related decline in appetite and energy intake in healthy, ambulant, noninstitutionalized people.[20] Healthy older persons are less hungry and more full before a meal, become more rapidly satiated after eating, and eat fewer snacks between meals than younger persons.[18,21] In cross-sectional studies, average daily energy intake decreases by approximately 30% between 20 and 80 years of age.[20,22] Similarly, longitudinal studies of older people have demonstrated reductions in energy intake of 19 to 72 kcal/d/y in women and 25 to 100 kcal/d/y in men, respectively, over 6 to 7 years.[23]

The physiologic reduction in appetite and energy intake has been termed "the anorexia of aging."[18] The causes are not fully understood, probably multiple, and have been reviewed elsewhere.[24,25] Likely causes include increased activity of satiety hormones, such as cholecystokinin; diminished activity of hormones stimulating appetite, such as opioids; reduced sense of smell[26] and hence taste and enjoyment of food; and changes in the gastrointestinal system that increase fullness and satiety.

Age-associated increases in the production or effect of satiating cytokines may contribute to the physiologic anorexia of aging.[27] Cytokines are secreted in response to significant stress, often because of malignancy or infection. The cytokines interleukin (IL)-1, IL-6, and tumor necrosis factor alpha (TNF-α) decrease food intake and reduce body weight via several central and peripheral pathways. Blockade of these cytokines attenuates weight loss in high-stress conditions associated with cachexia.

It is tempting to postulate that aging itself is a form of stress. It is associated with stresslike changes in circulating hormonal patterns: increased cortisol and catecholamines and decreased sex hormones and growth hormone, which in turn stimulate the release of IL-6 and TNF-α. IL-1 and IL-6 levels are elevated in older people with cachexia; whereas, plasma IL-6 concentrations apparently increase as a function of normal aging and correlate inversely with levels of functional ability in elderly people. Higher circulating levels of C-reactive protein and cytokine receptors also appear to be associated independently with physical dysfunction and disability.[28]

Pathologic Anorexia and Undernutrition in Older People

Protein-energy malnutrition is particularly likely to develop in an older person in the presence of pathologic factors, many of which become more common with increased age (see **Box 1**). Most factors are at least partly responsive to treatment, so recognition is important. Some of the more important factors are discussed later.

Depression is often associated with bereavement and the deterioration of social networks and is common in older people; it is present in 2% to 10% of community-dwelling older people and a much higher proportion of those in institutions.[29] Depression is more likely to manifest as reduced appetite and weight loss in older adults than in younger adults and is an important cause of weight loss and undernutrition in this group. Undernutrition per se may further worsen depression. Treatment of depression is effective in producing weight gain and improving other nutritional indices.[30]

Older people are more likely to live alone than young adults. Social isolation and loneliness have been associated with decreased appetite and energy intake in the elderly.[31] Elderly people tend to consume substantially more food (up to 50%) during a meal when eating in the company of friends than when eating alone. The simple measure of having older people eat in company rather than alone may be effective in increasing their energy intake.

Dementia may also contribute to reduced food intake in the elderly because individuals simply forget to eat. Up to 50% of institutionalized patients with dementia have been reported to suffer from protein-energy malnutrition.[32]

Immobility (eg, stroke), tremor (eg, Parkinson's disease), and impaired vision may reduce the capacity of an older person to shop for, prepare, and consume food. Many older people no longer have their own teeth. Poor dentition limits the type and quantity of food eaten. In one study of nursing home residents aged 60 to 101 years in Boston, half complained of problems with chewing, biting, and swallowing. Those with dentures were more likely to have poor protein intake than those with their own teeth.[33] Common medical conditions in the elderly, such as gastrointestinal disease, malabsorption syndromes, acute and chronic infection, and hypermetabolism (ie, hyperthyroidism), often cause anorexia, micronutrient deficiencies, and increased energy requirements.[18] Cancer and conditions, such as rheumatoid arthritis, that produce anorectic effects by releasing cytokines are also common.

The elderly are major users of prescription medications; several prescription medications can cause malabsorption of nutrients, gastrointestinal symptoms, and loss of appetite. For example, digoxin and some forms of chemotherapy can cause nausea, vomiting, and loss of appetite. The elderly often take multiple medications that increase the risk of drug interactions that can cause anorexia.

Cachexia

Cachexia is a complex metabolic syndrome associated with underlying illness and characterized by loss of muscle with or without loss of fat mass. The prominent clinical feature of cachexia is weight loss, but inflammation is also a key component. Anorexia, insulin resistance, and increased muscle protein breakdown are also frequently associated with cachexia. Although there is often overlap between them, cachexia and malnutrition are not the same. All patients with cachexia are malnourished but not all malnourished patients are cachectic.[34] Inflammation plays a major role in the pathogenesis of cachexia, with an absolute or relative increase in levels of inflammatory cytokines, such as TNF-α, IL-1, and IL-6.[34] Conditions that often afflict older people that are associated frequently with cachexia include cancer, cardiac failure, chronic obstructive pulmonary disease, and chronic renal failure.

DIAGNOSIS AND TREATMENT OF UNDERNUTRITION IN OLDER PEOPLE

These issues are covered in an articles by Rolland and colleagues and Jean Woo elsewhere in this issue for further exploration of this topics. A key point to be aware of is low body weight (BMI <22 kg/m2) or weight loss (particularly if unintentional and more than 5% of body weight) as markers of poor outcomes and the need for further assessment and treatment. These markers of poor outcomes are under-recognized or unrecognized in older people, and therefore not addressed.

DELIBERATE WEIGHT LOSS IN OVERWEIGHT AND OBESE OLDER PEOPLE
The Prevalence of Overweight and Obesity Among Older People

Many older people in developed countries are overweight by conventional criteria. In recent surveys, approximately 71% of Americans aged 60 years or older were overweight (BMI $\geq$25 kg/m^2) and approximately 32% of those aged 60 years or older were obese (BMI ≥30).[35,36] Obesity is becoming more common in older people, in line with the increasing rate in younger adults.[37,38]

Causes of Overweight and Obesity in Older People

On average, people do not usually gain weight during old age (see previous discussion), therefore, the high and increasing proportion of overweight in older people is mainly caused by the high and increasing proportion of adults who reach old age already overweight. The causes of obesity in the elderly are, therefore, largely the same causes of obesity in younger adults. There are some people who only become overweight or whose weight increases dramatically in later life because of conditions, such as osteoarthritis-induced immobility, cardiac failure, and increased food intake caused by corticosteroid use.

Consequences of Obesity in Older People

Obesity in older adults, as in younger adults, is associated with absolute and relative increases in both mortality and morbidity.[1] Functional capacity and mobility are significantly reduced in obese older adults compared with lean older adults.[39] This association is particularly strong in older adults in whom obesity is often associated with reduced muscle mass and hence with physical frailty.[10] Obese older people have increased difficulties performing activities of daily living,[40] are less likely to be pain free, and more likely to be homebound. Obesity is predictive of a greater rate of future disability, declines in functional status,[1] and an increased admission rate to nursing homes.[41] Obesity is associated with a reduced quality of life[42,43] and caused by multiple factors, including associated joint pain.[44] Obesity has been linked to depression, but study results are conflicting,[45,46] and there is some evidence for a link between obesity and the later development of Alzheimer-type dementia.[47]

Paradoxically, although obesity is a risk factor for the development of vascular diseases, when obese people develop vascular diseases, including hypertension, coronary artery disease, congestive cardiac failure, and peripheral arterial disease, they have better outcomes than their normal-weight counterparts. Mortality is up to 40% lower in people with heart failure who are obese compared with individuals without elevated BMIs.[48,49] This contradiction has been termed the "obesity paradox."[48,50–53] There is also evidence that overweight and obese people with end stage renal failure on dialysis, chronic obstructive airways disease, HIV/AIDS, and certain cancers, as well as after vascular and other surgery, have lower mortality than their normal-weight counterparts.[48,54,55] Several potential mechanisms for the protective effects of body fat and increased BMI have been proposed.[48]

Obesity in older people is also associated with increased bone density and reduced fracture rates.[56] When overweight adults of any age intentionally lose weight they also lose bone[1,57] and substantial unintentional weight loss in older people is associated with an increased risk of hip fracture.[58] Although it is reasonable to think there may be an increased fracture risk caused by bone loss in overweight older people who intentionally lose weight, this has not been established.

Mortality

The relationship between BMI and mortality is U-shaped, with an increase in mortality in people whose BMI is less than 18.5 to 19.0 kg/m^2[59,60] and at high BMIs. The body weight compatible with the greatest life expectancy increases with increasing age and the relative increase in the risk of death associated with being obese is not as great in older adults as it is in young adults. An assessment of 13 prospective studies of people older than 65 years[59] found an association between mortality and increased BMI in only a few, and then only for BMI of more than 27.0 to 28.5 kg/m², with little or no increase in mortality at any BMI for people older than 75 years. Where an optimum BMI could be identified, it was usually in the range of 27 to 30 kg/m². Other studies support this; for example, a combined analysis of the American National Health and Nutrition Examination Survey (NHANES) I to III (1974–2000) study results found no significant increase in mortality with any degree of overweight in people older than 70 years and an increased death rate only in those with a BMI greater than or equal to 35 kg/m² among those aged 60 to 69 years.[61] Furthermore, the adverse effects of obesity on life expectancy may have weakened over recent decades in all age groups, including the elderly, possibly because of improved medical care for the associated metabolic ill effects.[61]

Management of Obesity in Older People

Should overweight older people be advised to lose weight?

This question is difficult to answer. Obesity in older people is associated with increased morbidity and reduced life expectancy at high BMIs up to at least 70 years of age, and there is some evidence that weight loss by overweight older people is associated with improved quality of life.[62,63] On the other hand, weight loss has detrimental effects on muscle mass and bone density, and there is an association repeatedly detected in large population studies between all-cause weight loss and increased mortality in older people, even those who are initially overweight.[12,15,64–67] This finding is highlighted by the results of an intriguing study of 1114 Finnish men, sequentially examined at mean ages of 25, 47 (midlife), and 73 years (late life), and classified as to whether they were normal weight (BMI ≤25) or overweight (BMI >25) at these time points. The highest mortality was in the men who were overweight in midlife and then lost weight to be normal weight in late life (2 times greater than in both the constantly normal weight group and in the group normal weight in midlife and overweight in late life, $P<.001$).[53]

The increased mortality associated with weight loss in older people appears related to whether such weight loss is intentional and also to how weight loss is achieved. Although there seems little doubt that unintentional weight loss is not good for the elderly, available evidence suggests that intentional weight loss probably has no significant effect on mortality and even reduces mortality in the unhealthy obese and those with obesity-related risk factors.[15,68–70]

Although studies involving predominantly younger adults have found that intentional weight loss can reduce mortality in those with obesity-related health problems,[71] such studies have not been done in older people. Nevertheless, it is the opinion of the author that evidence suggests it is probably safe to recommend weight loss to overweight older people with obesity-related morbidities, particularly reduced mobility and function. There are few if any indications for recommending weight loss to older people based on their weight alone.

Effects of losing fat versus losing lean tissue in older people

A substantial amount of the tissue lost when older people lose weight is lean tissue (ie, muscle). Muscle loss is harmful; whereas, loss of fat tissue seems to be more beneficial. Prospective studies examining the independent effects of weight loss and fat loss[65] have shown weight loss to be associated with increased mortality; whereas, fat loss is associated with decreased mortality. This finding emphasizes the importance for older people to preserve lean tissue, if possible, when weight is intentionally lost.

Weight-loss measures for overweight older people
The ways that older people can deliberately lose weight, if this is considered appropriate, are the same as those in younger adults; changes in diet and exercise, medications, and surgery.[1] There is limited information about the effectiveness and safety of weight-loss treatments in older people.

Lifestyle measures Lifestyle interventions combining a reduced-energy diet (reduction of about 500–750 kcal/d) and exercise are at least as effective in producing weight loss in people older than 60 years as it is in younger adults.[1,72] An exercise component is important, particularly weight-bearing aerobic and resistance exercise. In the absence of an exercise program about 25%, and sometimes considerably more, of the diet-induced weight loss is accounted for by loss of lean tissue, essentially skeletal muscle.[73–75] The addition of an exercise program to a weight-loss diet reduces the loss of lean tissue, often dramatically.[74] In older people, exercise can also inhibit the loss of bone density that accompanies diet-induced weight loss, improves physical function by increasing muscle mass and fitness,[76,77] and reduces the risk of falls.[78] Multivitamin supplements together with adequate calcium and vitamin D (800–1000 IU/d) for bone protection should also be taken.

Medications There is little reported experience with weight-loss drugs in older people. Such drugs should be used with caution in older people, because of limited efficacy data, the possibility of interactions with other (multiple) medications, and potential side effects. The lipase inhibitor orlistat appears to be as effective in older adults as it is in young adults,[1] but can cause gastrointestinal side effects.

Surgery for weight loss There have been few reports of the results of bariatric surgery in people older than 60 years.[79] In 3 studies comparing the effects of gastric bypass surgery in 115 people older than 60 years to those in 3470 people younger than 60 years,[80–82] the perioperative death rate was slightly increased in the older group (0.86%) and there was possibly a slightly greater operative complication rate in the older subjects. The mean weight loss was 39 to 43 kg at 1 year in the older subjects, with a reduction in the number of obesity-related morbidities and medications needed to treat these subjects; both reductions were slightly but significantly less in older adults than in young adults. Similarly, studies involving laparoscopic banding have found slightly higher perioperative mortality in older subjects, comparable substantial reductions in obesity-related morbidities, and impressive but significantly smaller reductions in BMI in the older subjects than in the young subjects (approximately 12% vs 20%) at 1 year, $P<.05$.[83] The mean age of the older subjects in these studies has been quite young, however, between 63 to 65 years, and the results of surgery in older people remain to be determined. The numbers of surgically treated older people in such published studies are also still small, so caution should be exercised in recommending bariatric surgery to the very old. Nevertheless, available evidence suggests that bariatric surgery is an effective weight-loss option in older people, particularly those substantially disabled by complications of obesity.

SUMMARY

Weight loss is common in older people. It is associated with increased morbidity and mortality, particularly when unintentional, excessive (>5% body weight), or associated with low body weight (BMI <22 kg/m²). It is often unrecognized, the associated adverse effects not appreciated, and underlying causes not addressed. Intentional weight loss by overweight older people is probably appropriate only when functional problems have resulted from the excess weight. It is important to include, wherever possible, exercise in weight-loss measures to preserve skeletal muscle mass.

REFERENCES

1. Villareal DT, Apovian CM, Kushner RF, et al. Obesity in older adults: technical review and position statement of the American Society for Nutrition and NAASO, The Obesity Society. Am J Clin Nutr 2005;82(5):923–34.
2. Schoenborn CA, Adams PF, Barnes PM. Body weight status of adults: United States, 1997–98. Adv Data 2002;(330):1–15.
3. Stevens J, Cai J, Pamuk ER, et al. The effect of age on the association between body-mass index and mortality. N Engl J Med 1998;338(1):1–7.
4. Wallace JI, Schwartz RS, LaCroix AZ, et al. Involuntary weight loss in older outpatients: incidence and clinical significance. J Am Geriatr Soc 1995;43(4):329–37.
5. Prentice AM, Jebb SA. Beyond body mass index. Obes Rev 2001;2(3):141–7.
6. Beaufrere B, Morio B. Fat and protein redistribution with aging: metabolic considerations. Eur J Clin Nutr 2000;54(Suppl 3):S48–53.
7. Cree MG, Newcomer BR, Katsanos CS, et al. Intramuscular and liver triglycerides are increased in the elderly. J Clin Endocrinol Metab 2004;89(8):3864–71.
8. Janssen I, Baumgartner RN, Ross R, et al. Skeletal muscle cutpoints associated with elevated physical disability risk in older men and women. Am J Epidemiol 2004;159(4):413–21.
9. Roubenoff R. Sarcopenic obesity: the confluence of two epidemics. Obes Res 2004;12(6):887–8.
10. Villareal DT, Banks M, Siener C, et al. Physical frailty and body composition in obese elderly men and women. Obes Res 2004;12(6):913–20.
11. Baumgartner RN, Wayne SJ, Waters DL, et al. Sarcopenic obesity predicts instrumental activities of daily living disability in the elderly. Obes Res 2004;12(12): 1995–2004.
12. Newman AB, Yanez D, Harris T, et al. Weight change in old age and its association with mortality. J Am Geriatr Soc 2001;49(10):1309–18.
13. Somes GW, Kritchevsky SB, Shorr RI, et al. Body mass index, weight change, and death in older adults: the systolic hypertension in the elderly program. Am J Epidemiol 2002;156(2):132–8.
14. Rumpel C, Harris TB, Madans J. Modification of the relationship between the Quetelet index and mortality by weight-loss history among older women. Ann Epidemiol 1993;3(4):343–50.
15. Harrington M, Gibson S, Cottrell RC. A review and meta-analysis of the effect of weight loss on all-cause mortality risk. Nutr Res Rev 2009;22(1):93–108.
16. Milne AC, Potter J, Avenell A. Protein and energy supplementation in elderly people at risk from malnutrition. Cochrane Database Syst Rev 2005;2:CD003288.
17. Stessman J, Jacobs JM, Ein-Mor E, et al. Normal body mass index rather than obesity predicts greater mortality in elderly people: the Jerusalem longitudinal study. J Am Geriatr Soc 2009;57(12):2232–8.
18. Morley JE. Anorexia of aging: physiologic and pathologic. Am J Clin Nutr 1997; 66(4):760–73.
19. Cederholm T, Jagren C, Hellstrom K. Outcome of protein-energy malnutrition in elderly medical patients. Am J Med 1995;98(1):67–74.
20. Wurtman JJ, Lieberman H, Tsay R, et al. Calorie and nutrient intakes of elderly and young subjects measured under identical conditions. J Gerontol 1988;43(6):B174–80.

21. Clarkston WK, Pantano MM, Morley JE, et al. Evidence for the anorexia of aging: gastrointestinal transit and hunger in healthy elderly vs. young adults. Am J Physiol 1997;272(1 Pt 2):R243–8.
22. Briefel RR, McDowell MA, Alaimo K, et al. Total energy intake of the US population: the third National Health and Nutrition Examination Survey, 1988–1991. Am J Clin Nutr 1995;62(Suppl 5):1072S–80S.
23. Koehler KM. The New Mexico Aging Process Study. Nutr Rev 1994;52(8 Pt 2):S34–7.
24. Chapman IM. Nutritional disorders in the elderly. Med Clin North Am 2006;90(5): 887–907.
25. Chapman IM. Endocrinology of anorexia of ageing. Best Pract Res Clin Endocrinol Metab 2004;18(3):437–52.
26. Doty RL, Shaman P, Applebaum SL, et al. Smell identification ability: changes with age. Science 1984;226(4681):1441–3.
27. Yeh SS, Schuster MW. Geriatric cachexia: the role of cytokines. Am J Clin Nutr 1999;70(2):183–97.
28. Haren MT, Malmstrom TK, Miller DK, et al. Higher C-reactive protein and soluble tumor necrosis factor receptor levels are associated with poor physical function and disability: a cross-sectional analysis of a cohort of late middle-aged African Americans. J Gerontol A Biol Sci Med Sci 2010;65(3):274–81.
29. Evers MM, Marin DB. Mood disorders. Effective management of major depressive disorder in the geriatric patient. Geriatrics 2002;57(10):36–40 [quiz: 41].
30. Thomas P, Hazif-Thomas C, Clement JP. Influence of antidepressant therapies on weight and appetite in the elderly. J Nutr Health Aging 2003;7(3):166–70.
31. Walker D, Beauchene RE. The relationship of loneliness, social isolation, and physical health to dietary adequacy of independently living elderly. J Am Diet Assoc 1991;91(3):300–4.
32. Sandman PO, Adolfsson R, Nygren C, et al. Nutritional status and dietary intake in institutionalized patients with Alzheimer's disease and multi-infarct dementia. J Am Geriatr Soc 1987;35(1):31–8.
33. Sahyoun NR, Otradovec CL, Hartz SC, et al. Dietary intakes and biochemical indicators of nutritional status in an elderly, institutionalized population. Am J Clin Nutr 1988;47(3):524–33.
34. Muscaritoli M, Anker SD, Argiles J, et al. Consensus definition of sarcopenia, cachexia and pre-cachexia: joint document elaborated by Special Interest Groups (SIG) "cachexia-anorexia in chronic wasting diseases" and "nutrition in geriatrics". Clin Nutr 2010;29(2):154–9.
35. Li F, Fisher KJ, Harmer P. Prevalence of overweight and obesity in older U.S. adults: estimates from the 2003 Behavioral Risk Factor Surveillance System survey. J Am Geriatr Soc 2005;53(4):737–9.
36. Ogden CL, Carroll MD, Curtin LR, et al. Prevalence of overweight and obesity in the United States, 1999–2004. JAMA 2006;295(13):1549–55.
37. Flegal KM, Carroll MD, Ogden CL, et al. Prevalence and trends in obesity among US adults, 1999–2000. JAMA 2002;288(14):1723–7.
38. Mokdad AH, Bowman BA, Ford ES, et al. The continuing epidemics of obesity and diabetes in the United States. JAMA 2001;286(10):1195–200.
39. Jensen GL. Obesity and functional decline: epidemiology and geriatric consequences. Clin Geriatr Med 2005;21(4):677–87, v.
40. Peytremann-Bridevaux I, Santos-Eggimann B. Health correlates of overweight and obesity in adults aged 50 years and over: results from the Survey of Health, Ageing and Retirement in Europe (SHARE). Obesity and health in Europeans aged > or = 50 years. Swiss Med Wkly 2008;138(17/18):261–6.

41. Zizza CA, Herring A, Stevens J, et al. Obesity affects nursing-care facility admission among whites but not blacks. Obes Res 2002;10(8):816–23.
42. Kortt MA, Clarke PM. Estimating utility values for health states of overweight and obese individuals using the SF-36. Qual Life Res 2005;14(10):2177–85.
43. Jia H, Lubetkin EI. The impact of obesity on health-related quality-of-life in the general adult US population. J Public Health (Oxf) 2005;27(2):156–64.
44. Heo M, Allison DB, Faith MS, et al. Obesity and quality of life: mediating effects of pain and comorbidities. Obes Res 2003;11(2):209–16.
45. Simon GE, Ludman EJ, Linde JA, et al. Association between obesity and depression in middle-aged women. Gen Hosp Psychiatry 2008;30(1):32–9.
46. Ho RC, Niti M, Kua EH, et al. Body mass index, waist circumference, waist-hip ratio and depressive symptoms in Chinese elderly: a population-based study. Int J Geriatr Psychiatry 2008;23(4):401–8.
47. Salihu HM, Bonnema SM, Alio AP. Obesity: what is an elderly population growing into? Maturitas 2009;63(1):7–12.
48. Lavie CJ, Milani RV, Ventura HO. Obesity and cardiovascular disease: risk factor, paradox, and impact of weight loss. J Am Coll Cardiol 2009;53(21): 1925–32.
49. Fonarow GC, Srikanthan P, Costanzo MR, et al. An obesity paradox in acute heart failure: analysis of body mass index and in hospital mortality for 108,927 patients in the Acute Decompensated Heart Failure National Registry. Am Heart J 2007; 153(1):74–81.
50. McAuley P, Myers J, Abella J, et al. Body mass, fitness and survival in veteran patients: another obesity paradox? Am J Med 2007;120(6):518–24.
51. Uretsky S, Messerli FH, Bangalore S, et al. Obesity paradox in patients with hypertension and coronary artery disease. Am J Med 2007;120(10):863–70.
52. Galal W, van Gestel YR, Hoeks SE, et al. The obesity paradox in patients with peripheral arterial disease. Chest 2008;134(5):925–30.
53. Strandberg TE, Strandberg AY, Salomaa VV, et al. Explaining the obesity paradox: cardiovascular risk, weight change, and mortality during long-term follow-up in men. Eur Heart J 2009;30(14):1720–7.
54. Davenport DL, Xenos ES, Hosokawa P, et al. The influence of body mass index obesity status on vascular surgery 30-day morbidity and mortality. J Vasc Surg 2009;49(1):140–7, 147,e1 [discussion: 147].
55. Mullen JT, Moorman DW, Davenport DL. The obesity paradox: body mass index and outcomes in patients undergoing nonbariatric general surgery. Ann Surg 2009;250(1):166–72.
56. Schott AM, Cormier C, Hans D, et al. How hip and whole-body bone mineral density predict hip fracture in elderly women: the EPIDOS Prospective Study. Osteoporos Int 1998;8(3):247–54.
57. Ensrud KE, Fullman RL, Barrett-Connor E, et al. Voluntary weight reduction in older men increases hip bone loss: the osteoporotic fractures in men study. J Clin Endocrinol Metab 2005;90(4):1998–2004.
58. Langlois JA, Harris T, Looker AC, et al. Weight change between age 50 years and old age is associated with risk of hip fracture in white women aged 67 years and older. Arch Intern Med 1996;156(9):989–94.
59. Heiat A, Vaccarino V, Krumholz HM. An evidence-based assessment of federal guidelines for overweight and obesity as they apply to elderly persons. Arch Intern Med 2001;161(9):1194–203.
60. Willett WC, Dietz WH, Colditz GA. Guidelines for healthy weight. N Engl J Med 1999;341(6):427–34.

61. Flegal KM, Graubard BI, Williamson DF, et al. Excess deaths associated with underweight, overweight, and obesity. JAMA 2005;293(15):1861–7.
62. Villareal DT, Banks M, Sinacore DR, et al. Effect of weight loss and exercise on frailty in obese older adults. Arch Intern Med 2006;166(8):860–6.
63. Taylor CJ, Layani L. Laparoscopic adjustable gastric banding in patients > or =60 years old: is it worthwhile? Obes Surg 2006;16(12):1579–83.
64. Andres R, Muller DC, Sorkin JD. Long-term effects of change in body weight on all-cause mortality. A review. Ann Intern Med 1993;119(7 Pt 2):737–43.
65. Allison DB, Zannolli R, Faith MS, et al. Weight loss increases and fat loss decreases all-cause mortality rate: results from two independent cohort studies. Int J Obes Relat Metab Disord 1999;23(6):603–11.
66. Seidell JC, Visscher TL. Body weight and weight change and their health implications for the elderly. Eur J Clin Nutr 2000;54(Suppl 3):S33–9.
67. Wedick NM, Barrett-Connor E, Knoke JD, et al. The relationship between weight loss and all-cause mortality in older men and women with and without diabetes mellitus: the Rancho Bernardo study. J Am Geriatr Soc 2002;50(11):1810–5.
68. Yaari S, Goldbourt U. Voluntary and involuntary weight loss: associations with long term mortality in 9,228 middle-aged and elderly men. Am J Epidemiol 1998;148(6):546–55.
69. Wannamethee SG, Shaper AG, Lennon L. Reasons for intentional weight loss, unintentional weight loss, and mortality in older men. Arch Intern Med 2005; 165(9):1035–40.
70. Gregg EW, Gerzoff RB, Thompson TJ, et al. Intentional weight loss and death in overweight and obese U.S. adults 35 years of age and older. Ann Intern Med 2003;138(5):383–9.
71. Fontaine KR, Allison DB. Does intentional weight loss affect mortality rate? Eat Behav 2001;2(2):87–95.
72. Wing RR, Hamman RF, Bray GA, et al. Achieving weight and activity goals among diabetes prevention program lifestyle participants. Obes Res 2004;12(9): 1426–34.
73. Ryan AS, Nicklas BJ, Dennis KE. Aerobic exercise maintains regional bone mineral density during weight loss in postmenopausal women. J Appl Physiol 1998;84(4):1305–10.
74. Garrow JS, Summerbell CD. Meta-analysis: effect of exercise, with or without dieting, on the body composition of overweight subjects. Eur J Clin Nutr 1995; 49(1):1–10.
75. Pavlou KN, Steffee WP, Lerman RH, et al. Effects of dieting and exercise on lean body mass, oxygen uptake, and strength. Med Sci Sports Exerc 1985;17(4): 466–71.
76. Binder EF, Schechtman KB, Ehsani AA, et al. Effects of exercise training on frailty in community-dwelling older adults: results of a randomized, controlled trial. J Am Geriatr Soc 2002;50(12):1921–8.
77. Seguin R, Nelson ME. The benefits of strength training for older adults. Am J Prev Med 2003;25(3 Suppl 2):141–9.
78. Chang JT, Morton SC, Rubenstein LZ, et al. Interventions for the prevention of falls in older adults: systematic review and meta-analysis of randomised clinical trials. BMJ 2004;328(7441):680.
79. Miller ME, Kral JG. Surgery for obesity in older women. Menopause Int 2008; 14(4):155–62.
80. St Peter SD, Craft RO, Tiede JL, et al. Impact of advanced age on weight loss and health benefits after laparoscopic gastric bypass. Arch Surg 2005;140(2):165–8.

81. Sosa JL, Pombo H, Pallavicini H, et al. Laparoscopic gastric bypass beyond age 60. Obes Surg 2004;14(10):1398–401.

82. Sugerman HJ, DeMaria EJ, Kellum JM, et al. Effects of bariatric surgery in older patients. Ann Surg 2004;240(2):243–7.

83. Busetto L, Angrisani L, Basso N, et al. Safety and efficacy of laparoscopic adjustable gastric banding in the elderly. Obesity (Silver Spring) 2008;16(2): 334–8.

Medical Care in the Nursing Home

Debbie Tolson, MSc, PhD, RGN[a], John E. Morley, MB, BCh[b],*

KEYWORDS

- Nursing home • National recommendations • Quality of care
- Gerontologic nursing

With the aging of the baby boomers, the need to establish high-quality long-term health and social care provision for older people is increasing rapidly. One option for care in the last few years of life for frail older persons is nursing homes. Nursing homes can also function as skilled nursing facilities to provide the majority of rehabilitation given to persons discharged from hospitals. Nursing home provision in some countries including the United States, the United Kingdom, and Australia is mainly funded through commercial providers, with some charitable or public funded facilities. There is no universal model, and comparisons between countries reveal differences in the underlying care philosophy and culture, arrangements for physician involvement, and the skill mix of registered nurses to other practitioners.

In the United States 4.3% of persons older than 65 years live in nursing homes, with a mean of 100 individuals residing in each nursing home. Twenty-two percent of people older than 85 years live in care homes within Scotland. In the developed countries of the world there is enormous variability in the number of older persons living in nursing homes, ranging from 0.2% in Korea to 7.9% in Sweden. Care in nursing homes is generally provided by generalist primary care practitioners, either family practitioners or internists. In the Netherlands, the vast majority of nursing home care is delivered by nursing home specialists.[1] In the United States, it was found that nursing homes whose medical director had training in nursing home care, as signified by the American Medical Director Association's Certified Medical Director designation, had better outcomes than those that did not have a certified medical director.[2,3]

With the aging of the population, the importance of increasing the quality of nursing home care and the prestige and training of persons who work there cannot be overstated. For this reason, the International Association of Geriatrics and Gerontology (IAGG) in concert with the World Health Organization formed a task force to develop

[a] Scottish Centre for Evidence Based Care of Older People: A Collaborating Centre for the Joanna Briggs Institute, Glasgow Caledonian University, Cowcaddens Road, Glasgow G4 0BA, UK
[b] Division of Geriatric Medicine, Saint Louis University & GRECC VA Medical Center, 1402 South Grand Boulevard, M238, St Louis, MO 63104, USA
* Corresponding author.
E-mail address: morley@slu.edu

Med Clin N Am 95 (2011) 595–614
doi:10.1016/j.mcna.2011.02.007
0025-7125/11/$ – see front matter. Published by Elsevier Inc.

medical.theclinics.com

recommendations to improve nursing home care. The recommendations are summarized in **Box 1**.[4] These proposals examined 4 areas, namely, reputational enhancement and leadership, care quality essentials, practitioner education, and research. It is believed that following these recommendations will result in evidence-based quality care in nursing homes and enhance the status of nursing home carers among health professionals and the public.

Nursing home care, since it evolved from its rudimentary beginnings in ancient Turkey,[5] has evolved into a highly complex scientific endeavor involving a variety of high-touch and high-tech approaches.[6] This selective review highlights "hot topics" in nursing home practice that are central to the provision of safe and dignified care for older people, which is mindful of the relationships between practitioners, the individual, and family members. A key area is the ability to balance appropriate aggressive medical interventions that enhance quality of life with the ability to not carry out interventions that may theoretically produce small increases in longevity but at the expense of worsening quality of life. It is also important to recognize when a person in the nursing home is better served by hospice (palliative care) than regular medical care.[7]

CONTINUOUS QUALITY IMPROVEMENT

A high-quality administrative trio of administrator, director of nursing, and medical director is the key to good outcomes in the nursing home.[8] This group, together with the middle managers, should meet at least once a month to review quality indicators.[9,10] These indicators include focused reviews of problem areas, and range from falls and food service problems to laundry and cleaning services. This meeting ideally includes representatives from the certified nurse's aides who often have insights not seen by management. When problems are identified, a small task force should be designated to determine the cause or causes using a Paretto diagram and then institute a rapid cycle of repair, reporting back to the meeting next month.[11]

In the United States a Minimum Data Set (MDS) is routinely collected in nursing homes and then transmitted electronically to the state. The nursing home then receives regular reports comparing its performance to other nursing homes in the state and nationally (**Box 2**). The MDS is a tool designed to implement standardized assessment and improvement of care management in nursing homes. An updated version of the MDS, MDS 3.0, has now been developed. The MDS 3.0 is considered to be more reliable, accurate, and useful than the MDS 2.0.[12] It now directly involves the resident in the assessment.

Nurses with advanced practice knowledge make important contributions to the quality of care in nursing homes.[13,14] Advanced practice nurses (nurses with extra medical training) in the United States tend to be more available in facilities than physicians. These specialists greatly improve communication between physicians and nurses, and are ideal practice educators and developers key to driving quality improvements toward optimal standards.

Transitions from nursing homes to emergency departments and from hospitals to nursing homes represent an area fraught with difficulty.[15–18] A major problem concerns maintaining appropriate medication lists between one place and another. Lack of adequate knowledge of the resident's mental status and whether the present state represents delirium is another problematic area.[19,20] Laboratory tests obtained in the hospital often never find their way back to the nursing home patient chart. Failure to adequately communicate "do not resuscitate" orders and inappropriate insertion of

Box 1
Recommendations of the International Association of Gerontology and Geriatrics and World Health Association's Task Force for improving nursing home care

Recommendation 1. Effective leadership structures are established, that where possible, include an expert physician (medical director), and an expert registered nurse (nursing director) and skilled administrator.

Recommendation 2. An international alliance is formed to develop nursing home leadership capacity and capabilities.

Recommendation 3. To showcase international exemplars of excellence in nursing home practice to raise awareness of the demonstrable benefits for older people and high standards achieved through expert practice.

Recommendation 4. To create positive working conditions for nursing home practitioners with attractive career development opportunities, recognition, and similar rewards enjoyed by health care workers in comparable roles within the acute care services.

Recommendation 5. That nursing home quality indicators are developed that are sensitive to clinical and care needs and the right of older people to care that is dignified and respectful.

Recommendation 6. The use of physical and chemical restraints should be reduced to those that are absolutely indispensable.

Recommendations 7. That "meaningful activities" be offered to residents to provide physical and mental exercise and opportunities to participate within the nursing home and in community life, enhancing personal autonomy, social relationships (including intergenerational relationships), and social support.

Recommendation 8. That evidence-informed pain assessment and management programs are introduced into all nursing homes.

Recommendation 9. That evidence-informed end of life and palliative care programs are introduced into all nursing homes.

Recommendation 10. That national drug approval agencies consider requiring drug trials that are age appropriate and inclusive of nursing home residents before they are approved.

Recommendation 11. That IAGG develop international certification courses for nursing (care) home health professionals.

Recommendation 12. Pilot the use of "Community of Practice Models" as a practice improvement method for nursing homes; using both face-to-face interdisciplinary training and virtual team support.

Recommendation 13. That a universal ethical approach to obtaining informed consent and monitoring the appropriateness of research is developed.

Recommendation 14. Develop nursing home research capacity in developing nations.

Recommendation 15. An investment is made in research priorities that address major public health problems and inequalities that affect older people receiving long-term care. Research priorities for which a high need is recognized include:

- A worldwide survey of different models of care, nursing home structure, and issues in improving quality of care is undertaken.
- A worldwide survey of older persons and their families is undertaken to determine their preferences for long-term care.
- A cross-national, prospective epidemiologic study measuring function and quality of life in nursing homes is undertaken.
- Development of culturally appropriate standardized assessment instruments including those involving social participatory methods.
- A function-focused approach to the prevalence of geriatric syndromes, their impact on function, and development of strategies to improve care for these syndromes needs to be developed.
- Research that evaluates the impact of different models of care against trajectories of physical and cognitive function is conducted.

Box 2
Nursing home facility quality measurement/indicators: national average based on MDS 2.0 reporting

Domain/Measure Description	National Average (%)
Chronic Care Measures	
Accidents	
Incidence of new fractures	1.4
Prevalence of falls	13.0
Behavioral/Emotional Patterns	
Residents who have become more depressed or anxious	15.0
Prevalence of behavior symptoms affecting others: Overall	16.7
Prevalence of behavior symptoms affecting others: High risk	19.2
Prevalence of behavior symptoms affecting others: Low risk	6.8
Prevalence of symptoms of depression without antidepressant therapy	4.5
Clinical Management	
Use of 9 or more different medications	71.3
Cognitive Patterns	
Incidence of cognitive impairment	12.5
Elimination/Incontinence	
Low-risk residents who lost control of their bowels or bladder	50.8
Residents who have/had a catheter inserted and left in their bladder	6.2
Prevalence of occasional or frequent bladder or bowel incontinence without a toileting plan	51.8
	0.0
Prevalence of fecal impaction	
Infection Control	
Residents with a urinary tract infection	9.6
Nutrition/Eating	
Residents who lose too much weight	8.7
Prevalence of tube feeding	6.4
Prevalence of dehydration	0.1
Pain Management	
Residents who have moderate to severe pain	4.0
Physical Functioning	
Residents whose need for help with daily activities has increased	14.7
Residents who spend most of their time in bed or in a chair	4.6
Residents whose ability to move in and around their room got worse	12.1
Incidence of decline in range of motion	6.6
Psychotropic Drug Use	
Prevalence of antipsychotic use, in the absence of psychotic or related conditions: Overall	18.4 / 39.4
Prevalence of antipsychotic use, in the absence of psychotic or related conditions: High risk	15.6 / 23.3
Prevalence of antipsychotic use, in the absence of psychotic or related conditions: Low risk	5.5
Prevalence of antianxiety/hypnotic use	
Prevalence of hypnotic use more than 2 times in last week	
Quality of Life	
Residents who were physically restrained	2.7
Prevalence of little or no activity	5.4
Skin Care	
High-risk residents with pressure ulcers	12.0
Low-risk residents with pressure ulcers	2.4
Post-Acute Care (PAC) Measures	
Short-stay residents with delirium	1.5
Short-stay residents who had moderate to severe pain	19.0
Short-stay residents with pressure ulcers	12.1

feeding tubes are other problems. Continuous attention to transition problems is essential in enhancing care.

MEANINGFUL ACTIVITY

Maintaining meaningful physical and mental activity is a key to high quality of life for persons in nursing homes.[21,22] Physical activity programs have been shown to slow the decline in activities of daily living,[23] and also decrease aggressive behavior and improve mood.[24,25] Resistance exercise programs can decrease falls, as can balance exercises.[26,27] Dual tasking exercises can reduce the tendency to fall in persons with executive function impairment.[28] Dancing is an underused physical activity in nursing homes. "Wii" sports have also proved useful in rehabilitation.[29] Physical activity should be offered for at least 30 minutes daily, recognizing that most residents will only attend one or two sessions a week. In addition, activities need to be separately designed for persons of different cognitive abilities and also for wheelchair and ambulatory individuals.

Mental activities are also important and should be slightly challenging for the person's ability. Watching television and movies do not represent meaningful activities. Playing games and group sessions are key. Reminiscence groups can be useful at some stages of Alzheimer. Innovative approaches to providing social and cognitive stimulation tailored to persons of different abilities need to be explored. For some, this may include music therapy, pet therapy, or even the use of robotic dogs.[30,31]

POLYPHARMACY

Numerous studies show that once a person receives more than 5 to 7 drugs, the next drug is as likely to do harm as it will do good.[32–37] In many cases, the addition of the second drug borders on the ludicrous, for example, the addition of an anticholinergic for incontinence in someone on a cholinesterase inhibitor for dementia. Overtreatment of hypertension is rampant in nursing homes.[38,39] Statins are often given to persons with minimal or no evidence of atherosclerosis.[40] Drugs such as colace, which is ineffectual, are used to treat constipation, then the person receives 3 or 4 other drugs to treat constipation.[41]

WEIGHT LOSS

Weight loss remains one of the best indicators of poor outcome in nursing homes.[42–45] Weight loss is a major component of frailty.[46–48] The most common cause of weight loss in nursing homes is depression.[44,49,50] Medications represent another major cause of weight loss; for example, metformin causes anorexia and weight loss.[51] Other causes of weight loss that are reversible are listed in **Box 3**. Dysphagia can lead to both decreased food intake and weight loss, but its treatment with specific diets can actually create anorexia.[52,53] Mealtime ambience plays a role in the prevention of weight loss.[54] Therapeutic diets should be avoided in the majority of nursing home residents.[52]

Anorexia predicts weight loss and can be detected in nursing homes with the Simplified Nutrition Assessment Questionnaire.[55] The Mini Nutritional Assessment should be used to assess all persons with weight loss.[56]

Persons with cachexia should be carefully assessed for underlying causes of cytokine excess.[57,58] Dehydration needs to be considered in the differential diagnosis of weight loss.[59] Sarcopenia can be treated with a leucine-enriched essential amino

---

Box 3
MEALS-ON-WHEELS mnemonic for treatable causes of weight loss in older persons

Medications (eg, digoxin, theophylline, cimetidine)

Emotional (eg, depression)

Alcoholism, elder abuse, anorexia tardive

Late life paranoia

Swallowing problems

Oral factors

Nosocomial infections (eg, tuberculosis)

Wandering and other dementia-related factors

Hyperthyroidism, Hypercalcemia, Hypoadrenalism

Enteral problems (eg, gluten enteropathy)

Eating problems

Low salt, low cholesterol, and other therapeutic diets

Stones (cholecystitis)

---

acid supplement and resistance exercise.[60–62] The role of anabolic hormones in the management of muscle loss in the nursing home remains controversial.[63,64]

A logical approach to the diagnosis and management of weight loss in the nursing home has been published.[65] Caloric supplements should be given between meals and at least 2 hours before the next meal.[64] A best practice statement to improve nutrition in frail older persons also exists.[66]

HEARING LOSS AND COMMUNICATION IMPAIRMENT

Hearing loss is one of the most common and most neglected problems in nursing homes.[67,68] Hearing loss occurs in 70% to 80% of persons in nursing homes.[68] Hearing disability leads to dysphoria in older persons and an increase in carer burden.[69] A major barrier to hearing in nursing home residents is background noise which, even if the person is using a hearing aid, makes intelligible communication extremely difficult. Pocket talkers and particularly their use while listening to television, thus decreasing high-volume use of the radio and television, are rarely used. Improvement of the listening environment greatly enhances hearing aid use.[70] Adequate audiological testing has often not been performed in residents, and even when a hearing aid was available about 70% had problems with the device.[71] Most residents needed help with care of their hearing aids, yet less than half of the nursing aides have been trained in the use of hearing aids.

Cerumen impaction is common in nursing homes. Removal of wax from impacted ears improves hearing,[72] and was associated with an improvement in the Mini Mental Status Examination score of greater than 1. The authors have had a similar experience in the Saint Louis University associated nursing homes.

For many of the hearing impaired, lip reading becomes the major method by which they obtain oral information. Only 20% of nursing home residents have severe visual impairment, and many visual problems can be treated.[73] Thus, for communication it is essential that the room is well lit to allow the resident to see the face of the person with whom they are communicating. All health professionals and visitors need to be aware that they should only speak to a resident when the resident can see their face. Using a deeper tone may also help, but shouting actually is harmful to communication. A writing slate should be readily available to communicate with persons whose hearing handicap does not allow them to get the gist of the conversation.

In nursing homes there are numerous persons with dysphasia or aphasia. These individuals need to be provided with communication boards, which in the modern age should ideally be computer based. Classic examples of poor communication are persons who have "locked-in syndrome" from mid-brain cerebrovascular accidents. Health professionals need to have increased awareness that these individuals have intact understanding of events in their environment. Communication can be established by using blinking for simple "yes" and "no" answers, all the way through to completing a publishable book such as The Diving Bell and the Butterfly.[74] Communication with persons with communication handicaps is highly time consuming, and requires the use of special apparatus and the training of all health care professionals.

ORAL HEALTH

Poor oral health is a very common problem in institutionalized older persons,[75,76] more so in older persons with functional impairment and dementia. Persons with periodontal disease and other oral problems have a poor quality of life, develop anorexia and weight loss, have an increased incidence of aspiration pneumonia, have problems with speaking and social interaction, and are at risk for the cytokine-related aging process. Poor oral health increases mortality risk from pneumonia.[77] More than 100 systemic diseases can lead to oral problems. Despite this, physicians pay little attention to the state of the mouth.

Most oral health care is done by certified nursing aids. Teeth brushing occurs inconsistently, with the average resident having his or her teeth brushed from 16 to 50 seconds when it occurs.[78,79] Unfortunately, educational programs have made little impact on oral health care.[79] There is a major need to increase the number of dentists who focus on oral health care in older persons and nursing home residents.

PRESSURE ULCERS

The prevalence of pressure ulcers in nursing facilities in the United States is 11%. Pressure ulcers occur because external pressure and sheer forces interact with factors intrinsic to the patient that make the skin more vulnerable to these factors.[80] The intrinsic risk factors include local ischemia, local inflammation, poor nutrition to allow healing, and impaired lymphatic function. Thus while prevention and management of pressure ulcers requires a focus on pressure relief, it also requires an understanding of other factors involved. Pressure relief falls predominantly to the nursing staff, and involves frequent repositioning (every 2 hours) for bedfast individuals and encouraging persons to get out of bed. Australian standard medical sheepskins prevent pressure ulcers.[81] Higher specification foam mattresses provide better prevention than standard hospital mattresses. Low-air-loss beds and alternating pressure beds may have a small advantage. Only air-fluidized beds reduce pressure below the 32 mm Hg required to be less than capillary closing pressure.[82]

Debridement is necessary only to remove devitalized tissue. There are 5 different kinds of dressings: films, foams, hydrogels, alginates, and hydrocolloid. Topical therapies, such as silver dressings, can be used if the wound is infected. Systemic antibiotics should be used only when cellulitis is present. There is evidence for the efficacy of negative pressure wound therapy in diabetic ulcers, and perhaps in some other skin wounds.[83]

DIABETES MELLITUS

The approach to diabetes care in older persons is undergoing modification.[84,85] Recent studies have suggested that the ideal mortality outcomes for hemoglobin A_{1c} (HbA_{1c}) levels in diabetics occur between an HbA_{1c} of 7% to 8%.[86] Pneumonia is not more common in diabetics with HbA_{1c} greater than 7%.[87]

Given the data concerning thiazolidinediones and their propensity to cause edema, these should be avoided. A major need is to avoid hypoglycemia, making metformin the drug of choice unless the serum creatinine level is greater than 1.4 mg/dL. The restriction on using metformin in persons older than 80 years no longer exists. Combination drug therapy increases polypharmacy, and appears to show little benefit until the HbA_{1c} is greater than 7.5%. Insulin glarginine is becoming a popular long-acting insulin that in low doses has minimal hypoglycemia.[88] Where possible, insulin sliding scales should be avoided. Often the glucose levels are obtained after the resident has begun to eat, and this leads to spuriously high glucose levels with too much insulin being administered in response to the glucose. Diabetic therapeutic diets are no longer appropriate in nursing homes.[89]

High blood glucose levels (>200 mg/dL) are associated with a decline in cognition.[90,91] Thus it is advisable to try and maintain blood glucose levels below 200 mg/dL. Hypertriglyceridemia is also associated with cognitive impairment.[92] Pain perception is increased with elevated glucose levels.[93] Hyperglycosuria leads to zinc deficiency in diabetics.[94,95] For this reason diabetics with pressure or vascular ulcers should most probably receive zinc supplementation. Depression is more common in persons with diabetes and leads to poor outcomes.[96,97] For this reason, all persons with diabetes should be screened for depression and aggressively treated if it is present.

Overall, persons with diabetes have a greater prevalence of disability, which means that persons with diabetes are more likely to be in nursing homes. There are numerous unique components of the management of older diabetics.

FALLS

The fall rate in the nursing home is approximately 1.5 falls per bed per year, which is nearly 3 times the rate of falls seen in the community.[98–100] Paradoxically, falls occur more often in active persons with less disability. Falls are particularly common during the first few weeks after admission to a nursing home. Three-quarters of falls occur in the bedroom and the associated bathroom. Most falls occur during standing or sitting. Fall-related injuries are the most common reason for lawsuits in the United States.

Several interdisciplinary approaches have been shown to reduce falls.[101] The approach to fall prevention demands a focus on both the environment and the intrinsic factors. Environmental modifications need to be resident focused. For example, chair height needs to be adjusted to the resident, rather than having "one size fits all." Optimized lighting is different for a person with age-related macular degeneration than for a person with cataracts, where the lighting may increase the glare. Grab bars and raised toilet seats represent relatively easy environmental modifications. Shock-absorbing floor surfaces are now being tested in high-risk areas, for example, bathroom and bedroom.[102] New footwear that should reduce fall risk is being developed. Beds at floor level can be useful for some individuals. Alarm devices can be used for high-risk fallers. Wheelchair maintenance and safety is important.

In persons at risk for falls, a variety of specific exercise (rehabilitation) programs are necessary. Basic strengthening of leg muscles needs to be coupled with balance exercises. In persons with executive function decline, dual tasking exercises can be useful. Residents can also be taught how to fall in a manner less likely to produce injury. Provision of appropriate assistive mobility devices also can help in fall reduction. By itself, exercise does not decrease falls in nursing homes. Maintaining mobility is a key component of high quality of life. For this reason physical restraints should never be used. Studies suggest that there is a decrease in falls when physical restraints are not used.[103] Merry walkers, which increase mobility, should not be considered restraints.

Resident-specific factors to reduce falls include a full medical examination. Medication review is key. Psychoactive drugs are associated with a high risk of falls and often are of minimal benefit. Many medications cause orthostatic hypotension, a key cause of falls.[104] All residents who fall need to have standing blood pressure measured. Postprandial hypotension occurs 30 minutes to 2 hours following a meal,[105] caused by the release of a vasodilatory peptide, calcitonin gene-related peptide, which causes peripheral vasodilation.[106] Postprandial hypotension can be treated with the α1-glucosidase inhibitors miglitol and acarbose, which increase glucagon-like peptide and slow gastric emptying.[107] High anticholinergic burden is commonly associated with falls and recognizes the key role of anticholinergic medicines in producing falls.[108] Delirium should be considered as a diagnosis in all persons with new-onset falls. Anemia is commonly associated with falls.[109] When a fall occurs, whether a loss of consciousness has occurred needs to be determined. In such a case seizures or syncope needs to be considered. In syncopal persons carotid sinus massage can determine the need for a pacemaker. Persons with atrial fibrillation and recurrent falls should receive either coumadin or dabigatrin, as their falls are often caused by small strokes.

Decline in 25(OH) vitamin D is common in most nursing home residents.[110,111] Vitamin D deficiency is associated with sarcopenia, falls, functional decline, and hip fracture.[112] Vitamin D should be replaced to a level of about 30 ng/mL 25(OH) vitamin D.

Hip and pelvic fractures are much more common in nursing homes than in the community.[113,114] While calcium replacement is important, it should not be given with other medicines. A 6-ounce (170 g) carton of yogurt is an excellent way to provide adequate calcium replacement. The use of bisphosphonates should be limited to those with at least a 6-month estimated survival. Denusomab is inappropriate in nursing home residents in view of the increased risk of serious infections. Hip pads are protective in frequent fallers, but adherence is often difficult to obtain.[115,116] Not all hip protectors are of adequate design to reduce the impact of the fall sufficiently to prevent hip fractures.[117]

While decreasing falls and injuries in the nursing home requires an interdisciplinary approach, nursing staff play a key role in implementing change and adherence. High-quality nursing practice is very important. Lack of nursing support or ambivalence creates a high probability that fall prevention programs will fail. Nursing communication with physicians and other health professionals is essential to maximize outcomes.

BEHAVIORAL SYMPTOMS AND DEMENTIA

The cognitive status of all residents in the nursing home should be assessed, using a formal tool such as the Veterans Administration St Louis University Mental Status Examination (**Fig. 1**).[118,119] Behavioral symptoms in persons with dementia include apathy (27%), depression (21%), and agitation/aggression (24%).[120–122] Paranoia, delusions, illusions, and hallucinations are also not rare in demented persons.

VAMC
SLUMS EXAMINATION
Questions about this assessment tool? E-mail aging@slu.edu

Name_____ Age_____

Is the patient alert?_____ Level of education_____

_/1	**1. What day of the week is it?**
_/1	**2. What is the year?**
_/1	**3. What state are we in?**
	4. Please remember these five objects. I will ask you what they are later. Apple Pen Tie House Car
_/3	**5. You have $100 and you go to the store and buy a dozen apples for $3 and a tricycle for $20.** ❶ How much did you spend? ❷ How much do you have left?
_/3	**6. Please name as many animals as you can in one minute.** ❶ 0-4 animals ❶ 5-9 animals ❷ 10-14 animals ❸ 15+ animals
_/5	**7. What were the five objects I asked you to remember? 1 point for each one correct.**
_/2	**8. I am going to give you a series of numbers and I would like you to give them to me backwards. For example, if I say 42, you would say 24.** ❶ 87 ❶ 648 ❶ 8537
_/4	**9. This is a clock face. Please put in the hour markers and the time at ten minutes to eleven o'clock.** ❷ Hour markers okay ❷ Time correct ❶ **10. Please place an X in the triangle.**
_/2	❶ Which of the above figures is largest?
_/8	**11. I am going to tell you a story. Please listen carefully because afterwards, I'm going to ask you some questions about it.** Jill was a very successful stockbroker. She made a lot of money on the stock market. She then met Jack, a devastatingly handsome man. She married him and had three children. They lived in Chicago. She then stopped work and stayed at home to bring up her children. When they were teenagers, she went back to work. She and Jack lived happily ever after. ❷ What was the female's name? ❷ What work did she do? ❷ When did she go back to work? ❷ What state did she live in?

_____ TOTAL SCORE

SCORING		
HIGH SCHOOL EDUCATION		**LESS THAN HIGH SCHOOL EDUCATION**
27-30	NORMAL	25-30
21-26	MILD NEUROCOGNITIVE DISORDER	20-24
1-20	DEMENTIA	1-19

_____   _____   _____
CLINICIAN'S SIGNATURE   DATE   TIME

Fig. 1. The Veterans Administration St Louis University Mental Status Examination. (*From* Tariq SH, Tumosa N, Chibnall JT, Perry HM III, Morley JE. Comparison of the Saint Louis University Mental Status Examination and the Mini-Mental State Examination for detecting dementia and mild neurocognitive disorder – a pilot study. Am J Geriatr Psych 2006;14:903; with permission.)

Persons who have illusions, hallucinations, and socially inappropriate behaviors are more likely to have Lewy body dementia. Classic aggressive behavior symptoms include verbal or physical aggression, resistiveness to care, and sundowning or elopement.[123] When persons in nursing homes have agitated behavior, the possibility that it is caused by delirium or pain should always be considered.[124–126]

Antipsychotics have marginal benefit in persons with dementia,[127] whereas they play a major role in increasing aspiration pneumonia and hip fracture.[128,129] Antipsychotics also increase mortality and functional decline.[130–132]

Several nonpharmacologic treatments have been developed for treating agitation, including:

- Brief psychological therapy
- Continuous activity programming
- Namaste care (meaningful activities, loving touch, soft music, low light, aromatherapy)
- Snoezelen (multisensory stimulation)
- Musical therapy (but only during sessions)
- Education and support systems for staff and caregivers.

Other pharmacologic agents have been tried. Their effectiveness in double-blind trials is at best borderline, and often the high doses needed come with side effects. These drugs include carbamazepine, sodium valproate, trazodone, and citalopram. The large trial using cholinesterase inhibitors was negative. Memantine improves behavior by 12% compared with 8% for placebo, perhaps because its effect on N-methyl-D-aspartate reduces pain. The authors have seen numerous patients on memantine who have developed hypotension and have falls.

Depression occurs in about 30% of nursing home residents,[133] but is often undetected.[134] Depression should be treated in all persons with cognitive impairment. The finding that selective serotonin reuptake inhibitors cause osteoporosis and hip fractures is causing concern about the long-term treatment of depression in nursing homes.

Overall, management of abnormal behaviors in nursing home residents is enormously difficult. Regular exercise programs have the best outcomes. Again, this is an area where high-quality nursing is a key to good outcomes.

URINARY INCONTINENCE

Urinary incontinence represents one of the most frustrating problems to manage in the nursing home, because cognitive and mobility impairment adds to the real difficulties of managing the other causes of incontinence. In addition, the drugs used to treat urge incontinence decrease cognition. Drugs used to treat lower urinary tract symptomatology produce hypotension and orthostasis. Constipation also increases urinary incontinence. Thus, it is not surprising that urinary incontinence occurs in 50% to 65% of persons receiving long-term care.[135–137]

The key to continence maintenance is frequent, regular toileting and prompted voiding. Prompted voiding is particularly important in persons with cognitive dysfunction. If prompted voiding is successful in the first 3 days of a trial, its effect will be maintained over a long period of time.[138] Providing fluid at an appropriate time in juxtaposition to the toileting time as determined by incontinence diaries is also helpful.[139] More sophisticated biofeedback programs including Kegel exercises can benefit residents who are reasonably cognitively intact.

Of residents with incontinence, only 7% received a medication.[140] Similarly, whereas the use of urethral sphincters is now becoming more common in community dwellers, their use in nursing homes remains rare.[141] Catheter use should be avoided wherever possible, and straight catheterization on a regular schedule is preferred to the use of an indwelling catheter.[142] Like indwelling catheters, condom catheters also increase the likelihood of urinary tract infections.

Even with an excellent toileting program, many of the nursing home residents will need to use absorbent briefs or pads.[143] Disposable pull-ups are preferred by women, but are the most expensive. Regular diapers were preferred by men, and were better than inserts as well as being cheaper. Only some men found regular washable diapers acceptable at night. While these are the least expensive design, they are unacceptable to women. In all nursing home residents preferences for absorbent products should be determined, and these may vary between day and night. Combinations of products can be better and more cost effective.

The appropriate care of urinary incontinence is highly time intensive and present reimbursement in the nursing homes is most probably insufficient to provide adequate staffing. An advanced practice nurse specializing in incontinence care can further improve outcomes for residents.

RELATIONAL ASPECTS OF CARE

The idea of people, especially those with long-term conditions, being partners in their care is not new and has long been promoted in the academic literature.[144] Making this work in practice has its challenges, and Nolan and colleagues[145] have long advocated that family carers and, where possible, frail older people should also be viewed as coexperts. Promoting partnerships between the cared-for person, the family, and staff within nursing home practice has been recognized as a strategy for improving quality.[144] Achievement of a practice culture that is safe, dignified, and respectful within nursing home care thus becomes a blend of case knowledge (eg, condition management such as stroke), patient knowledge (eg, functional, cognitive abilities), and person knowledge (eg, life history, meaningful relationships, preferences, and aspirations). Blending these different types of knowledge allows us to move beyond person-centered care toward relational care that is focused on providing the best care for an individual within the context of nursing home life. The SENSES Framework, originally suggested by Nolan in 1997 and developed over several years,[146–149] has proved particularly helpful in terms of influencing the culture of care and enriching the practice learning environment in Europe. Nolan and colleagues[150] suggest that staff working in nursing homes should create an environment in which older people, family, and staff experience 6 senses, namely sense of security, sense of belonging, sense of continuity, sense of purpose, sense of achievement, and sense of significance.

As the matrix by Brown and colleagues[144] indicates, the idea of "interdependence" rather than independence is central to enriching the relational care environment within nursing homes. A prerequisite for relationship-centered care is effective communications and trust between all staff, older persons, and family members. It is easy to overlook the voice of individuals, and research has shown that this influences perceptions of care experience and affects staff morale.[148,149] Practice toolkits (short questionnaires) to determine how the SENSES are created can be useful, and help identify priorities for change.[144]

TRUTH TELLING

One of the key determinants of trust between staff and older people is truth telling within care. As Tuckett[151] observes, communication exerts a powerful influence over relationships with others, and for older people who reside in nursing homes the way practitioners communicate is a function of the caring culture within that home as much at it has to do with individual traits. It is well known that oversimplification and patronizing talk can diminish an older person, as can talking to the visitor and talking over an individual. Information sharing in health care is linked to perceptions of honesty, and several studies have revealed that older people rate "staff being honest with them" as one of the most important caring behaviors.[152] An Australian study recently described nursing homes as "places of suspicious awareness and mutual pretence" in which relatives, staff, and older people conspire to protect each other, resulting in a web of often unhelpful but well-intended deception designed to protect either patients or their kin.[153]

Obtaining informed consent for procedures is predicated on truth-telling processes that acknowledge the potential risk associated with procedures. As noted in the introduction, sometimes decisions not to use aggressive medical management are appropriate. To uphold the principles of truth telling, advanced conversations about such possibilities should be held as soon as possible and individual preferences noted in accordance with local guidelines.

Practitioners often rationalize their truth-telling practices in terms of their assumptions about what an older person "would or would not wish to know" set against their professional judgments about what people "need to know." What is ethically right in a given situation is of course a matter of opinion, and a recent review concluded that the most reasonable stance to take is to directly ask those with the capacity to respond about their preferences for information and truth, rather than to rely on assumptions or make relatives information gatekeepers.[154]

SUMMARY

Nursing home care is extraordinarily complex, and requires a high level of interdisciplinary care and expert practice. On the whole, health professionals working in nursing homes worldwide have been undervalued. There is a need for increased translational research and improved services in nursing homes as the numbers of people who require long-term care place increasing demands on the nursing home sector.

REFERENCES

1. Schols JM, Crebolder HF, van Weel C. Nursing home and nursing home physician: the Dutch experience. J Am Med Dir Assoc 2004;5:207–12.
2. Rowland FN, Cowles M, Dickstein C, et al. Impact of medical director certification on nursing home quality of care. J Am Med Dir Assoc 2009;10:431–5.
3. Morley JE. Having a CMD is associated with improved nursing home quality of care. J Am Med Dir Assoc 2009;10:515.
4. Tolson D, Rolland Y, Andrieu S, et al. International Association of Gerontology and Geriatrics: a global agenda for clinical research and quality of care in nursing homes. J Am Med Dir Assoc 2011;12:184–9.
5. Morley JE. A brief history of geriatrics. J Gerontol A Biol Sci Med Sci 2004;59: 1132–52.
6. Morley JE. Clinical practice in nursing homes as a key for progress. J Nutr Health Aging 2010;14:586–93.
7. Cruz-Oliver DM, Sanford AM, Paniagua MA. End-of-life care in the nursing home. J Am Med Dir Assoc 2010;11:461–4.
8. Levenson SA. The basis for improving and reforming long-term care, part 1: the foundation. J Am Med Dir Assoc 2009;10:459–65.
9. Levenson SA. The basis for improving and reforming long-term care, part 2: clinical problem solving and evidence-based care. J Am Med Dir Assoc 2009;10:520–9.
10. Levenson SA. The basis for improving and reforming long-term care, part 4: identifying meaningful improvement approaches (segment 1). J Am Med Dir Assoc 2010;11:84–91.
11. Morley JE. Rapid cycles (continuous quality improvement), an essential part of the medical director's role. J Am Med Dir Assoc 2008;9:535–8.
12. Centers for Medicare and Medicaid Services (CMS), HHS. Medicare Program; prospective payment system and consolidated billing for skilled

nursing facilities for HY 2010; Minimum Data Set, version 3.0 for skilled nursing facilities and Medicaid nursing facilities. Final Rule. Fed Regist 2009;74(153):40287–395.

13. American Medical Directors Association ad hoc Work Group on Role of Attending Physician and Advanced Practice Nurse Collaborators. Collaborative and supervisory relationships between attending physicians and advanced practice nurses in long-term care facilities. J Am Med Dir Assoc 2011;12:12–8.

14. Philpot C, Tolson D, Morley JE. Advanced practice nurses and attending physicians: a collaboration to improve quality of care in the nursing home. J Am Med Dir Assoc 2011;12:161–5.

15. Shah F, Burack O, Boockvar KS. Perceived barriers to communication between hospital and nursing home at time of patient transfer. J Am Med Dir Assoc 2010; 11:239–45.

16. Morley JE. Transitions. J Am Med Dir Assoc 2010;11:607–11.

17. Murray LM, Laditka SB. Care transitions by older adults from nursing homes to hospitals: implications for long-term care practice, geriatrics education, and research. J Am Med Dir Assoc 2010;11:231–8.

18. Steinberg KE. Reducing unnecessary hospitalizations: apple pie! J Am Med Dir Assoc 2009;10:595–6.

19. Flaherty JH, Rudolph J, Shay K, et al. Delirium is a serious and under-recognized problem: why assessment of mental status should be the sixth vital sign. J Am Med Dir Assoc 2007;8:273–5.

20. Eeles E, Rockwood K. Delirium in the long-term care setting: clinical and research challenges. J Am Med Dir Assoc 2008;9:157–61.

21. Morley JE. The magic of exercise. J Am Med Dir Assoc 2008;9:375–7.

22. O'Konski M, Bane C, Hettinga J, et al. Comparative effectiveness of exercise with patterned sensory enhanced music and background music for long-term care residents. J Music Ther 2010;47:120–36.

23. Rolland Y, Abellan van Kan G, Vellas B. Physical activity and Alzheimer's disease: from prevention to therapeutic perspectives. J Am Med Dir Assoc 2008;9:390–405.

24. Aman E, Thomas DR. Supervised exercise to reduce agitation in severely cognitively impaired persons. J Am Med Dir Assoc 2009;10:271–6.

25. Morley JE. Managing persons with dementia in the nursing home: high touch trumps high tech. J Am Med Dir Assoc 2008;9:139–46.

26. Rose DJ, Hernandez D. The role of exercise in fall prevention for older adults. Clin Geriatr Med 2010;26:706–31.

27. Liu H, Frank A. Tai Chi as a balance improvement exercise for older adults: a systematic review. J Geriatr Phys Ther 2010;33:103–9.

28. Plotnik M, Dagan Y, Gurevich T, et al. Effects of cognitive function on gait and dual tasking abilities in patients with Parkinson's disease suffering from motor response fluctuations. Exp Brain Res 2011;208:169–79.

29. Saposnik G, Teasell R, Mamdani M, et al. Effectiveness of virtual reality using Wii gaming technology in stroke rehabilitation: a pilot randomized clinical trial and proof of principle. Stroke 2010;41:1477–84.

30. Banks MR, Wiloughby LM, Banks WA. Animal-assisted therapy and loneliness in nursing homes: use of robotic versus living dogs. J Am Med Dir Assoc 2008;9: 173–7.

31. Colberg SR, Somma CT, Sechrist SR. Physical activity participation may offset some of the negative impact of diabetes on cognitive function. J Am Med Dir Assoc 2008;9:434–8.

32. Fitzgerald SP, Bean NG. An analysis of the interactions between individual co-morbidities and their treatments—implications for guidelines and polypharmacy. J Am Med Dir Assoc 2010;11:475–84.

33. Morley JE. Polypharmacy in the nursing home. J Am Med Dir Assoc 2009;10:289–91.

34. Verrue CL, Mehuys E, Somers A, et al. Medication administration in nursing homes: pharmacists' contribution to error prevention. J Am Med Dir Assoc 2010;11:275–83.

35. Flaherty JH, Perry HM 3rd, Lynchard GS, et al. Polypharmacy and hospitalization among older home care patients. J Gerontol A Biol Sci Med Sci 2000;55:M554–9.

36. Miles RW. A conversation: polypharmacy in the nursing home. J Am Med Dir Assoc 2010;11:296–7.

37. Gokce Kutsal Y, Barak A, Atalay A, et al. Polypharmacy in the elderly: a multicenter study. J Am Med Dir Assoc 2009;10:486–90.

38. Morley JE. Hypertension: is it overtreated in the elderly? J Am Med Dir Assoc 2010;11:147–52.

39. Simonson W, Han LF, Davidson HE. Hypertension treatment and outcomes in US nursing homes: results from the US National Nursing Home Survey. J Am Med Dir Assoc 2011;12:44–9.

40. Taylor F, Ward K, Moore TH, et al. Statins for the primary prevention of cardiovascular disease. Cochrane Database Syst Rev 2011;1:CD004816.

41. Tariq SH. Constipation in long term care. J Am Med Dir Assoc 2007;8:209–18.

42. Morley JE. Weight loss in older persons: new therapeutic approaches. Curr Pharm Des 2007;13:3637–47.

43. Bourdel-Marchasson I. How to improve nutritional support in geriatric institutions. J Am Med Dir Assoc 2010;11:13–20.

44. Morley JE, Kraenzle D. Causes of weight loss in a community nursing home. J Am Geriatr Soc 1994;42:583–5.

45. Morley JE. Anorexia, sarcopenia, and aging. Nutrition 2001;17:660–3.

46. Morley JE. Developing novel therapeutic approaches to frailty. Curr Pharm Des 2009;15:3384–95.

47. Abellan van Kan G, Rolland Y, Bergman H, et al. The I.A.N.A. Task Force on frailty assessment of older people in clinical practice. J Nutr Health Aging 2008;12:29–37.

48. Gobbens RJ, van Assen MA, Luijkx KG, et al. The Tilburg Frailty Indicator: psychometric properties. J Am Med Dir Assoc 2010;11:344–55.

49. Landi F, Laviano A, Cruz-Jentoft AJ. The anorexia of aging: is it a geriatric syndrome? J Am Med Dir Assoc 2010;11:153–6.

50. Landi F, Russo A, Liperoti R, et al. Anorexia, physical function, and incident disability among the frail elderly population: results from the ilSIRENTE study. J Am Med Dir Assoc 2010;11:268–74.

51. Lee A, Morley JE. Metformin decreases food consumption and induces weight loss in subjects with obesity with type II non-insulin-dependent diabetes. Obes Res 1998;6:47–53.

52. Coyle JL, Davis LA, Easterling C, et al. Oropharyngeal dysphagia assessment and treatment efficacy: setting the record straight (response to Campbell-Taylor). J Am Med Dir Assoc 2009;10:62–6.

53. Gottfred C. Oropharyngeal dysphagia in long-term care: response from ASHA. J Am Med Dir Assoc 2009;10:78.

54. Nijs K, de Graaf C, van Staveren WA, et al. Malnutrition and mealtime ambiance in nursing homes. J Am Med Dir Assoc 2009;10:226–9.

55. Wilson MM, Thomas DR, Rubenstein LZ, et al. Appetite assessment: simple appetite questionnaire predicts weight loss in community-dwelling adults and nursing home residents. Am J Clin Nutr 2005;82:1074–81.

56. Vellas B, Villars H, Abellan G, et al. Overview of the MNA—its history and challenges. J Nutr Health Aging 2006;10:456–63.

57. Evans WJ, Morley JE, Argiles J, et al. Cachexia: a new definition. Clin Nutr 2008; 27:793–9.

58. Argiles JM, Anker SD, Evans WJ, et al. Consensus on cachexia definitions. J Am Med Dir Assoc 2010;11:229–30.

59. Thomas DR, Cote TR, Lawhorne L, et al. Understanding clinical dehydration and its treatment. J Am Med Dir Assoc 2008;9:292–301.

60. Rolland Y, Czerwinski S, Abellan van Kan G, et al. Sarcopenia: its assessment, etiology, pathogenesis, consequences and future perspectives. J Nutr Health Aging 2008;12:433–50.

61. Morley JE, Argiles JM, Evans WJ, et al. Society for Sarcopenia, Cachexia and Wasting Disease. Nutritional recommendations for the management of sarcopenia. J Am Med Dir Assoc 2010;11:391–6.

62. van Wetering CR, Hoogendoorn M, Broekhuizen R, et al. Efficacy and costs of nutritional rehabilitation in muscle-wasted patients with chronic obstructive pulmonary disease in a community-based setting: a prespecified subgroup analysis of the INTERCOM trial. J Am Med Dir Assoc 2010;11:179–87.

63. Morley JE. Anabolic steroids and frailty. J Am Med Dir Assoc 2010;11:533–6.

64. Wilson MM, Purushothaman R, Morley JE. Effect of liquid dietary supplements on energy intake in the elderly. Am J Clin Nutr 2002;75:944–7.

65. Thomas DR, Ashmen W, Morley JE, et al. Nutritional management in long-term care: development of a clinical guideline. Council for Nutritional Strategies in Long-Term Care. J Gerontol A Biol Sci Med Sci 2000;55:M725–34.

66. Booth J, Alex L, Francis M, et al. Implementing a best practice statement in nutrition for frail older people: part 1. Nurs Older People 2005;16:26–8.

67. Tolson D, Nolan M. Gerontological nursing. Gerontological nursing 4: age-related hearing explored. Br J Nurs 2000;9:205–8.

68. Cohen-Mansfield J, Taylor JW. Hearing aid use in nursing homes. Part 1: Prevalence rates of hearing impairment and hearing aid use. J Am Med Dir Assoc 2004;5:283–8.

69. Tolson D, Swan I, Knussen C. Hearing disability: a source of distress for older people and carers. Br J Nurs 2002;11:1021–5.

70. Tolson D, McIntosh J. Listening in the care environment—chaos or clarity for the hearing-impaired elderly person. Int J Nurs Stud 1997;34:173–82.

71. Cohen-Mansfield J, Taylor JW. Hearing aid use in nursing homes. Part 2: Barriers to effective utilization of hearing AIDS. J Am Med Dir Assoc 2004;5: 289–96.

72. Moore AM, Voytas J, Kowalski D, et al. Cerumen, hearing, and cognition in the elderly. J Am Med Dir Assoc 2002;3:136–9.

73. Carcenac G, Herard ME, Kergoat MJ, et al. Assessment of visual function in institutional elderly patients. J Am Med Dir Assoc 2009;10:45–9.

74. Bauby J-D. The diving bell and the butterfly. A memoir of life in death. Paris: Vintage International; 1997.

75. Haimschild MS, Haumschild RJ. The importance of oral health in long-term care. J Am Med Dir Assoc 2009;10:667–71.

76. Awano S, Ansai T, Takata Y, et al. Oral health and mortality risk from pneumonia in the elderly. J Dent Res 2008;87:334–9.

77. Coleman P, Watson NM. Oral care provided by certified nursing assistants in nursing homes. J Am Geriatr Soc 2006;54:138–43.
78. Gammack JK, Pulisetty S. Nursing education and improvement in oral care delivery in long-term care. J Am Med Dir Assoc 2009;10:658–61.
79. Soini H, Suominen MH, Muurinen S, et al. Long-term care and oral health. J Am Med Dir Assoc 2009;10:512–4.
80. Thomas DR. Does pressure cause pressure ulcers? An inquiry into the etiology of pressure ulcers. J Am Med Dir Assoc 2010;11:397–405.
81. Ochs RF, Horn SD, van Rijswijk L, et al. Comparison of air-fluidized therapy with other support surfaces used to treat pressure ulcers in nursing home residents. Ostomy Wound Manage 2005;51:38–68.
82. Mistiaen PJ, Jolley DJ, McGowan S, et al. A multilevel analysis of three random-ized controlled trials of the Australian Medical Sheepskin in the prevention of sacral pressure ulcers. Med J Aust 2010;193:638–41.
83. Damiani G, Pinnarelli L, Sommella L, et al. Vacuum-assisted closure therapy for patients with infected sternal wounds: a meta-analysis of current evidence. J Plast Reconstr Aesthet Surg 2011. [Epub ahead of print].
84. Meyers RM, Reger L. Diabetes management in long-term care facilities: a prac-tical guide. J Am Med Dir Assoc 2009;10:354–60.
85. Feldman SM, Rosen R, DeStasio J. Status of diabetes management in the nursing home setting in 2008: a retrospective chart review and epidemiology study of diabetic nursing home residents and nursing home initiatives in dia-betes management. J Am Med Dir Assoc 2009;10:354–60.
86. Mazza AD, Morley JE. Update on diabetes in the elderly and the application of current therapeutics. J Am Med Dir Assoc 2007;8:489–92.
87. Chen LK, Peng LN, Lin MH, et al. Diabetes mellitus, glycemic control, and pneu-monia in long-term care facilities: a 2-year, prospective cohort study. J Am Med Dir Assoc 2011;12:33–7.
88. Pandya N, Nathanson E. Managing diabetes in long-term care facilities: benefits of switching from human insulin to insulin analogs. J Am Med Dir Assoc 2010;11:171–8.
89. Tariq SH, Karcic E, Thomas DR, et al. The use of no-concentrated-sweets diet in the management of type 2 diabetes in nursing homes. J Am Diet Assoc 2001;101:1463–6.
90. Mooradian AD, Perryman K, Fitten J, et al. Cortical function in elderly non-insulin dependent diabetic patients. Behavioral and electrophysiologic studies. Arch Intern Med 1988;148:2369–72.
91. Flood JF, Mooradian AD, Morley JE. Characteristics of learning and memory in streptozocin-induced diabetic mice. Diabetes 1990;39:1391–8.
92. Farr SA, Yamada KA, Butterfield DA, et al. Obesity and hypertriglyceridemia produce cognitive impairment. Endocrinology 2008;149:2628–36.
93. Morley GK, Mooradian AD, Levine AS, et al. Mechanism of pain in diabetic peripheral neuropathy. Effect of glucose on pain perception in humans. Am J Med 1984;77:79–82.
94. Kinlaw WB, Levine AS, Morley JE, et al. Abnormal zinc metabolism in type II dia-betes mellitus. Am J Med 1983;75:273–7.
95. Mooradian AD, Morley JE. Micronutrient status in diabetes mellitus. Am J Clin Nutr 1987;45:877–95.
96. Rosenthal MJ, Fajardo M, Gilmore S, et al. Hospitalization and mortality of dia-betes in older adults. A 3-year prospective study. Diabetes Care 1998;21:231–5.

97. Morley JE. Diabetes and aging: epidemiologic overview. Clin Geriatr Med 2008; 24:395–405.

98. Quigley P, Bulat T, Kurtzman E, et al. Fall prevention and injury protection for nursing home residents. J Am Med Dir Assoc 2010;11:284–93.

99. Beauchet O, Dubost V, Revel Delhom C, et al. How to manage recurrent falls in clinical practice: guidelines of the French society of geriatrics and gerontology. J Nutr Health Aging 2011;15:79–84.

100. Messinger-Rapport BJ, Thomas DR, Gammack JK, et al. Clinical update on nursing home medicine: 2009. J Am Med Dir Assoc 2009;10:530–53.

101. Messinger-Rapport B, Dumas LG. Falls in the nursing home: a collaborative approach. Nurs Clin North Am 2009;44:187–95.

102. Becker C, Rapp K. Fall prevention in nursing homes. Clin Geriatr Med 2010;26: 693–704.

103. Wang WW, Moyle W. Physical restraint use on people with dementia: a review of the literature. Aust J Adv Nurs 2005;22:46–52.

104. Vu MW, Weintraub N, Rubenstein LZ. Falls in the nursing home: are they preventable? J Am Med Dir Assoc 2006;7(Suppl 3):S53–8.

105. Morley JE. Editorial: postprandial hypotension—the ultimate Big Mac attack. J Gerontol A Biol Sci Med Sci 2001;56:M741–3.

106. Edwards BJ, Perry HM 3rd, Kaiser FE, et al. Relationship of age and calcitonin gene-related peptide to postprandial hypotension. Mech Ageing Dev 1996;87: 61–73.

107. Lee A, Patrick P, Wishart J, et al. The effects of miglitol on glucagon-like peptide-1 secretion and appetite sensations in obese type 2 diabetics. Diabetes Obes Metab 2002;4:329–35.

108. Kolanowski A, Fick DM, Campbell J, et al. A preliminary study of anticholinergic burden and relationship to a quality of life indicator, engagement in activities, in nursing home residents with dementia. J Am Med Dir Assoc 2009;10:252–7.

109. Dharmarajan TS. Falls and fractures linked to anemia, delirium, osteomalacia, medications, and more: the path to success is strewn with obstacles! J Am Med Dir Assoc 2007;8:549–50.

110. Braddy KK, Imam SN, Palia KR, et al. Vitamin D deficiency/insufficiency practice patterns in a veterans health administration long-term care population: a retrospective analysis. J Am Med Dir Assoc 2009;10:653–7.

111. Drinka PJ, Krause PF, Nets LJ, et al. Determinants of vitamin D levels in nursing home residents. J Am Med Dir Assoc 2007;8:76–9.

112. Morley JE. Vitamin D redux. J Am Med Dir Assoc 2009;10:591–2.

113. Morley JE. Hip fractures. J Am Med Dir Assoc 2010;11:81–3.

114. Young Y, Fried LP, Kuo RH. Hip fractures among elderly women: longitudinal comparison of physiological function changes and health care utilization. J Am Med Dir Assoc 2010;11:100–5.

115. Cameron ID, Kurrle SE, Quine S. Improving adherence with the use of hip protectors among older people living in nursing care facilities: a cluster randomized trial. J Am Med Dir Assoc 2011;12:50–7.

116. Zimmerman S, Magaziner J, Birge SJ, et al. Adherence to hip protectors and implications for U.S. long-term care settings. J Am Med Dir Assoc 2010;11: 106–15.

117. Rubenstein LZ. Hip protectors in long-term care: another confirmatory trial. J Am Med Dir Assoc 2008;9:289–90.

118. Tariq SH, Tumosa N, Chibnall JT, et al. Comparison of the Saint Louis University mental status examination and the mini-mental state examination for detecting

dementia and mild neurocognitive disorder—a pilot study. Am J Geriatr Psychiatry 2006;14:900–10.

119. Cruz-Oliver DM, Morley JE. Early detection of cognitive impairment: do screening tests help? J Am Med Dir Assoc 2010;11:1–6.

120. Volicer L, Van der Steen JT, Frijters DH. Modifiable factors related to abusive behaviors in nursing home residents with dementia. J Am Med Dir Assoc 2009;10:617–22.

121. Ishii S, Weintraub N, Mervis JR. Apathy: a common psychiatric syndrome in the elderly. J Am Med Dir Assoc 2009;10:381–93.

122. Volicer L. Culture change for residents with dementia. J Am Med Dir Assoc 2008;9:459.

123. Morley JE. Alzheimer's disease: future treatments. J Am Med Dir Assoc 2011;12: 1–7.

124. Tait RC, Chibnall JT. Under-treatment of pain in dementia: assessment is key. J Am Med Dir Assoc 2008;9:372–4.

125. Cervo FA, Bruckenthal P, Chen JJ, et al. Pain assessment in nursing home residents with dementia: psychometric properties and clinical utility of the CNA Pain Assessment Tool (CPAT). J Am Med Dir Assoc 2009;10:505–10.

126. Voyer P, Richard S, Doucet L, et al. Detecting delirium and subsyndromal delirium using different diagnostic criteria among demented long-term care residents. J Am Med Dir Assoc 2009;10:181–8.

127. Schneider LS, Tariot PN, Dagerman KS, et al. Effectiveness of atypical antipsychotic drugs in patients with Alzheimer's Disease. N Engl J Med 2006;355: 1525–38.

128. Jalbert JJ, Eaton CB, Miller SC, et al. Antipsychotic use and the risk of hip fracture among older adults afflicted with dementia. J Am Med Dir Assoc 2010;11: 120–7.

129. Trifiro G, Spina E, Gambassi G. Use of antipsychotics in elderly patients with dementia: do atypical and conventional agents have a similar safety profile? Pharmacol Res 2009;59:1–12.

130. Cabrera MA, Dellroza MS, Trelha CS, et al. Psychoactive drugs as risk factors for functional decline among noninstutionalized dependent elderly people. J Am Med Dir Assoc 2010;11:519–22.

131. Ballard C, Creese B, Corbett A, et al. Atypical antipsychotics for the treatment of behavioral and psychological symptoms in dementia, with a particular focus on longer term outcomes and mortality. Expert Opin Drug Saf 2011;10:35–43.

132. Cohen-Mansfield J, Jensen B. Nursing home physicians' knowledge of and attitudes toward nonpharmacological interventions for treatment of behavioral disturbances associated with dementia. J Am Med Dir Assoc 2008;9:491–8.

133. Morley JE. Depression in nursing home residents. J Am Med Dir Assoc 2010;11: 301–3.

134. Damian J, Pastor-Barriuso R, Valderrama-Gama E. Descriptive epidemiology of undetected depression in institutionalized older people. J Am Med Dir Assoc 2010;11:312–9.

135. Lawhorne LW, Ouslander JG, Parmelee PA. Urinary Incontinence Work Group of the AMDA-F LTC Research Network. Clinical practice guidelines, process improvement teams, and performance on a quality indicator for urinary incontinence: a pilot study. J Am Med Dir Assoc 2008;9:504–8.

136. Fink HA, Taylor BC, Tacklind JW, et al. Treatment interventions in nursing home residents with urinary incontinence: a systematic review of randomized trials. Mayo Clin Proc 2008;83:1332–43.

137. Ouslander JG. Quality improvement initiatives for urinary incontinence in nursing homes. J Am Med Dir Assoc 2007;8(Suppl 3):S6–11.

138. Schnelle JF, Leung FW, Rao SS, et al. A controlled trial of an intervention to improve urinary and fecal incontinence and constipation. J Am Geriatr Soc 2010;58:1504–11.

139. Leung FW, Schnelle JF. Urinary and fecal incontinence in nursing home residents. Gastroenterol Clin North Am 2008;37:697–707.

140. Narayanan S, Cerulli A, Kahler KH, et al. Is drug therapy for urinary incontinence use optimally in long-term care facilities? J Am Med Dir Assoc 2007;8:98–104.

141. Mohammed A, Khan A, Shaikh T, et al. The artificial urinary sphincter. Expert Rev Med Devices 2007;4:567–75.

142. Warren JW. Catheter-associated urinary tract infections. Infect Dis Clin North Am 1997;11:609–22.

143. Fader M, Cottenden A, Getliffe K, et al. Absorbent products for urinary/faecal incontinence: a comparative evaluation of key product designs. Health Technol Assess 2008;12:iii–iiv, ix–185.

144. Brown J, Robb Y, Lowndes A, et al. Understanding relationships within care. In: Tolson D, Booth J, Schofield I, editors. Evidence informed nursing with older people. London: Wiley Blackwell; 2011. p. 38–54. Chapter 3.

145. Nolan MR, Hanson E, Grant G, et al. User participation in health and social care research: voices, values and evaluation. Buckingham (UK): Open University Press; 2007.

146. Davies S, Nolan M, Brown J, et al. Dignity on the ward: promoting excellence in care. London: Help the Aged; 1999.

147. Nolan MR, Brown J, Davies S, et al. The Senses Framework: improving care for older people through a relationship-centred approach. Getting Research into Practice (GRIP) Series No. 2. Sheffield (UK): University of Sheffield; 2006.

148. Brown J, Nolan M, Davies S. Bringing caring and competence into focus in gerontological nursing: a longitudinal, multi-method study. Int J Nurs Stud 2007;45:654–67.

149. Brown J, Nolan M, Davies S, et al. Transforming students' views of gerontological nursing: Realising the potential of 'enriched' environments of learning and care: a multi-method longitudinal study. Int J Nurs Stud 2008;45:1214–32.

150. Nolan MR, Davies S, Grant G. Working with older people and their families: key issues in policy and practice. Buckingham (UK): Open University Press; 2001.

151. Tuckett A. The care encounter: pondering caring, honest communication and control. Int J Nurs Pract 2005;11:77–84.

152. Tuckett A, Hughes K, Schluter P, et al. Validation of CARE-Q in residential aged-care. Rating of importance of caring behaviours from an e-cohort sub-study. J Clin Nurs 2009;18:1501–9.

153. Tuckett A. The meaning of nursing-home: 'Waiting to go up to St. Peter, OK! Waiting house, sad but true'—An Australian perspective. J Aging Stud 2007; 21:119–33.

154. Tuckett AG, Tolson D. Truth telling and the evidence. In: Tolson D, Booth J, Schofield I, editors. Evidence informed nursing with older people. London: Wiley Blackwell; 2011. p. 55–67. Chapter 4.

Diabetes and Insulin Resistance in Older People

Adie Viljoen, MBChB, MMed, FCPath(SA), FRCPath, MBA[a,b],
Alan J. Sinclair, MSc, MD, FRCP[a,*]

KEYWORDS

- Diabetes mellitus • Aged elderly • Insulin resistance
- Diagnosis • Metabolic syndrome

KEY POINTS

Diabetes mellitus is very common in the older adults.

There is interplay between hyperglycemia, significant cardiovascular risk, marked propensity to comorbid illness, and the aging process.

The diagnostic criteria for diabetes have recently changed and now include testing for glycated hemoglobin (HbA_{1c}).

Insulin resistance is an important feature of type 2 diabetes mellitus (T2DM), is associated with a wide spectrum of aging factors, and increases the risk of cardiovascular disease (CVD) and the metabolic syndrome.

Disorders of lipids in T2DM occur commonly and are associated with an increasing evidence base of benefit with statin therapies.

Diabetes is a common condition in older people. About 10% to 25% of older individuals in Europe, North America, and Australia have diabetes.[1] In the United States, the prevalence of diabetes in people aged 70 to 74 years, 75 to 79 years, 80 to 84 years, and older than 85 years was 20%, 21%, 20%, and 17%, respectively.[2] In Western Europe, 1 in 2 diabetic subjects was found to be older than 65 years.[3,4] Of even greater concern is that the prevalence of diabetes is expected to increase further, because of a true increase in incidence (due to an increase in obesity and aging of the general population), better screening, and increased life expectancy of diabetic patients.[5] Diabetes significantly lowers the chances of successful aging, and notably increases functional limitations and impairs quality of life.[6] Functional impairments are

[a] Beds & Herts Postgraduate Medical School, Institute of Diabetes for Older People, University of Bedfordshire, Bedfordshire, Putteridge Bury Campus, Hitchin Road, Luton LU2 8LE, UK
[b] Department of Chemical Pathology, Lister Hospital, Coreys Mill Lane, Stevenage SG1 4AB, UK
* Corresponding author. Beds & Herts Postgraduate Medical School, Institute of Diabetes for Older People, University of Bedfordshire, Putteridge Bury Campus, Hitchin Road, Luton LU2 8LE, UK.
E-mail address: Sinclair.5@btinternet.com

Med Clin N Am 95 (2011) 615–629
doi:10.1016/j.mcna.2011.02.003
0025-7125/11/$ – see front matter © 2011 Published by Elsevier Inc.

medical.theclinics.com

largely due to specific diabetic complications, but these can also be caused by or aggravated by diabetes-related comorbidities. Diabetes in older persons represents significant medical, human, and socioeconomic burden (**Fig. 1**).

PATHOPHYSIOLOGY

Diabetes mellitus is a complex metabolic disorder that manifests primarily with derangements related to glucose homeostasis. It is classified into 2 clinical types, namely: type 1 diabetes and T2DM. Essentially, type 1 diabetes is caused by autoimmune destruction of the beta cells of the pancreas with an absolute insulin deficiency and T2DM is characterized by insulin resistance with a compensatory increased insulin secretion and an eventual failure of beta cell secretion of insulin. The absolute lack of insulin or the inability to respond to insulin signaling leads to hyperglycemia. Insulin recruits the GLUT-4 transmembrane glucose transporter in the muscle and adipose tissue, and this reduced glucose uptake leads to glucose-poor muscle and adipose tissue despite excess glucose levels in the plasma—the so-called poverty amongst plenty. In many ways, diabetes in the elderly is metabolically distinct. Most older persons with diabetes have T2DM. The Oxford diabetes community study reported that 95% of older persons with diabetes had T2DM. Nonetheless, studies conducted in Denmark and the United States reported the incidence of type 1 diabetes to be similar in patients aged 30 to 80 years.[7,8] The high prevalence of diabetes in the elderly is related to several factors, including genetics, coexisting illness, age-related decreased insulin secretion, age-related insulin resistance, adiposity, decreased physical activity, and concomitant medication.

Diabetes is much more common in the elderly in certain ethnic groups, while the likelihood that an elderly identical twin will develop diabetes if the sibling is affected is more than 80%.[9] The mechanisms that contribute to the dysglycemia of aging include impaired glucose-induced insulin secretion and resistance to insulin-mediated glucose uptake.[10,11] The most important of these mechanisms is resistance to insulin-mediated glucose disposal. It is debated whether the insulin resistance of the elderly is intrinsic to the aging process itself or is the result of lifestyle factors commonly associated with aging. Despite the strong genetic component, it is clear that environmental and lifestyle factors can influence the likelihood of a predisposed genetic susceptibility. Here, coexisting conditions may act as important contributors. These conditions include the fact that many older people take multiple drugs such as thiazide diuretics, which may precipitate diabetes.[12] Obesity, in particular central obesity, and reduced physical activity are well-established factors associated with disturbed carbohydrate metabolism. Both these factors are associated with increasing age and are independently linked to T2DM. Several age-related comorbid conditions of the muscular-skeletal (eg, arthritis), pulmonary (eg, chronic obstructive airways disease), and cardiovascular systems (eg, heart failure, stroke) may lead to decreased mobility, insulin resistance, and an increased risk to develop T2DM.

Distinct differences in the metabolic profiles and hypoglycemia responses exist between older and younger diabetic subjects. The principal defect in lean elderly diabetic subjects is impaired glucose-induced insulin secretion, whereas in obese elderly subjects, the principal defect is insulin resistance. Healthy older subjects have an impaired glucose counterregulation response such that they demonstrate an impaired glucagon and growth hormone response to hypoglycemia when compared with younger subjects. This impairment of response is further accentuated in older diabetic subjects.[13] In addition to the reduced counterregulatory response to hypoglycemia, older subjects are more prone to hypoglycemia because of a reduced

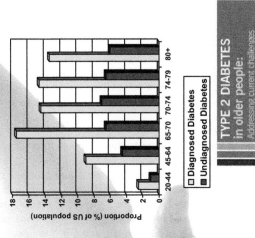

INTERACTIVE WEBCAST SERIES

TYPE 2 DIABETES
in older people:
Addressing current challenges

- Ongoing cross-sectional survey of non-institutionalised people in the US
- Study population consisted of 3,765 (aged 40-64y) and 2,809 (aged ≥ 65y) individuals
- Prevalence of diagnosed diabetes in the elderly cohort was 15.3% (about 60% diagnosed between 40-64y of age – middle age onset), and prevalence of undiagnosed was 6.9%
- Other results

Elderly people with middle age onset differ from those of elderly onset:

Mean age 71.7 v 76.5y, p <.0001

Proportion with HbA1c > 7.0% = 50.9% v 41.6%, p = .005

More likely to be treated with insulin alone, 31.7% v 6.9%, p <.0001

More likely to be treated for BP (71.7 v 59.3%, p = .001)

Fig. 1. Prevalence of diagnosed and undiagnosed diabetes by age—NHANES, 1999–2002. (*From* Sinclair A. Type 2 diabetes and the older adult: Why should we care? SB Communications. Available at http://www.sbcommswebcasts.com/register.php?eventId=4&page=alan-presentation.)

knowledge and awareness of warning symptoms and an altered psychomotor performance. Based on these pathophysiologic differences between older and younger subjects, different treatment options are preferred when treating older diabetic subjects.

DIAGNOSIS

Because of the lack of a unique biological marker, the diagnosis of diabetes is based exclusively on the consequences of disrupted carbohydrate metabolism, namely hyperglycemia.[14] At present, diabetes mellitus can be diagnosed by using 3 different investigations that demonstrate dysglycemia. The diagnostic criteria are the same for children, adults, and older subjects. Different tests will not necessarily identify the same subjects, and each investigation has its specific limitations and strengths. **Table 1** summarizes the diagnostic criteria and the relative merits and limitations of these investigations.

Because there have been recent changes in the diagnostic criteria for diabetes, it is worth considering the background to this. Circulating glucose levels may be considered as a part of a continuum. Persons destined to develop type 2 diabetes progress along this continuum over time from having blood glucose concentrations that are physiologic to those in some intermediate but asymptomatic range to glucose concentrations that are frankly increased and often associated with acute symptoms and chronic complications of the disease.[15] The diagnostic criteria for diabetes have changed several times in the last few decades. In the late 1970's, the National Diabetes Data Group (NDDG) developed consensus diagnostic criteria for diabetes based on population distributions of glucose concentrations (despite a clear bimodal distribution and demarcation between those with and without the disease).[16] These diagnostic criteria included a fasting plasma glucose (FPG) level greater than 7.8 mmol/L (140 mg/dL) and a 120-minute glucose level after administration of 75 g of glucose (oral glucose tolerance test [OGTT]) of greater than 11.1 mmol/L (200 mg/dL). In the late 90s, population data for retinopathy in 3 distinct populations were examined, and it was noted that the 120-minute glucose cutpoint after OGTT of 11.1 mmol/L (200 mg/dL) seemed to be appropriate for determining the emergence of retinopathy. However, it was also recognized that the NDDG FPG cutpoint of 140 mg/dL (7.8 mmol/L) was less sensitive (ie, diagnosing far fewer people than the 120-minute cutpoint). The FPG cutpoint of 7.8 mmol/L (140 mg/dL) was also clearly more than the point at which retinopathy prevalence was observed to increase. This group recommended 126 mg/dL (7.0 mmol/L) as the FPG cutpoint to diagnose diabetes, and this concentration subsequently became the worldwide FPG standard for a diagnosis of diabetes.[15,16] Following progress in assay standardization, the diagnostic ability of HbA_{1c} has come to the fore. Following an expert committee recommendation,[17] the American Diabetes Association adopted HbA_{1c} as part of its diagnostic criteria in 2010,[18] using a cutpoint of greater than 6.5%, and this has been followed by the World Health Organization adoption of these criteria in 2011.[19] The clinical utility of performing these different investigations in older people remains understudied (see **Table 1**).

Development of the Metabolic Syndrome

Insulin resistance has been linked to the development of the metabolic syndrome, and older people with diabetes seem to have many of its key features. The poor outcome in terms of increased cardiovascular morbidity and mortality in this syndrome should prompt physicians to gain a better understanding to systematically plan management strategies.

Table 1
Diagnostic investigations for diabetes mellitus

Investigation	Normal	Prediabetes	Diabetes	Strength	Limitations
HbA$_{1c}$	<5.6% <38 mmol/mol	5.7%–6.4% 39–47 mmol/mol	>6.5% >48 mmol/mol	Requires no fasting Stable Reproducible	Costly Influenced by abnormal red cell turnover, pregnancy, hemoglobinopathies
Glucose (fasting) levels	<5.5 mmol/L	5.6–6.9 mmol/L	>7 mmol/L	Cheap Allows accurate measurement	Requires fasting
Glucose (random)	—	—	>11.1 mmol/L		—
OGTT (120-min glucose)	<7.8 mmol/L	7.9–11.0 mmol/L	>11.1 mmol/L	More sensitive Previously considered gold standard	Costly Poor repeatability Time consuming

Abbreviations: HbA$_{1c}$, glycated hemoglobin; OGTT, oral glucose tolerance test.

Several definitions of the metabolic syndrome have been proposed (**Table 2**), including those of the World Health Organization, National Cholesterol Education Program and the International Diabetes Federation.[20–22] In the United States, the metabolic syndrome is present in more than 5% of individuals aged between 20 and 30 years, in more than 20% of individuals aged between 40 and 50 years, and in more than 40% persons older than 60 years.[23] This condition is more common in men than women, and more recently, a central role of visceral (intra-abdominal) obesity has become more recognized. Other areas for targeting new research in older people are vitamin D and testosterone, in males, both of which decrease with aging and may be associated with adverse cardiovascular outcomes.[24]

Various cellular and inflammatory processes have been implicated in contributing to the insulin resistance of the metabolic syndrome, including increased levels of mesenteric and omental adipose tissue lipolysis, inflammatory cytokine secretion, and reduced levels of adiponectin, an insulin-sensitizing hormone. Free fatty acids released from visceral adipose tissue pass directly into the portal circulation, enhancing lipid synthesis and gluconeogenesis as well as producing insulin resistance in the liver.

Environmental factors, such as poor physical activity and excess calorie intake (especially sucrose), may increase the risk of developing insulin resistance. Stress and factors that increase catecholamine levels, such as disturbances in sleep patterns because of obesity or obstructive lung disease, can lead to increased lipolysis, especially from visceral fat depots.

VASCULAR COMPLICATIONS OF DIABETES

The complications of diabetes can be broadly categorized into microvascular (retinopathy, neuropathy, and nephropathy) and macrovascular (coronary heart disease [CHD], stroke, and peripheral arterial disease) complications.

Diabetic Eye Disease

Diabetic retinopathy (DR) is the most common microvascular complication of diabetes, the leading cause of blindness in the developed world, and one of the leading causes of blindness in the developing world. DR is clinically characterized by microaneurysms, exudates, and hemorrhages and less commonly by neovascularization. Poor glycemic control and elevated blood pressure are the principal risk factors for developing DR and progressive disease. Clinical trials have demonstrated the effectiveness of photocoagulation, vitrectomy, and control of hyperglycemia and hypertension for DR.[25] At present, the most effective medical treatment to slow the progression of DR is glycemic control. The Diabetes Control and Complications Trial (DCCT) and the United Kingdom Prospective Diabetes Study (UKPDS) are 2 randomized clinical trials that conclusively showed the efficacy of glycemic control in preventing DR.[26,27] The UKPDS study group also reported the effectiveness of tight blood pressure control.[28] Diabetes-related complications are only one part of the many ophthalmologic disorders affecting older people.[29] Visual problems in the elderly amplify frailty and are risk factors for depression, multiple morbidities, and mortality. A comprehensive eye examination is advisable because screening methods based on simple retinal photography are more often inadequate in elderly patients. Cataract surgery in older diabetic patients can lead to worsening of their retinopathy or to infection. This surgery should be performed under conditions of good glycemic and blood pressure controls to minimize these risks.[1]

Table 2
Comparison of 3 different definitions of the metabolic syndrome

Source	Central Obesity	Dyslipidemia	Hypertension	Glucose Level	Microalbuminuria
WHO (1999) Presence of diabetes mellitus, impaired glucose tolerance, impaired fasting glucose levels, or insulin resistance, AND 2 of central obesity, dyslipidaemia, HT, glucose level, and microalbuminuria	Waist: hip ratio >0.90 (men); >0.85 (women), and/or body mass index >30 kg/m²	TG levels≥1.695 HDL-C levels ≤0.9 (men) ≤1.0 (women)	BP ≥140/90 mm Hg	—	Urinary albumin excretion ratio ≥20 mg/min or albumin:creatinine ratio ≥30 mg/g
The NCEP Adult Treatment Panel III (2001) requires at least 3 of the following	Waist circumference >88 cm or >102 cm (Asian WHO criteria ≥80 cm and ≥90 cm) in women and men, respectively	Fasting plasma TG levels ≥1.69 mmol/L Fasting HDL-C levels <1.04 mmol and <1.29 mmol in men and women, respectively	BP ≥130/85 mm Hg	Fasting glucose levels ≥6.1 mmol/L	—
IDF (2005) Person has a central obesity (defined as waist circumference with ethnicity-specific values) plus any 2 of the following	—	TG levels ≥1.7 mmol/L, HDL-C levels <1.03 mmol/L (men); <1.29 (women) mmol/L, or on specific treatment for both	Systolic BP ≥130 mm Hg and diastolic BP ≥85 mm Hg or on specific treatment for this	Fasting glucose levels ≥5.6 mmol/L or previously diagnosed with type 2 diabetes	—

Abbreviations: BP, blood pressure; HDL-C, high-density-lipoprotein cholesterol; IDF, International Diabetes Federation; NCEP, National Cholesterol Education Program; TG, triglyceride; WHO, World Health Organization.

Neuropathy and the Diabetic Foot

Neuropathies are among the most common of the long-term complications of diabetes, affecting up to 50% of patients. Neuropathies are characterized by a progressive loss of nerve fibers, which may affect both principle divisions of the peripheral nervous system.[30] Several studies have confirmed the major contribution of prolonged hyperglycemia in the pathogenesis of neuropathy and neuropathic pain. The degree of hyperglycemia and the duration of diabetes have been identified as risk factors in both epidemiologic studies and clinical trials. Diabetic neuropathy, which includes sensorimotor and autonomic neuropathies, is one of the main causes of foot problems in diabetes. The other causes include peripheral vascular disease, foot pressure abnormalities, and limited joint mobility. The risks of foot ulcers and amputation increase considerably with age. Depending on the diabetes duration, the risk of amputation can be as high as 0.5%/patient/year in people older than 80 years. The reduced mobility and visual impairment of older subjects hampers their ability to inspect their feet, which is a fundamental component of diabetic foot care. The most common triggering factors for a foot ulcer are inappropriate footwear, direct injury, bathroom surgery, walking barefoot at home, and reduced mobility. Attention needs to be paid to shoes and fitting, cutting nails, ulcers, callouses, and infections, and patient education is crucial to the prevention of complications. Once foot abnormality is established, it leads to significant of morbidity and mortality, which is accentuated in elderly diabetic patients.

Diabetic Kidney Disease

Diabetic nephropathy occurs in 20% to 40% of patients with diabetes and is the single leading cause of end-stage renal disease.[31] Diabetic nephropathy is independently associated with increased cardiovascular risk. The earliest indicator of renal disease in diabetes is microalbuminuria. Persistent albuminuria in the range of 30 to 300 mg/24 h (microalbuminuria) has been shown to be the earliest stage of diabetic nephropathy in type 1 diabetes and a marker for development of nephropathy in T2DM. Several interventions have demonstrated the reduction in risk and slowing of progression of renal disease. Large prospective randomized studies (DCCT and UKPDS) have shown that optimal glycemic control can delay the onset of microalbuminuria and the progression of microalbuminuria to macroalbuminuria (>300 mg/24 h) in patients with type 1 diabetes and T2DM.[30] Several authoritative studies, UKPDS in T2DM[27] and type 1 diabetes,[32] have shown the value of optimal blood pressure control in reducing the risk of nephropathy. In addition, angiotensin-converting enzyme (ACE) inhibitors have been shown to reduce major CVD outcomes (ie, myocardial infarction, stroke, and death) in patients with diabetes, thus further supporting the use of these agents in patients with microalbuminuria, a CVD risk factor.[33] Other drugs, such as diuretics, calcium channel blockers, and β-blockers, should be used as additional therapy to further lower blood pressure in patients already treated with ACE inhibitors or angiotensin receptor blockers.[34]

CVD

The magnitude of T2DM as a CVD risk factor is substantial, with the increase in cardiovascular risk being 2- to 4-fold. Many guidelines regard diabetes as a CHD risk equivalent.[21,35,36] CVD is the largest cause of morbidity and mortality for individuals with diabetes and the primary contributor to the direct and indirect costs of diabetes. The common conditions coexisting with T2DM (eg, hypertension and dyslipidemia) are clear risk factors for CVD, and diabetes itself confers independent risk. Numerous studies have shown the efficacy of controlling individual cardiovascular risk factors in preventing or slowing CVD in people with diabetes.[31] The most notable of these cardiovascular risk factors shows the substantial benefit to controlling blood pressure and lipid abnormalities. Despite the well-established association between blood glucose levels and atherosclerosis, risk reductions for myocardial infarction and death from any cause were observed only with extended posttrial follow-up of UKPDS[37] and DCCT[38] and are in contrast to the prospective studies ADVANCE (Action in Diabetes and Vascular Disease: Preterax and Diamicron Modified Release Controlled Evaluation)[39] and ACCORD (Action to Control Cardiovascular Risk in Diabetes),[40] each including in excess of 10,000 participants. These studies could not show a significant beneficial effect on CVD outcome when targeting near-normal glucose levels in and an HBA_{1c} of less than 6.5%.

TARGETING MODIFIABLE RISK FACTORS

The main modifiable risk factors that are the focus of clinical care include control of glycemia, blood pressure, and lipids. These factors should be individualized by setting treatment goals for each individual patient. These individualized goals are of particular importance in older diabetic subjects because the clinical treatment decisions are often more complex. Ideally, care should be administered by a multidisciplinary team, which would include the primary care physician, nurse, social worker, dietician, optometrist, ophthalmologist, endocrinologist, and geriatrician, and this should also be done in a coordinated manner to avoid confusion. Several additional factors that are of less clinical relevance in younger individuals need to be considered in the older diabetic, including factors such as life expectancy and expectancy of manifestation of complications, comorbidities, side effects of medication, and frailty. Frailty could be defined as an intermediate state between successful aging, with complete functional autonomy, and irreversible dependence and pathologic aging. Multiple clinical disorders, polypharmacy, depression, mild cognitive impairment, and geriatric syndromes indicate frailty. Frailty not only has a medical component but also has a social component and includes familial and socioeconomic difficulties. Expectedly, age has a continuous impact on frailty in subjects older than 65 years.[1] Once a decision is made to intervene medically, the following modifiable risk factors should be considered: blood pressure, lipids, and glycemic control.

Lifestyle

The nonpharmacologic treatment of diabetes combines diet and physical activity. Combining these 2 is time consuming because it requires counseling, education, and motivation of the patient, their relatives, and caregivers, including the health care professional. Because of the physical and mental effort required, this aspect often gets neglected. However, the benefits of diet and physical activity can be significant and include improving glycemic control, restoring or maintaining muscle mass, improving functional independence, improving dyslipidemia and reducing blood pressure, and improving overall well-being, all of which increase the likelihood of successful aging.[41] Aspects specifically relevant in older persons such as mobility, motor and sensory impairment, and injury prevention, such as by preventing falls, must be considered.

Glucose Control

There are no outcome data on the long-term effects of tight glycemic control in older people with diabetes, so the benefits demonstrated in younger individuals are assumed to be similar for older people. Glycemic targets need to be individualized by allowing for frailty and its consequences. The European Diabetes Working Party for Older People[1] recommended that the glucose control targets for frail patients is an HbA_{1c} of 7.5% to 8.5% and an FPG level between 7.50 and 9.00 mmol/L and for nonfrail patients and those with an absence of comorbidities is an HbA_{1c} of 7.0% to 7.5% and an FPG level between 6.5 and 7.5 mmol/L. However, in their revised executive summary in 2011 (available on www.instituteofdiabetes.org) these recommendations have been revised. The first-choice drug is often metformin. It is efficacious, and inexpensive, and its use is well validated. It can have gastrointestinal side effects, so gradual dose titration is recommended to minimize these effects. Metformin should be used with caution in patients with impaired renal function and should be stopped if the serum creatinine level is greater than 150 μmol/L or the estimated glomerular filtration rate (eGFR) is less than 30 mL/min/1.73 m^2. After withdrawal of metformin, or in cases of intolerance to it, several drug classes may be considered. The sulfonylureas are well-established drugs and have the advantage of being rapidly effective and inexpensive. However, they cause weight gain and hypoglycemia. Long-acting sulfonylureas such as glibenclamide and chlorpropamide are to be avoided, and caution should be exercised when using sulfonylureas in patients with impaired renal function. Gliclazide modified release and glimepiride are alternative sulfonylureas, with a lower risk of hypoglycemia. The 2 newer drug classes, dipeptidyl-peptidase-IV (DPP-IV) inhibitors or gliptins (sitagliptin, vildagliptin, and saxagliptin) and glucagon-like peptide 1 (GLP-1) analogues (exenatide and liraglutide), are either weight neutral (in the case of gliptins) or have the potential to cause weight loss (GLP-1 analogues). Additional DPP-IV inhibitors and GLP-1 analogues are in development. Data in older subjects receiving these medications remain limited, with the most extensively researched medication in the population older than 75 years, which included 301 patients, being the DPP-IV inhibitor Vildagliptin.[42] Both classes of drugs may have some advantages in older people, such as low risk of weight gain and no hypoglycemia, and several additional drugs in these 2 classes are being evaluated. The thiazolidinedione pioglitazone does not cause hypoglycemia but does have several side effects, including fluid retention, heart failure, and increased risk of bone fractures. It does have an advantageous effect on the lipid profile compared with the recently suspended rosiglitazone.[43] Insulin is efficacious, and it can improve the nutritional status of older diabetic patients. Premixed insulin and prefilled insulin pens have the advantage of reducing dosage errors. Insulin's most-feared side effect is hypoglycemia. Symptoms of hypoglycemia in older people may differ from those seen in younger people. Residents of care homes who have diabetes are particularly vulnerable. The most common symptoms consist of nonspecific neurologic signs, notably vertigo, disorientation, falls, or sudden changes in behavior. The most important risk factors for hypoglycemia are reduced food intake because of intercurrent disease, a change in the setting of care, or a recent stay in hospital.

Some comorbidities are also risk factors for hypoglycemia, and these include renal failure, cognitive and psychiatric disorders (leading to errors in medication or food intake), and polypharmacy.[44]

Blood Pressure

The benefits of treating hypertension seem even greater and manifest sooner than targeting glucose control in preventing both microvascular and macrovascular complications.[28,31,32] Several major trials of antihypertensive treatment in the elderly (>65 years old), conducted with thiazide diuretics, calcium channel blockers, or ACE inhibitors have shown that antihypertensive treatment reduces the risk of cardiovascular mortality, stroke, and heart failure to a similar or even greater extent in older people than in younger people, and subgroup analyses have indicated that the absolute benefit is even greater in diabetic patients. The benefits are also realized in patients older than 80 years.[45] The benefits of controlling blood pressure in older diabetic patients are substantial and the evidence for this is well established. Most official guidelines recommend starting antihypertensive treatment in older diabetic patients if the blood pressure exceeds 140/80 mm Hg, and even 130/80 mm Hg. In older patients who are frail or who have multiple disorders, a target of 150/90 mm Hg could be acceptable.[1]

Lipids

Control of lipid parameters is one of the fundamental interventions necessary to reduce the cardiovascular risk in diabetic patients. As opposed to hyperglycemia, targeting dyslipidemia has proven much more effective in preventing the macrovascular complications of diabetes.[46] The excess risk that diabetic subjects carry is also in part related to the disturbances in their lipid metabolism. The reasons for this excess risk are numerous and varied and in part relate to the lipid abnormalities seen in diabetes. Enhanced glycation of lipoproteins has direct effects on lipoprotein metabolism because these glycated lipoproteins are handled differently by lipoprotein receptors, particularly of the scavenger group, thus promoting atherogenesis. Enhanced glycation also amplifies the effects of oxidative stress on lipoproteins, and this therefore implicates patients with type 1 and 2 diabetes.[46] Low-density-lipoprotein cholesterol (LDL-C) is identified as the primary target of lipid-lowering therapy. For many years, the benefits of intervention on lipoproteins as cardiovascular risk factors in diabetes were uncertain. The principal reason was that patients with diabetes were excluded from trials of lipid-lowering therapies. Thus, virtually no data exist from studies using earlier medications such as bile acid sequestrants, fibrates, or nicotinic acid. Even early statin trials either excluded or included very few diabetic subjects. In the last decade, a wealth of evidence has accumulated after several targeted randomized control trials were conducted using statin therapy, which specifically included diabetic subjects. **Table 3** depicts the most notable statin studies, providing information on the number of diabetic patients as well as the age distributions.[47] A meta-analysis that evaluated the efficacy of cholesterol-lowering therapy in 18,686 people with diabetes in 14 randomized trials of statins reported a 9% proportional reduction in all-cause mortality and a 21% proportional reduction in major vascular events per 1 mmol/L reduction in LDL-C.[48] This level of evidence for statins has lead most guidelines to recommend statin treatment for diabetic patients 40 years and younger if additional risk factors are present.[21,35,36] This benefit is also apparent in older patients who have a higher absolute cardiovascular risk. A meta-analysis of 90,056 patients which included 14 randomized trials showed that those older than 65 years (n = 6446) had a 19% reduction in the risk of major cardiovascular events, a benefit similar to the 22% reduction in risk experienced by those younger than 65 years (n = 7902). Although statins form the cornerstone of pharmacologic CVD prevention, many other agents can be useful as add-on therapies.[49] One such agent is ezetimibe, a cholesterol absorption inhibitor, which has been widely used in combination with a statin to given an additional LDL-C–lowering effect. Used as monotherapy, ezetimibe is associated with a reduction in LDL-C by around one-fifth.[50] In making management decisions, clinicians must make an individual assessment of the potential risks and benefits of intervention. The evidence base for treating older patients with lipid-lowering agents, particularly statins, is becoming increasingly robust. However, many of these trials were based on populations of healthy older patients with few comorbidities who

Table 3
Notable statin trials

Year	1994	1995	1996	1998	2002	2002	2004	2008
Study	4S	WOSCOPS	CARE	LIPID	HPS	PROSPER	CARDS	JUPITER
Setting	Secondary prevention	Primary prevention	Secondary prevention	Secondary prevention	Combined	Combined	T2DM	Primary prevention
Statin	Simvastatin	Pravastatin	Pravastatin	Pravastatin	Simvastatin	Pravastatin	Atorvastatin	Rosuvastatin
Number of Patients	4444	6595	4159	9014	20,536	5804	2838	17,802
Diabetic Patients (%)	202 (4.5)	76 (1)	586 (14)	1077 (12)	5963 (29)	623 (11)	2838 (100)	0 (0)
Follow-up (mean in y)	5.4	4.9	5	5	5	3.2	3.9	1.9
LDL-C Lowering (%)	36	26	28	25	31	34	40	50
Age Group (y)	35–70	45–64	21–75	31–75	40–80	70–82	40–75	60–71
% Older Than 65 y	23	0	31	39	52	100	40	32[a]
Primary End Point	Reduced total mortality from 12%–8%	Reduced CHD mortality or nonfatal MI from 8%–5.5%	Reduced CHD mortality or nonfatal MI from 13%–10%	Reduced total CHD mortality from 12%–8%	Reduced total mortality from 15%–13%	Reduced CHD mortality or nonfatal MI or fatal or nonfatal stroke from 16%–14%	Reduction in acute CHD event or stroke from 9%–6%	Reduction in acute coronary heart disease event, or stroke from 1.8%–0.9%

Abbreviations: 4S, Scandinavian Simvastatin Survival Study; CARDS, Collaborative Atorvastatin Diabetes Study; CARE, Cholesterol and Recurrent Events; HPS, Heart Protection Study; JUPITER, Justification for the Use of statins in prevention: an intervention Trial Evaluating Rosuvastatin; LIPD, Long-term Intervention with Pravastatin in Ischemic Disease; MI, Myocardial Infarction; PROSPER, Prospective Study of Pravastatin in the Elderly at Risk; WOSCOPS, West of Scotland Coronary Prevention Study.

[a] Percentage subjects in the JUPITER trial older than 70 years and not 65 years.

Data from Viljoen A. A practical approach to lipid management in the elderly. J Nutr Health Aging 2011;15:65–70.

may have been on minimal additional medication. In addition, patients older than 80 years have not been widely studied.[47] Thus, clinical trial data are not always representative of older patients in general. A focus on quality of life and patient choice is also important. Multiple medications can be burdensome to take and poor compliance can often be a consequence, but the improved quality of life because of lower vascular event rates remains the important alternative perspective. In summary, although multiple other lipid-lowering agents exist, none have been evidenced to be as successful as statins at reducing cardiovascular events and mortality.

SUMMARY

Multiple interventions are now available to treat patients with diabetes. The evidence base for this has become increasingly robust. For older patients, however, fewer data are available and clinicians often have to extrapolate the potential benefits demonstrated in trials that included younger populations. As the health of our society improves, individuals have a better likelihood of long and active life than ever before. However, microvascular and macrovascular complications associated with diabetes remain a significant cause of morbidity and mortality in older patients. Clinicians have to weigh the risks and benefits of the treatments available to prevent these complications.

REFERENCES

1. Fagot-Campagna A, Bourdel-Marchasson I, Simon D. Burden of diabetes in an aging population: prevalence, incidence, mortality, characteristics and quality of care. Diabetes Metab 2005;31(Spec No 2):5S35–35S52.
2. McBean AM, Li S, Gilbertson DT, et al. Differences in diabetes prevalence, incidence, and mortality among the elderly of four racial/ethnic groups: whites, blacks, hispanics, and asians. Diabetes Care 2004;27(10):2317–24.
3. Diabetes UK. Diabetes in the UK 2004. London: Diabetes UK; 2004.
4. Ubink-Veltmaat LJ, Bilo HJ, Groenier KH, et al. Prevalence, incidence and mortality of type 2 diabetes mellitus revisited: a prospective population-based study in The Netherlands (ZODIAC-1). Eur J Epidemiol 2003;18:793–800.
5. The International Diabetes Federation atlas. 4th edition. 2009. Available at: http://www.diabetesatlas.org/content/regional-overview. Accessed March 21, 2011.
6. Bourdel-Marchasson I, Helmer C, Fagot-Campagna A, et al. Disability and quality of life in elderly people with diabetes. Diabetes Metab 2007;33(Suppl 1):S66–74.
7. Neil HA, Thompson AV, Thorogood M, et al. Diabetes in the elderly: the Oxford Community Diabetes Study. Diabet Med 1989;6:608–13.
8. Melton LJ 3rd, Palumbo PJ, Chu CP. Incidence of diabetes mellitus by clinical type. Diabetes Care 1981;4(5):547–50.
9. Mølbak AG, Christau B, Marner B, et al. Incidence of insulin-dependent diabetes mellitus in age groups over 30 years in Denmark. Diabet Med 1994;11(7):650–5.
10. Lipton RB, Liao Y, Cao G, et al. Determinants of incident non-insulin-dependent diabetes mellitus among blacks and whites in a national sample. The NHANES I Epidemiologic Follow-up Study. Am J Epidemiol 1992;136:503–12.
11. Ferrannini E, Vichi S, Beck-Nielsen H, et al. Insulin action and age. European Group for the Study of Insulin Resistance (EGIR). Diabetes 1996;45:947–53.
12. Pandit MK, Burke J, Gustafson AB, et al. Drug-induced disorders of glucose tolerance. Ann Intern Med 1993;118(7):529–39.
13. Meneilly GS, Cheung E, Tuokko H. Counterregulatory hormone responses to hypoglycemia in the elderly patient with diabetes. Diabetes 1994;43(3):403–10.

14. Sacks DB, Fonseca V, Goldfine AB. Diabetes: advances and controversies. Clin Chem 2011;57:147–9.
15. Kirkman MS, Kendall DM. HemoglobinA1c to diagnose diabetes: why the controversy over adding a new tool? Clin Chem 2011;57:255–7.
16. Expert Committee on the Diagnosis and Classification of Diabetes Mellitus. Report of the Expert Committee on the diagnosis and classification of diabetes mellitus. Diabetes Care 1997;20:1183–97.
17. International Expert Committee. International Expert Committee report on the role of the A1C assay in the diagnosis of diabetes. Diabetes Care 2009;32:1327–34.
18. American Diabetes Association. Diagnosis and classification of diabetes mellitus. Diabetes Care 2010;33(Suppl 1):S62–9.
19. Use of Glycated Haemoglobin (HbA1c) in the Diagnosis of Diabetes Mellitus. Abbreviated report of a WHO Consultation. Available at: http://www.who.int/diabetes/publications/report-hba1c_2011.pdf. Accessed March 21, 2011.
20. World Health Organization. Definition, diagnosis and classification of diabetes mellitus and its complications. Report of a WHO consultation 1999. Available at: http://whqlibdoc.who.int/hq/1999/who_ncd_ncs_99.2.pdf. Accessed March 21, 2011.
21. Expert Panel on detection, evaluation, and treatment of high blood cholesterol in adults. Executive summary of the Third Report of The National Cholesterol Education Program (NCEP) Expert Panel on detection, evaluation, and treatment of high blood cholesterol in adults (Adult Treatment Panel III). JAMA 2001;285:2486–97.
22. Alberti KG, Zimmet P, Shaw J. Metabolic syndrome-a new world-wide definition. A Consensus statement from the International Diabetes Federation. Diabet Med 2006;23(5):469–80.
23. Morley JE. The metabolic syndrome and aging. J Gerontol A Biol Sci Med Sci 2004;59:139–42.
24. Morley JE, Sinclair AJ. The metabolic syndrome in older persons: a loosely defined constellation of symptoms or a distinct entity? Age Ageing 2009;38:494–7.
25. Fong DS, Aiello LP, Ferris FL 3rd, et al. Diabetic retinopathy. Diabetes Care 2004;27:2540–53.
26. The effect of intensive treatment of diabetes on the development and progression of long-term complications in insulin-dependent diabetes mellitus. The Diabetes Control and Complications Trial Research Group. N Engl J Med 1993;329:977–86.
27. Intensive blood-glucose control with sulphonylureas or insulin compared with conventional treatment and risk of complications in patients with type 2 diabetes (UKPDS 33). UK Prospective Diabetes Study (UKPDS) Group. Lancet 1998;352:837–53.
28. Tight blood pressure control and risk of macrovascular and microvascular complications in type 2 diabetes: UKPDS 38. BMJ 1998;317:703–13.
29. Massin P, Kaloustian E. The elderly diabetic's eyes. Diabetes Metab 2007;33(Suppl 1):S4–9.
30. Boulton AJ, Malik RA, Arezzo JC, et al. Diabetic somatic neuropathies. Diabetes Care 2004;27:1458–86.
31. American Diabetes Association. Standards of medical care in diabetes–2011. Diabetes Care 2011;34(Suppl 1):S11–61.
32. Effect of intensive therapy on the development and progression of diabetic nephropathy in the Diabetes Control and Complications Trial. The Diabetes Control and Complications (DCCT) Research Group. Kidney Int 1995;47:1703–20.

33. Effects of ramipril on cardiovascular and microvascular outcomes in people with diabetes mellitus: results of the HOPE study and MICRO-HOPE substudy. Heart Outcomes Prevention Evaluation Study Investigators. Lancet 2000;355:253–9.

34. Lewis EJ, Hunsicker LG, Bain RP, et al. The effect of angiotensin-converting-enzyme inhibition on diabetic nephropathy. The Collaborative Study Group. N Engl J Med 1993;329:1456–62.

35. Graham I, Atar D, Borch-Johnsen K, et al. European guidelines on cardiovascular disease prevention in clinical practice: full text. Fourth Joint Task Force of the European Society of Cardiology and other societies on cardiovascular disease prevention in clinical practice (constituted by representatives of nine societies and by invited experts). Eur J Cardiovasc Prev Rehabil 2007;14(Suppl 2):S1–113.

36. British Cardiac Society, British Hypertension Society, Diabetes UK, et al. JBS 2: the Joint British Societies' guidelines for prevention of cardiovascular disease in clinical practice. Heart 2005;91(Suppl V):v1–52.

37. Holman RR, Paul SK, Bethel MA, et al. 10-year follow-up of intensive glucose control in type 2 diabetes. N Engl J Med 2008;359:1577–89.

38. Nathan DM, Cleary PA, Backlund JY, et al. Intensive diabetes treatment and cardiovascular disease in patients with type 1 diabetes. N Engl J Med 2005; 353:2643–53.

39. Patel A, MacMahon S, Chalmers J, et al. Intensive blood glucose control and vascular outcomes in patients with type 2 diabetes. N Engl J Med 2008;358: 2560–72.

40. Gerstein HC, Miller ME, Byington RP, et al. Effects of intensive glucose lowering in type 2 diabetes. N Engl J Med 2008;358:2545–59.

41. Constans T, Lecomte P. Non pharmacological treatments in elderly diabetics. Diabetes Metab 2007;33(Suppl 1):S79–86.

42. Schweizer A, Dejager S, Foley JE, et al. Clinical experience with vildagliptin in the management of type 2 diabetes in a patient population ≥75 years: a pooled analysis from a database of clinical trials. Diabetes Obes Metab 2011;13:55–64.

43. Viljoen A, Sinclair A. Safety and efficacy of rosiglitazone in the elderly diabetic patient. Vasc Health Risk Manag 2009;5:389–95.

44. Sinclair AJ. Diabetes in old age. In: Holt R, Cockram CS, Flyvberg A, et al, editors. Textbook of diabetes. 4th edition. Oxford (UK): Wiley-Blackwell; 2010. p. 13–8. Chapter 54.

45. Beckett NS, Peters R, Fletcher AE, et al. HYVET Study Group. Treatment of hypertension in patients 80 years of age or older. N Engl J Med 2008;58:1887–98.

46. Viljoen A, Wierzbicki AS. Cardiovascular risk factors – Dyslipidaemia diabetes lipid therapies. In: Holt R, Cockram CS, Flyvberg A, et al, editors. Textbook of diabetes. 4th edition. Oxford (UK): Wiley-Blackwell; 2010. p. 672–83. Chapter 40.

47. Viljoen A. A practical approach to lipid management in the elderly. J Nutr Health Aging 2011;15:65–70.

48. Kearney PM, Blackwell L, Collins R, et al. Efficacy of cholesterol-lowering therapy in 18,686 people with diabetes in 14 randomised trials of statins: a meta-analysis. Lancet 2008;371:117–25.

49. Cholesterol Treatment Trialists' (CTT) Collaborators. Efficacy and safety of cholesterol-lowering treatment: prospective meta-analysis of data from 90,056 participants in 14 randomised trials of statins. Lancet 2005;366:1267–78.

50. Viljoen A, Wierzbicki AS. Enhanced LDL-C reduction: lower is better. Does it matter how? Int J Clin Pract 2008;62(4):518–20.

Index

Note: Page numbers of article titles are in **boldface** type.

A

ABCDE mnemonic, for secondary hypertension, 528–529
Absorptive undergarments, for urinary incontinence, 549
ACCOMPLISH (Avoiding Cardiovascular events through COMbination therapy
    in Patients LIving with Systolic Hypertension), 532
ACCORD study, for diabetes mellitus, 623
Acne, in testosterone replacement, 518
α-Adrenergic antagonists, for urinary incontinence, 548–549
ADVANCE study, for diabetes mellitus, 623
Aggressive behavior, in nursing homes, 603–605
Aging Male Symptoms Scale, 508–509
Agitation, in nursing homes, 603–605
Alfuzosin, for urinary incontinence, 548
ALLHAT (Antihypertensive and Lipid-Lowering Treatment to Prevent Heart Attack Trial),
    532–534
Alzheimer's disease, prevention of. See Brain, revitalization of.
American College of Sport and Medicine, physical activity recommendations of, 431
American Geriatrics Society, physical activity recommendations of, 431
American Heart Association, physical activity recommendations of, 431
Amino acids, for sarcopenia, 428–430
Amisulpride, for delirium, 569
Androgen Deficiency in Aging Male questionnaire, 508–509
Androgens
    deficiency of. See Hypogonadism.
    for osteoporosis, 499
Anemia, testosterone replacement effects on, 516
Anesthesia, delirium in, 556
Angiotensin receptor blockers
    for heart failure, 457
    for hypertension, 532–533
Angiotensin-converting enzyme inhibitors
    for heart failure, 457
    for hypertension, 532–533
    for sarcopenia, 432
    urinary incontinence due to, 542
Anorexia, 582
    in nursing homes, 599
    in sarcopenia, 428
Anthocyanins, in black rice, 484
Anthropometric values, 478–479

Med Clin N Am 95 (2011) 631–646
doi:10.1016/S0025-7125(11)00035-6
0025-7125/11/$ – see front matter © 2011 Elsevier Inc. All rights reserved.

medical.theclinics.com

Moving?

Make sure your subscription moves with you!

To notify us of your new address, find your **Clinics Account Number** (located on your mailing label above your name), and contact customer service at:

Email: journalscustomerservice-usa@elsevier.com

800-654-2452 (subscribers in the U.S. & Canada)
314-447-8871 (subscribers outside of the U.S. & Canada)

Fax number: 314-447-8029

Elsevier Health Sciences Division
Subscription Customer Service
3251 Riverport Lane
Maryland Heights, MO 63043

*To ensure uninterrupted delivery of your subscription,
please notify us at least 4 weeks in advance of move.

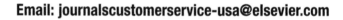

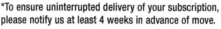

Printed and bound by CPI Group (UK) Ltd, Croydon, CR0 4YY

03/10/2024

01040460-0004